Autoimmune Diseases

Munther A. Khamashta • Manuel Ramos-Casals

(Editors)

Autoimmune Diseases

Acute and Complex Situations

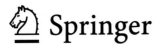 Springer

Editors
Munther A. Khamashta, MD, FRCP, PhD
Lupus Research Unit
The Rayne Institute
St. Thomas' Hospital
London
UK

Manuel Ramos-Casals, MD, PhD
Department of Autoimmune Diseases
Laboratory of Autoimmune Diseases
Josep Font, Institut d'Investigacions
Biomèdiques August Pi i Sunyer (IDIBAPS)
Hospital Clinic, Barcelona
Spain

ISBN 978-0-85729-357-2   e-ISBN 978-0-85729-358-9
DOI 10.1007/978-0-85729-358-9
Springer London Dordrecht Heidelberg New York

British Library Cataloguing in Publication Data
A catalogue record for this book is available from the British Library

Library of Congress Control Number: 2011921945

Cover design: eStudioCalamar, Figueres/Berlin

Printed on acid-free paper

Springer is part of Springer Science+Business Media (www.springer.com)

This book is dedicated to the memory of our friend and inspirational leader, Dr. Josep Font.

Contents

Contributors

Howard Amital
Department of Medicine 'B', Chaim Sheba
Medical Centre, Tel-Hashomer, Israel

Emmanuel Andrès
Service de Médecine Interne, Diabète et
Maladies Métaboliques, Clinique Médicale
B, Hôpital Civil, Hôpitaux Universitaires
de Strasbourg, Strasbourg Cedex,
France

Alejandro Balsa
Rheumatology Unit, Hospital Universitario
La Paz, Madrid, Spain

Robert P. Baughman
Department of Medicine, University of
Cincinnati Medical Center, Cincinnati,
OH, USA

Maria Laura Bertolaccini
Lupus Unit, The Rayne Institute,
St. Thomas' Hospital, London, UK

Gema Bonilla
Rheumatology Unit, Hospital Universitario
La Paz, Madrid, Spain

Xavier Bosch
Department of Internal Medicine, ICMD
Hospital Clinic, Barcelona, Spain

Albert Bové Boada
Department of Autoimmune Diseases,
Laboratory of Autoimmune Diseases
Josep Font, Institut d'Investigacions
Biomèdiques August Pi i Sunyer
(IDIBAPS), Hospital Clinic, Barcelona,
Spain

Pilar Brito-Zerón
Department of Autoimmune Diseases,
Laboratory of Autoimmune Diseases
Josep Font, Institut d'Investigacions
Biomèdiques August Pi i Sunyer
(IDIBAPS), Hospital Clinic, Barcelona,
Spain

Ana Campar
Internal Medicine Department,
Santo António Hospital, Porto, Portugal

Maria J. Cuadrado
Lupus Unit, The Rayne Institute,
St. Thomas' Hospital, London, UK

David P. D'Cruz
The Louise Coote Lupus Unit, Guys'
and St. Thomas' Hospital NHS Foundation
Trust, Gassiott House, St. Thomas' Hospital,
Lambeth Palace Road, London, UK

Christopher P. Denton
Center for Rheumatology, Royal Free
Campus, University College Medical
School, London, UK

Cándido Díaz-Lagares
Laboratory of Autoimmune Diseases
Josep Font, Institut d'Investigacions
Biomèdiques August Pi i Sunyer
(IDIBAPS), Hospital Clinic, Barcelona,
Spain

Petros V. Efthimiou
Rheumatology Division, Lincoln Medical
and Mental Health Center, New York, NY,
USA
Department of Clinical Medicine, Weill
Cornell Medical College, New York, NY,
USA

Rosa M. Fernández-Torres
Department of Dermatology, Hospital
Universitario de La Coruña, La Coruña,
Spain

Eduardo Fonseca
Department of Dermatology, Hospital
Universitario de La Coruña, La Coruña,
Spain

Helen Fothergill
Service de Médecine Interne, Diabète et
Maladies métaboliques, Clinique médicale
B, Hôpital Civil, Hôpitaux Universitaires
de Strasbourg, Strasbourg Cedex, France

Miriam García-Arias
Rheumatology Unit, Hospital Universitario
La Paz, Madrid, Spain

Duvuru Geetha
Division of Nephrology, Johns Hopkins
Bayview Medical Center, Johns Hopkins
University, Baltimore, MD, USA

Luis Gómez-Carreras
Pneumology Unit, Hospital Universitario
La Paz, Madrid, Spain

Patrick Gordon
Department of Rheumatology, King's
College London, London, UK

Loïc Guillevin
Department of Internal Medicine,
National Referral Center for Rare
Systemic and Autoimmune Diseases:
Vasculitides and Scleroderma, Hôpital
Cochin, Assistance Publique–Hôpitaux de
Paris, University Paris Descartes, Paris,
France

Gary S. Hoffman
Department of Rheumatic and
Immunologic Diseases, Cleveland Clinic,
Lerner College of Medicine, Cleveland,
OH, USA

David A. Isenberg
University College London, Centre for
Rheumatology, London, UK

Rotem Kedar
Department of Medicine 'D', Meir
Medical Center, Tel-Aviv University,
Kfar-Saba, Tel-Aviv, Israel
Department of Medicine 'B' and Center
for Autoimmune Diseases, Sheba Medical
Center, Tel-Aviv University,
Tel-Hashomer, Tel-Aviv, Israel

Aharon Kessel
Division of Clinical Immunology and
Allergy, Bnai-Zion Medical Center,
affiliated with the Technion Faculty of
Medicine, Haifa, Israel

Munther A. Khamashta
Lupus Research Unit, The Rayne Institute,
St. Thomas' Hospital, London, UK

Manil Kukar
Rheumatology Division, Lincoln Medical
and Mental Health Center, New York, NY,
USA

Ingrid E. Lundberg
Rheumatology Unit, Department of
Medicine, Karolinska Institutet,
Karolinska University Hospital, Solna,
Stockholm, Sweden

Kathleen Maksimowicz-McKinnon
Division of Rheumatology and Clinical
Immunology, University of Pittsburgh,
Pittsburgh, PA, USA

Spilios Manolakopoulos
Assistant Professor of Gastroenterology-
Hepatology, Department of Medicine,
Athens University School of Medicine,

Hippokration General Hospital, Athens, Greece

Mustapha Mecili
Service de Médecine Interne, Diabète et Maladies métaboliques, Clinique médicale B, Hôpital Civil, Hôpitaux Universitaires de Strasbourg, Strasbourg Cedex, France

Hilario Nunes
Service de Pneumologie, Hôpital Avicenne, Assistance Publique – Hôpitaux de Paris, Bobigny, France

Ashish S. Patel
Academic Department of Surgery, Cardiovascular Division, King's College London, St. Thomas' Hospital, London, UK

Michelle Petri
Department of Medicine, Division of Rheumatology, Johns Hopkins University School of Medicine, Baltimore, MD, USA

Olga Petryna
Internal Medicine Resident, Lincoln Medical and Mental Health Center, New York, NY, USA

Edward Pringle
Department of Clinical Ophthalmology, Medical Eye Unit, St. Thomas' Hospital, London, UK

Gregory Pugnet
Department of Internal Medicine, Toulouse Purpan University Hospital, Toulouse, France

Niamh P. Quillinan
Centre for Rheumatology, Royal Free Campus, University College Medical School, London, UK

Manuel Ramos-Casals
Department of Autoimmune Diseases, Laboratory of Autoimmune Diseases Josep Font, Institut d'Investigacions Biomèdiques August Pi i Sunyer (IDIBAPS), Hospital Clinic, Barcelona, Spain

Soledad Retamozo
Department of Autoimmune Diseases, Laboratory of Autoimmune Diseases Josep Font, Institut d'Investigacions Biomèdiques August Pi i Sunyer (IDIBAPS), Barcelona, Spain

Guillermo Ruiz-Irastorza
Autoimmune Disease Research Unit, Department of Internal Medicine, Hospital de Cruces, University of the Basque Country, Barakaldo, Bizkaia, Spain

Giovanni Sanna
Lupus Unit, The Rayne Institute, St. Thomas' Hospital, London, UK

Emire Seyahi
Cerrahpaşa Medical Faculty, Department of Internal Medicine, Division of Rheumatology, University of Istanbul, Istanbul, Turkey

Philip Seo
Division of Rheumatology, Johns Hopkins Vasculitis Center, Johns Hopkins University, Baltimore, MD, USA

Yehuda Shoenfeld
Department of Medicine 'B' and Center for Autoimmune Diseases, Sheba Medical Center, Tel-Aviv University, Tel-Hashomer, Tel-Aviv, Israel

Antoni Sisó-Almirall
Primary Care Center Les Corts, GESCLINIC, Institut d'Investigacions Biomèdiques August Pi i Sunyer (IDIBAPS), Barcelona, Spain

Miles Stanford
Department of Clinical Ophthalmology, Medical Eye Unit, St. Thomas' Hospital, London, UK

Koray Tascilar
Cerrahpaşa Medical Faculty, Department
of Internal Medicine, Division of
Rheumatology, University of Istanbul,
Istanbul, Turkey

Elias Toubi
Division of Clinical Immunology and
Allergy, Bnai-Zion Medical Center,
affiliated with the Technion Faculty of
Medicine, Haifa, Israel

Zahava Vadasz
Division of Clinical Immunology and
Allergy, Bnai-Zion Medical Center,
affiliated with the Technion Faculty of
Medicine, Haifa, Israel

Dimitrios Vassilopoulos
Associate Professor of Medicine-
Rheumatology, 2nd Department of Medicine,
Athens University School of Medicine,
Hippokration General Hospital, Athens,
Greece

Salvatore de Vita
Clinic of Rheumatology, DPMSC,
Azienda Ospedale Universitario S. Maria
della Misericordia, Udine,
Italy

Matthew Waltham
Academic Department of Surgery,
Cardiovascular Division, King's College
London, St. Thomas' Hospital, London,
UK

Duncan L. A. Wyncoll
Adult Intensive Care Unit, Guys' and
St. Thomas' Hospital NHS Foundation
Trust, St. Thomas' Hospital, Lambeth
Palace Road, London,
UK

Hasan Yazici
Cerrahpaşa Medical Faculty, Department
of Internal Medicine, Division of
Rheumatology, University of Istanbul,
Istanbul, Turkey

Assessment and Management of the Rheumatological Patient in the Critical Care Unit

1

David P. D'Cruz and Duncan L.A. Wyncoll

Abstract Musculoskeletal diseases are common and may result in significant morbidity and mortality especially in the context of the multisystem autoimmune rheumatic disorders. Patients with rheumatological disorders present acutely to emergency rooms, and the cause of the sudden deterioration may be due to complications of the underlying disorder, sepsis, or an iatrogenic effect resulting from an acute adverse event from therapy. Given the complexity of these patients, it is not surprising that outcome can be poor with in-hospital mortality rates of 40%. This introductory chapter is aimed at the admitting physician presented with an acutely ill patient with a rheumatological disorder who is deteriorating rapidly and needs admission to a critical care unit.

Keywords Critical care assessment and management • Immunosuppression • Multiorgan failure • Multisystem autoimmune rheumatic disorders • Sepsis

1.1
Introduction

Musculoskeletal diseases are common in the community and represent a major health care burden. These disorders may result in significant morbidity and mortality especially in the context of the less common multisystem autoimmune connective tissue disorders. From the patient's perspective, the risk of disability, economic loss because of inability to work and consequent dependence on benefits, poor quality of life, and loss of confidence and self-esteem can be life-changing.

D.P. D'Cruz (✉)
The Louise Coote Lupus Unit, Guys' and St. Thomas' Hospital NHS Foundation Trust,
Gassiott House, St. Thomas' Hospital, Lambeth Palace Road, London SE1 7EH, UK
e-mail: david.d'cruz@kcl.ac.uk

M.A. Khamashta and M. Ramos-Casals (eds.), *Autoimmune Diseases*,
DOI: 10.1007/978-0-85729-358-9_1, © Springer-Verlag London Limited 2011

While many of the musculoskeletal disorders including degenerative diseases, such as osteoarthritis, are associated with the normal aging process, some of these conditions will reduce life expectancy. For example, many of the inflammatory arthropathies are associated with an increased risk of premature mortality from cardiovascular disease. In other conditions such as systemic lupus erythematosus and the systemic vasculitides, renal disease and infections associated with immunosuppression are common causes of death.

There has been a revolution in the treatment of the inflammatory arthropathies. A decade or two ago, there were few effective treatments, and these were only used when nonsteroidal anti-inflammatory drugs had failed. The modern approach is to aim for an early diagnosis and to commence disease-modifying therapy immediately in order to prevent damage and disability. However, immunosuppressive agents and the biologics are extremely effective therapies but carry a significant burden of toxicity.

Patients with rheumatological disorders present acutely to emergency rooms, and the cause of the sudden deterioration may be due to complications of the underlying disorder, sepsis, or an iatrogenic effect resulting from an acute adverse event from therapy. Rheumatoid arthritis is the most common rheumatic disease seen in critical care units, followed by systemic lupus erythematosus and scleroderma, and these three conditions may account for up to 75% of patients with rheumatic disorders admitted to critical care services.[1] Given the complexity of these patients, it is perhaps not surprising that outcome can be poor with in-hospital mortality rates of 30–40% or more.[2]

This introductory chapter is aimed at the admitting physician presented with an acutely ill patient with a rheumatological disorder who is deteriorating rapidly and needs admission to a critical care unit. There have been major advances in the care of critically ill patients, including the way critical care units are run, moving from the previous "open" model of care to a "closed" system of multidisciplinary care and these will also be reviewed.

1.2
Initial Assessment of the Acutely Ill Patient

Early recognition that a patient's condition is deteriorating is essential, and in those patients who are severely unwell, immediate action is frequently required to correct abnormal physiology before a full history and examination can be carried out. If appropriate action is delayed, then there is a risk of further damage to vital organs, such as the brain and kidneys. Increasingly, it is being recognized that most in-hospital cardiorespiratory arrests are preventable if timely decision making is made, and relatively simple interventions such as antibiotics, fluids, oxygen administration, vasopressors, and appropriate intubation were carried out earlier.

Clinical severity may be obvious from the end of the bed, such as in a patient who presents with a massive pulmonary embolus, or a cerebral hemorrhage. In this situation, organ damage may well have occurred, but prompt intervention gives the best chance of recovery and prevents further secondary organ damage. Progressive insidious deterioration is less easy to spot, and often the hardest decision for an acute physician is to determine the precise point at which to refer a patient to critical care. Currently, the best approach is to monitor the basic physiological variables (respiratory and heart rate, blood pressure, urine output, oxygen saturation, and conscious level), and then by using a scoring system, agreed levels for referral to a "patient-at-risk," "outreach" or "medical emergency" team can be locally determined – these are often known as "Track and Trigger" systems. Around the world, use of these scoring systems, allied with support teams has been shown to expedite admission to critical care facilities and to prevent unnecessary in-hospital cardiac arrests.

Critical care units should no longer be viewed upon as "ventilation units," but should be utilized as the best places to take patients who are at high-risk of deterioration, since all the expertise and equipment is available "on tap" in a specifically designed location.

Initial assessment of the acutely unwell patient should be systematic, and the ABCD approach is a useful tool:

- **A**irway
- **B**reathing
- **C**irculation
- **D**isability

Airway obstruction (partial or complete) is a medical emergency leading to hypoxia, coma, and death within a few minutes if left uncorrected. It can result from aspiration, edema, bronchospasm, or most commonly reduced upper airway tone in patients who are obtunded. Simple airway maneuvers such as head tilt and chin lift, or a jaw thrust are usually effective; suction can remove blood, vomit, or foreign bodies. Intubation should be undertaken if the precipitant is unlikely to be resolved speedily.

The respiratory rate (<8 or >25/min) is widely thought of as the most sensitive marker of a deteriorating patient; central cyanosis and a fall in oxygen saturations may occur late. Oxygen should be administered early, and a clinical assessment made of the respiratory system. If time allows, arterial blood gas analysis and a chest radiograph can help determine further management. Traditionally, textbooks have given levels of PaO_2 and $PaCO_2$ that are absolute indications for ventilatory support (either invasive or noninvasive), but increasingly, these are not relied upon, and referral to a critical care specialist for an opinion is advised.

Hypovolemia and a low cardiac output are extremely common in acutely unwell patients. The heart rate is often falsely low because of medication (e.g., beta-blockers or digoxin), and many patients compensate well initially with increased peripheral resistance. Significant hypovolemia is relatively easy to detect, but occult hypovolemia (of up to 20%) is frequently overlooked. A mild metabolic acidosis and a raised lactate (>1.6 mmol/L), with cool peripheries and a prolonged capillary refill time, suggest the need for urgent intravenous fluids. A challenge of at least 20 mL/kg of a balanced crystalloid (such as Hartmann's) over 30–60 min is the best start, unless there is obvious heart failure. Further fluid resuscitation can be determined after response to the initial challenge, and after placement of a urinary catheter.

The neurological status can be rapidly determined by the Glasgow Coma Scale (GCS). In those who have a decreased conscious level, an early CT scan of the brain is indicated. Again, practice has changed in recent years, with patients being intubated for airway protection at less severely abnormal levels of consciousness, rather than waiting until the GCS is ≤8. Earlier intubation allows clear imaging, and prevents complications such as seizures and aspiration pneumonia occurring in a dark CT scanning suite. Hypoglycemia and drug intoxication should also be considered as well as ischemia and cerebral infection.

A thorough history and a fuller patient assessment can then be undertaken once stability has been achieved. Further information often then comes to light, as trends in measured physiological parameters are much more useful than single static measurements. Other investigations can then be prioritized, and a plan should be communicated to the whole team.

The management of acutely unwell patients, especially those with rheumatological conditions, frequently involves many teams, such as intensive care, nephrology, hematology, cardiology, respiratory, gastroenterology, and neurology. The outcome is likely to be optimal when these teams work together in a seamless process and cooperate and communicate well. As in all aspects of medicine, strong clinical leadership is an essential component of good team working.

There are two main systems/models of care that are used in critical care units throughout the world – these are known as "open" and "closed." In an open unit, each specialist can give patient care directions, order investigations, and prescribe new treatments for a patient. In a closed unit, specialists continue to visit frequently, but all recommended aspects of care by the different specialists who are consulting are authorized/signed-off by the attending intensive care specialist. The closed model has been shown to better control costs, and results in significantly better patient outcomes. This is perhaps most relevant for extremely complex patients who have multisystem involvement where recommended therapies for one organ may have a detrimental effect on a different system. Intensive care specialists often have significant expertise in understanding physiology and pharmacology as it relates to critically ill patients – especially those with multiple organ failure.

1.3
Specific Assessments of the Critically Ill Rheumatological Patient

It is vitally important to evaluate the rheumatological patient with multiorgan disease with a detailed history and physical examination as these patients often have complex medical problems and are on multiple medications. A referral letter from the primary care physician, if written well, can save much time in the emergency room. It is obviously helpful if the patient is already known to the hospital and the previous records are available and these should provide useful information on the diagnosis and current treatments. Previous investigations if available are especially helpful in terms of looking for changes in radiological appearances, biochemistry, hematology and acute phase markers.

The patient is often able to give a detailed account of the onset of their symptoms. Patients with chronic conditions such as inflammatory arthritis, lupus or systemic vasculitis can often tell the clinician whether the current symptoms represent a flare of the underlying condition, whether there are complications such as infection, or if the presentation represents new or a recurrence of organ involvement such as glomerulonephritis, pulmonary hemorrhage, or a thrombotic manifestation. The patient may also inform the admitting clinician if any new therapies have recently been commenced that may have resulted in a serious adverse effect. If a detailed history from the patient is not possible because they are too unwell, every effort should be made to speak to any accompanying relatives for as much information on the history as possible, assuming that the patient is able to give consent for the relatives to speak on their behalf.

When the patient has been referred from another hospital, a phone call or e-mail to the referring clinician may give a lot more information than a referral letter. In the age of electronic media, it is often possible for data on imaging studies, for example, to be sent directly between hospitals, reducing the need for unnecessary repetition of imaging, reducing radiation exposure, and giving a baseline for comparison with further imaging studies.

Once the patient has been stabilized as described above, a thorough history should be obtained followed by a detailed examination of all organ systems to rapidly prioritize the most seriously affected organs. During the examination, a careful assessment of all areas of the body is important. Close attention to the hands may, for example, reveal multiple splinter hemorrhages, which could point toward bacterial endocarditis, systemic lupus erythematosus, systemic vasculitis, or antiphospholipid syndrome. Cutaneous vasculitis can range from subtle periungual and digital infarction through to widespread palpable purpura and severe necrotizing ulceration. Livedo reticularis, especially if it is widespread and with a broken pattern on the forearms and legs – so-called livedo racemosa – may be a powerful clue to a diagnosis of antiphospholipid syndrome or systemic vasculitis such as polyarteritis nodosa. Examination of the hands will also show the extent of any damage from rheumatoid arthritis, and nodule formation may be seen over the fingers or at the elbows. The finding of periungual erythema with macroscopic nailfold capillary loops, Raynauds' phenomenon, and sclerodactyly with digital ulcers is pathognomonic for systemic sclerosis. Similarly, in a patient with respiratory failure, the presence of Gottron's sign and a heliotrope rash may indicate severe respiratory muscle weakness due to an inflammatory myopathy such as dermatomyositis.

Careful examination of the scalp may reveal discoid lesions with scarring alopecia of lupus. Examining the ears for skin lesions such as discoid lupus, cutaneous vasculitis, and fluid levels/tympanic membrane perforations may yield useful diagnostic information. Large nasal polyps in the context of late-onset asthma may point toward a diagnosis of Churg–Strauss syndrome. Schirmer's test for dry eyes is easily performed at the bedside and can be surprisingly helpful where an autoimmune connective tissue disorder is part of the differential diagnosis.

Cardiovascular examination for cardiac murmurs, signs of cardiac failure, absent or diminished peripheral pulses, and vascular bruits including listening for abdominal bruits may be helpful. Respiratory examination may reveal crepitations, signs of consolidation, or pleurisy. Stridor may indicate subglottic stenosis in Wegener's granulomatosis or tracheal collapse in relapsing polychondritis. However, clinical examination can be misleading. For example, patients with acute flares of Wegener's granulomatosis may have multiple cavitating pulmonary nodules that are not detected by simple bedside clinical methods. Likewise, patients with pulmonary hemorrhage often do not have obvious hemoptysis and there may be few if any detectable clinical signs in the lung fields.

Abdominal examination including rectal examination when appropriate in a patient with acute intestinal or mesenteric vasculitis may reveal signs of an acute abdomen or gastrointestinal hemorrhage due to bowel perforation or organ infarction. A careful neurological examination for motor or sensory deficits, which can be subtle, is essential.

A pattern of nerve damage suggesting mononeuritis multiplex or cranial neuropathies is a strong pointer to a vasculitic disorder. Likewise, lower limb long tract signs with bladder or bowel dysfunction may indicate transverse myelopathy in a patient with systemic lupus erythematosus. Fundoscopy should be performed wherever possible even in the absence of visual symptoms for signs of retinal vasculitis or hypertensive retinopathy as seen in patients with scleroderma renal crisis or a rapidly progressive glomerulonephritis.

In the locomotor system, the presence of an inflammatory arthropathy should be documented and the pattern of the arthritis can be useful diagnostically – there are only a few causes of a symmetrical inflammatory arthropathy: rheumatoid arthritis, systemic lupus erythematosus, and less commonly psoriatic arthritis. A monoarthritis in the context of a febrile patient should always be aspirated to investigate possible joint sepsis. A patient with acute urinary retention, bowel dysfunction, saddle anesthesia, and acute low back pain suggesting a large lumbar disk protrusion is a neurosurgical emergency.

This list is not exhaustive and the examination will be guided to large extent by the history and the patient's diagnosis if this is already known. It is therefore important for the clinician to have a thorough knowledge of the acute presenting features of the major multisystem rheumatic disorders and these will be described in detail in subsequent chapters of this book.

1.3.1
Investigations

At this stage, a diagnosis or a short differential diagnosis is usually possible allowing the clinician to discuss urgent investigations with colleagues. Simple investigations such as a full blood count, biochemistry, acute phase markers such as the erythrocyte sedimentation rate (ESR) and C-reactive protein (CRP) and a urine dip test for blood, protein, glucose, and leucocytes and a peak flow or simple spirometry at the bedside will provide useful information rapidly. In patients with autoimmune disorders such as lupus, a low CRP is very helpful as it lessens the likelihood of major bacterial infection. Likewise, a pancytopenia in a patient with previously normal blood counts could suggest either a lupus flare or bone marrow suppression from a cytotoxic drug. The presence of proteinuria and hematuria in the context of impaired renal function should lead to a search for dysmorphic red cells and granular casts in patients with systemic rheumatic diseases such as lupus or vasculitis where glomerulonephritis can lead rapidly to renal failure.

In patients with extensive skin manifestations, the differential diagnosis between a drug reaction and a cutaneous flare of lupus or systemic vasculitis can be difficult and a dermatology opinion and a skin biopsy may be helpful.

Imaging investigations need to be carefully selected to maximize clinical information gathering, balancing the risks of the investigation carefully. For example, in a patient with severe neurological manifestations, magnetic resonance imaging can yield critical information but this has to be set against the risk of contrast reactions and the possibility of nephrogenic dermal fibrosis due to gadolinium in patients with renal failure. Likewise, intra-arterial angiography in a patient with lupus, accelerated atherosclerosis, and gangrene may be combined with angioplasty or stent placement, but these procedures should be undertaken in centers with vascular surgery support. New-generation spiral computed tomography scanners now offer the ability to rapidly acquire good quality vascular imaging to identify arterial bleeding or thrombosis relatively noninvasively and may in time replace conventional arteriography as the initial investigation of choice.[3]

1.3.2
Treatment Approaches

The most important urgent treatments are those outlined above to rapidly stabilize the patient and allow transfer either directly to the critical care unit or to a larger center with expertise in the management of complex rheumatological patients. The diagnosis of the immediate clinical problem and the underlying rheumatological diagnosis will dictate the treatment approach. The specific management of the individual disease and treatment complications will be covered in later chapters, but before commencing treatment, it is worth considering the following points:

- A number of diseases can mimic the autoimmune rheumatic disorders. Good examples include infections such as subacute bacterial endocarditis (SBE) mimicking vasculitis, especially as low titer autoantibodies commonly occur in SBE. Other mimics include malignancy, atrial myxomas, and viral infections such as HIV which can mimic both lupus and Sjogren's syndrome.
- There should never be a rush to commence immunosuppressive agents until a thorough evaluation for infection has been performed. If the patient is overtly septic and has a rapidly progressive autoimmune rheumatic disorder such as lupus or systemic vasculitis, intravenous immunoglobulin, if available, can be useful as a short-term measure.
- Patients should be assessed frequently on the critical care unit for the development of unexpected complications including adverse effects from therapy and new organ disease manifestations of the underlying disorder.
- Failure to respond to a treatment protocol should lead to a reevaluation of the diagnosis.

1.3.3
Complications from Prolonged Immobilization

Patients with rheumatic disorders are even more likely than usual to develop complications from prolonged in-patient admissions and immobility. Attention should be paid to the risk of muscle wasting and joint contractures with early assessments and interventions from a physiotherapist and occupational therapist. Patients may be at risk of critical care neuropathies and these should be distinguished from the neuropathies that may occur for example in rheumatoid arthritis, lupus, or the vasculitides. Decubitus ulcer is a particular problem in patients who have been on long-term corticosteroid therapy where the skin has become thin and friable – intensive nursing care is essential in the prevention of these difficult-to-treat ulcers. Immobility will also exacerbate the risk of osteoporosis in these patients, and specific therapies such as calcium and vitamin D supplementation and bisphosphonates should be considered. Nutrition can be a problem in patients with systemic sclerosis who have dysphagia or malabsorption due to bowel involvement. Autoimmune rheumatic patients are at increased risk of venous thromboembolism, and the presence of antiphospholipid antibodies together with traditional cardiovascular risk factors will exacerbate this risk. It is vital therefore that these patients should be assessed for the risk of thrombosis on admission and managed accordingly.

1.3.4
End-of-Life Decisions

Critical care units are faced with decisions about withdrawal of active interventions on a daily basis. While patients with rheumatic disorders are usually young women of child-bearing age, many patients with systemic vasculitis and rheumatoid arthritis are older with multiple comorbidities. The decision to withdraw active treatment from a young patient with little or no hope of recovery from advanced scleroderma, for example, can be difficult. However, guidelines and specific training programs exist for open discussion of these issues with patients and their carers in a sensitive manner and to ensure that a high standard of care continues to be delivered in the last days and hours of the patient's life.

1.4
Conclusion

In summary, patients with autoimmune rheumatic disorders often present acutely and may need admission to a critical care unit. The outcome of these patients is still poor but will be significantly enhanced if clinicians have a good working knowledge of the often nonspecific presentations of these patients together with the ability to rapidly assess patients and liaise with colleagues in formulating a management plan and determining the ideal environment in which to deliver critical care.

References

1. Janssen NM, Karnad DR, Guntupalli KK. Rheumatologic diseases in the intensive care unit: epidemiology, clinical approach, management, and outcome. *Crit Care Clin.* 2002;18:729-748.
2. Godeau B, Mortier E, Roy PM, et al. Short and longterm outcomes for patients with systemic rheumatic diseases admitted to intensive care units: a prognostic study of 181 patients. *J Rheumatol.* 1997;24:1317-1323.
3. Seamon MJ, Smoger D, Torres DM, et al. A prospective validation of a current practice: the detection of extremity vascular injury with CT angiography. *J Trauma.* 2009;67:238-243.

Life-Threatening Complications of Systemic Lupus Erythematosus

2

Michelle Petri

Abstract The major cause of death in longstanding lupus is accelerated atherosclerosis leading to cardiovascular disease. Early in lupus, the major causes of death are active lupus and infection. Life-threatening or organ-threatening lupus is not rare. Multiple organs including skin (necrosis), hematologic (thrombocytopenia, hemolytic anemia, neutropenia, catastrophic antiphospholipid syndrome, and thrombotic thrombocytopenic purpura), heart (pericardial tamponade, myocarditis), lung (alveolar hemorrhage, pulmonary hypertension), gastrointestinal (vasculitis, pancreatitis), adrenal insufficiency, and neurologic (myelitis) may be encountered.

Keywords Catastrophic antiphospholipid syndrome • Hemolytic anemia • Myelitis • Myocarditis • Pancreatitis • SLE • Thrombocytopenia • Vasculitis

2.1
Introduction

Systemic lupus erythematosus (SLE) is the prototypic systemic autoimmune disease. It has a strong female predominance (9:1) and predominantly is diagnosed in the 20's and 30's. SLE and its treatment lead to important morbidity and mortality. Because SLE is a multisystem disease, the following chapter will divide emergencies by organ system. For each emergency, the manifestation will be described, its evaluation detailed, and initial treatment discussed.

M. Petri
Department of Medicine, Division of Rheumatology, Johns Hopkins University School of Medicine, 1820 E. Monument St., Ste. 7500, Baltimore, MD 21205, USA
e-mail: mpetri@jhmi.edu

M.A. Khamashta and M. Ramos-Casals (eds.), *Autoimmune Diseases*,
DOI: 10.1007/978-0-85729-358-9_2, © Springer-Verlag London Limited 2011

2.2
Cutaneous Digital Gangrene

Digital gangrene in SLE may start as small ischemic lesions but can quickly progress to digital gangrene. In the largest series, long disease duration, Raynaud's phenomenon, and elevated serum CRP were independent risk factors.[1] The differential diagnosis includes severe Raynaud's phenomenon, thromboembolic (i.e., antiphospholipid syndrome [APS]), and lupus vasculitis. Evaluation requires the assessment of antiphospholipid antibodies (lupus anticoagulant, anticardiolipin, and anti-beta$_2$-glycoprotein I), cardiac echocardiogram, and often arteriogram.

Treatment of digital gangrene is multifactorial. If vasospasm (Raynaud's) is involved, calcium channel blockers will be given. Other vasodilators, including topical nitrates, may be tried, as well. Intravenous prostacyclin may be needed. To prevent and treat thrombosis, low-dose aspirin (81 mg) and therapeutic doses of heparin are needed. If lupus vasculitis is present, intravenous methylprednisolone pulse therapy (1,000 mg daily for 3 days, given over 90 min), followed by high-dose oral prednisone (1 mg/kg) is started. Digital sympathectomy, if an experienced surgeon is available, may be considered. The goal is to save as much ischemic tissue as possible. Once tissue demarcation has occurred, a hand or vascular surgeon may amputate the gangrenous areas to relieve pain and improve cosmetic appearance.

2.3
Cutaneous Necrosis

Widespread cutaneous necrosis is rare in SLE. It can occur from antiphospholipid syndrome,[2] SLE vasculitis, and can be induced by warfarin in patients who are Protein C deficient (because warfarin further reduces Protein C and Protein S levels). Evaluation will include assessment of antiphospholipid antibodies (lupus anticoagulant, anticardiolipin, and anti-beta$_2$-glycoprotein I) and biopsy of the edge of a necrotic area (to detect vasculitis). If the necrosis is due to APS, therapeutic doses of heparin are started. If necrosis is due to SLE vasculitis, IV methylprednisolone pulse therapy (1,000 mg daily for 3 days, given over 90 min) is given, followed by high-dose oral prednisone (1 mg/kg).

2.4
Thrombocytopenia

Thrombocytopenia is common in SLE and is one of the American College of Rheumatology classification criteria for SLE.[3] In the Hopkins Lupus Cohort, 21% have had thrombocytopenia defined as a platelet count less than 100,000/mm^3. Most thrombocytopenia in SLE is not life-threatening, and, in fact, may be over-treated. It is rare for patients to bleed unless the platelet count is below 10,000; treatment usually is not needed unless the platelet count falls below 30,000/mm^3. An exception is made in an anti-coagulated patient, in whom the goal is to keep the platelet count above 50,000/mm^3. Evaluation of thrombocytopenia in an SLE patient includes assessment of antiphospholipid antibodies (lupus anticoagulant, anticardiolipin, and anti-beta$_2$-glycoprotein I), antiplatelet antibodies, drug toxicity, and infection. Rituximab can cause a very rare thrombocytopenia, with recovery usually within 2 weeks.

Treatment of serious thrombocytopenia requires intravenous methylprednisolone (1,000 mg daily for 3 days, given over 90 min) followed by high-dose oral prednisone (1 mg/kg). Some patients, however, may not respond. Intravenous immunoglobulin, 400 mg/kg over 5 days, is usually the next step; it may be necessary to increase the dose to 1 kg/kg to see a response. In those who still do not respond, rituximab can be considered. Maintenance therapy with azathioprine or mycophenolate is usually needed. Platelet transfusions can be given to patients who are actually bleeding, but the SLE patient's autoantibodies will rapidly destroy them. A patient who responds to intravenous immunoglobulin, but frequently relapses, is a candidate for splenectomy. Although it should not be considered a cure, most patients do improve postsplenectomy. A patient who is not a surgical candidate can be considered for splenectomy by radiation. Newer agents for thrombocytopenia, such as Promacta® (eltrombopag), have not been adequately assessed in SLE, and would not be routine in an emergent situation.

2.5
Autoimmune Hemolytic Anemia (AIHA)

AIHA is rare in SLE, occurring in only 11% of the Hopkins Lupus Cohort. Evaluation for AIHA would include a search for other causes of anemia (ferritin, B12, hemoglobinopathy, schistocytes) as well as tests to confirm hemolytic anemia (direct Coombs test, low haptoglobin, high LDH, high reticulocyte count).

Treatment of AIHA includes intravenous methylprednisolone (1,000 mg daily for 3 days, given over 90 min) followed by high-dose oral prednisone (1 mg/kg). Maintenance therapy with azathioprine or mycophenolate mofetil[4] is then given. Danazol has been used.[5] Refractory AIHA may require rituximab[6,7] or splenectomy.[8]

2.6
Neutropenia

Leukopenia in SLE is common and is part of the American College of Rheumatology classification criteria. Most leukopenia in SLE is lymphopenia; neutropenia from SLE is rare, but reported.[9,10] Evaluation of neutropenia in SLE would include anti-neutrophil antibodies and drug toxicity (usually cyclophosphamide or other immunosuppressive drugs). Rituximab can cause both an immediate and a late neutropenia.

Neutropenia in SLE is usually not an emergency; it is often over-treated. As long as the total neutrophil count is above 1,000/mm³, the risk of infection is small, and no treatment is necessary. If the patient becomes neutropenic due to cyclophosphamide, or other immunosuppressive drug, it is sufficient to stop the cyclophosphamide and allow the neutrophils to recover. Granulocyte colony stimulating factor (G-CSF) should not be given to the stable patient because of the risk of SLE flares (including fatal flares).[11] G-CSF should be reserved for the neutropenic patient with sepsis.

2.7
Catastrophic Antiphospholipid Syndrome (CAPS)

CAPS is a rare manifestation of APS. About 40% of CAPS patients have SLE; 10% another rheumatic disease; and 50% no history of autoimmune disease. Common precipitants include infection, surgery, trauma, pregnancy, oral contraceptives, and cessation of warfarin in an APS patient. "Definitive" CAPS requires three organ involvement, and demonstration of thrombosis in the setting of antiphospholipid antibodies. "Probable" CAPS requires involvement of two organs. CAPS manifestations differ from APS. In CAPS, 48% have primary APS, 40% have SLE, and 12% have secondary APS due to another cause.[12] Evaluation of CAPS involves assessment of antiphospholipid antibodies (lupus anticoagulant, anticardiolipin, and anti-beta$_2$-glycoprotein I), examination of the peripheral smear for microangiopathic hemolytic anemia and documentation of thrombosis.[13]

Treatment is truly an emergency, as mortality is as high as 50%. Treatment has three goals: to settle the "cytokine storm" (intravenous methylprednisolone pulse), treat and prevent further thrombosis (intravenous heparin), and reduce the antiphospholipid antibody burden (plasmapheresis or intravenous immunoglobulin).[13] In recalcitrant cases, rituximab may be helpful.

2.8
Thrombotic Thrombocytopenic Purpera (TTP)

Past series of TTP in SLE may have included some patients with CAPS, as the two can present in similar fashion.[14,15] Genetic or autoantibody-induced deficiency of the metalloproteinase ADAMTS13 is part of the pathogenesis. Classic TTP includes fever, thrombocytopenia, microangiopathic hemolytic anemia, renal dysfunction, and neurologic involvement.[16] Evaluation would include a peripheral blood smear for schistocytes, exclusion of infection, and drug toxicity.

Treatment of TTP in SLE is plasmapheresis or plasma exchange.[17] Intravenous cyclophosphamide and rituximab have also been used.[18,19]

2.9
Pericardial Tamponade

Pericarditis is frequent in SLE, occurring in 22% of the Hopkins Lupus Cohort. Serositis is one of the ACR classification criteria of SLE. Pericardial tamponade, however, is rare. It can occur as a presenting manifestation of SLE.[20] Typically, pericarditis is positional, such that the patient feels dyspneic lying flat and feels better leaning forward. Patients with tamponade may present with ascites and edema.[21] Evaluation would include physical examination findings including pericardial rub, distant heart sounds, pulsus paridoxus, and confirmatory cardiac echocardiogram.

Treatment of life-threatening pericardial tamponade will require a pericardial tap or pericardial window. Treatment of the underlying SLE activity would include intravenous methylprednisolone pulse therapy (1,000 mg daily for 3 days, given over 90 min) followed by high-dose oral prednisone (1 mg/kg).

2.10
Myocarditis

SLE myocarditis is rare, occurring in 14% in one series.[22] It may be associated with myositis.[23] Patients with SLE myocarditis often present with congestive heart failure. Evaluation would include cardiac echocardiogram, which would show hypokinesis, and coronary arteriogram to rule out atherosclerosis or coronary vasculitis. On occasion, a right ventricular biopsy confirms myocarditis.[24]

Treatment of myocarditis would include intravenous methylprednisolone pulse therapy (1,000 mg daily for 3 days, given over 90 min) followed by high-dose oral prednisone (1 mg/kg).[25] Pulse cyclophosphamide therapy may be needed.[26]

2.11
Pulmonary Alveolar Hemorrhage

Alveolar hemorrhage is extremely rare in SLE, with only a few case series.[27-29] It presents as dyspnea, fever, hemophysis, and chest pain. Evaluation would include chest CT and bronchoscopy.

Treatment of alveolar hemorrhage in SLE is plasmapheresis and intravenous methylprednisolone pulse therapy (1,000 mg daily for 3 days, given over 90 min) followed by high-dose oral prednisone (1 mg/kg).

2.12
Pulmonary Hypertension

Pulmonary hypertension in SLE can be severe, with a poor prognosis.[30] Dyspnea is the most common presenting symptom. Evaluation of an SLE patient with acute severe pulmonary hypertension would require cardiac echocardiogram followed by right heart catheterization. The immediate concern is whether it is due to thromboembolic disease or due to SLE activity.

Treatment of pulmonary hypertension due to thromboembolic disease may require surgical embolectomy or thrombolytic agent or heparin. Severe pulmonary hypertension due to active SLE is treated with intravenous methylprednisolone pulse therapy (1,000 mg daily for 3 days, given over 90 min) followed by high-dose oral prednisone (1 mg/kg). Chronic pulmonary hypertension can be treated in a fashion similar to idiopathic pulmonary hypertension, including sildenafil, bosentan, and intravenous prostacyclin.[31]

2.13
Pancreatitis

Pancreatitis is a rare manifestation of SLE. In the largest review, only 4% of SLE patients had pancreatitis attributed to SLE.[32] Patients present with abdominal pain, fever, and electrolyte disturbances. It can be fatal, especially in pediatric patients.[33] A multivariate model found that hypertriglyceridemia, psychosis, pleurisy, gastritis, and anemia were associated with a history of pancreatitis.[32] Although antiphospholipid antibodies can occur, they do not appear to be causative.

Although high-dose corticosteroids can cause pancreatitis, when SLE pancreatitis occurs, intravenous methylprednisolone 1,000 mg daily for 3 days remains the treatment of choice.

2.14
Adrenal Insufficiency

Adrenal insufficiency is a very rare manifestation of SLE. It appears in conjunction with antiphospholipid syndrome, or more commonly, in catastrophic antiphospholipid syndrome (CAPS), in whom 26% had adrenal involvement in one series.[12,34] In CAPS, adrenal involvement is usually bilateral, due to adrenal venous infarction. Adrenal insufficiency usually presents acutely, with flank pain, nausea, vomiting, hypotension, and electrolyte abnormalities.

Treatment of CAPS is reviewed elsewhere in this chapter. Management of adrenal insufficiency is both acute, in terms of steroid, volume and electrolyte management, and chronic, with adrenal replacement, with low-dose prednisone and fluorinated steroids.

2.15
Mesenteric Vasculitis

Mesenteric vasculitis is a very rare manifestation of SLE. Patients present with fever, abdominal pain, diarrhea, vomiting, and sepsis.[35,36] Early in the course, swollen layers of bowel may be present on abdominal CT.[37] A mesenteric arteriogram may show vasculitis. Occasionally, biopsy during colonoscopy may reveal vasculitis. The differential diagnosis would include atherosclerosis, pancreatitis, peptic ulcer, peritonitis, bowel infarction, and infection (such as *C. difficile* or cytomegalovirus).

Management requires both surgical resection of dead bowel and suppression of vasculitis by intravenous methylprednisolone pulse therapy (1,000 mg daily for 3 days, given over 90 min).

2.16
Myelitis

Longitudinal myelitis in SLE occurs in two forms, one affecting gray matter (that occurs in an acute catastrophic form) and one involving white matter (that clearly resembles neuromyelitis optica).[38] Myelitis presents as pain, weakness, and sphincteric defects. Patients with gray matter involvement will have flaccidity and hyporeflexia, while patients with white matter dysfunction will have spasticity and hyperreflexia. Patients with gray matter dysfunction may have a prodrome of fever and urinary retention. Those with white matter involvement are more likely to have had antiphospholipid antibodies.

Treatment for SLE myelitis needs to be given within a short time after symptom onset, with intravenous methylprednisolone pulse therapy (1,000 mg daily for 3 days, given over 90 min), followed by high-dose oral corticosteroids. There may be a role for rituximab, as well.

References

1. Liu A, Zhang W, Tian X, Zhang X, Zhang F, Zeng X. Prevalence, risk factors and outcome of digital gangrene in 2684 lupus patients. *Lupus*. 2009;18(12):1112-1118.
2. Frances C, Tribout B, Boisnic S. Cutaneous necrosis associated with the lupus anticoagulant. *Dermatologica*. 1989;178:194-201.
3. Tan EM, Cohen AS, Fries JF, et al. The 1982 revised criteria for the classification of systemic lupus erythematosus. *Arthritis Rheum*. 1982;25:1271-1277.
4. Alba P, Karim MY, Hunt BJ. Mycophenolate mofetil as a treatment for autoimmune haemolytic anaemia in patients with systemic lupus erythematosus and antiphospholipid syndrome. *Lupus*. 2003;12(8):633-635.
5. Cervera H, Jara LJ, Pizarro S, et al. Danazol for systemic lupus erythematosus with refractory autoimmune thrombocytopenia or Evans' syndrome. *J Rheumatol*. 1995;22(10):1867-1871.

6. Abdwani R, Mani R. Anti-CD20 monoclonal antibody in acute life threatening haemolytic anaemia complicating childhood onset SLE. *Lupus*. 2009;18(5):460-464.

7. Gomard-Mennesson E, Ruivard M, Koenig M, et al. Treatment of isolated severe immune hemolytic anaemia associated with systemic lupus erythematosus: 26 cases. *Lupus*. 2006; 15(4):223-231.

8. Gruenberg JC, VanSlyck EJ, Abraham JP. Splenectomy in systemic lupus erythematosis. *Am Surg*. 1986;52(7):366-370.

9. Keeling DM, Isenberg DA. Haematological manifestations of systemic lupus erythematosus. *Blood Rev*. 1993;7(4):199-207.

10. Martinez-Banos D, Crispin JC, Lazo-Langner A, Sanchez-Guerrero J. Moderate and severe neutropenia in patients with systemic lupus erythematosus. *Rheumatology (Oxford)*. 2006;45(8):994-998.

11. Vasiliu IM, Petri MA, Baer AN. Therapy with granulocyte colony-stimulating factor in systemic lupus erythematosus may be associated with severe flares. *J Rheumatol*. 2006; 33(9):1878-1880.

12. Asherson RA, Cervera R, Piette JC, et al. Catastrophic antiphospholipid syndrome. Clinical and laboratory features of 50 patients. *Medicine*. 1998;77(3):195-207.

13. Asherson RA, Cervera R, de Groot PG, et al. Catastrophic antiphospholipid syndrome: international consensus statement on classification criteria and treatment guidelines. *Lupus*. 2003;12(7):530-534.

14. Asherson RA, Cervera R, Font J. Multiorgan thrombotic disorders in systemic lupus erythematosus: a common link? *Lupus*. 1992;1(4):199-203.

15. Musio F, Bohen EM, Yuan CM, Welch PG. Review of thrombotic thrombocytopenic purpura in the setting of systemic lupus erythematosus. *Semin Arthritis Rheum*. 1998;28(1):1-19.

16. Kwok SK, Ju JH, Cho CS, Kim HY, Park SH. Thrombotic thrombocytopenic purpura in systemic lupus erythematosus: risk factors and clinical outcome: a single centre study. *Lupus*. 2009;18(1):16-21.

17. Nesher G, Hanna VE, Moore TL, Hersh M, Osborn TG. Thrombotic microangiopathic hemolytic anemia in systemic lupus erythematosus. *Semin Arthritis Rheum*. 1994;24:165-172.

18. Miyamura T, Watanabe H, Takahama S, et al. Thrombotic thrombocytopenic purpura in patients with systemic lupus erythematosus. *Nihon Rinsho Meneki Gakkai Kaishi*. 2008;31(3):159-165.

19. Letchumanan P, Ng HJ, Lee LH, Thumboo J. A comparison of thrombotic thrombocytopenic purpura in an inception cohort of patients with and without systemic lupus erythematosus. *Rheumatology (Oxford)*. 2009;48(4):399-403.

20. Rosenbaum E, Krebs E, Cohen M, Tiliakos A, Derk CT. The spectrum of clinical manifestations, outcome and treatment of pericardial tamponade in patients with systemic lupus erythematosus: a retrospective study and literature review. *Lupus*. 2009;18(7):608-612.

21. Kahl LE. The spectrum of pericardial tamponade in systemic lupus erythematosus: report of ten patients. *Arthritis Rheum*. 1992;35:1343-1349.

22. Badui E, Garcia-Rubi D, Robles E, et al. Cardiovascular manifestations in systemic lupus erythematosus. Prospective study of 100 patients. *Angiology*. 1985;36:431-441.

23. Borenstein DG, Fye WB, Arnett FC, Stevens MB. The myocarditis of systemic lupus erythematosus: association with myositis. *Ann Intern Med*. 1978;89:619-624.

24. Fairfax MJ, Osborn TG, Williams GA, Tsai CC, Moore TL. Endomyocardial biopsy in patients with systemic lupus erythematosus. *J Rheumatol*. 1988;15:593-596.

25. Gottenberg JE, Roux S, Assayag P, Clerc D, Mariette X. Specific cardiomyopathy in lupus patients: report of three cases. *Joint Bone Spine*. 2004;71(1):66-69.

26. Law WG, Thong BY, Lian TY, Kong KO, Chng HH. Acute lupus myocarditis: clinical features and outcome of an oriental case series. *Lupus*. 2005;14(10):827-831.

27. Koh WH, Thumboo J, Boey ML. Pulmonary haemorrhage in Oriental patients with systemic lupus erythematosus. *Lupus*. 1997;6(9):713-716.

28. Canas C, Tobon GJ, Granados M, Fernandez L. Diffuse alveolar hemorrhage in Colombian patients with systemic lupus erythematosus. *Clin Rheumatol.* 2007;26(11):1947-1949.

29. Zamora MR, Warner ML, Tuder R, Schwarz MI. Diffuse alveolar hemorrhage and systemic lupus erythematosus. Clinical presentation, histology, survival, and outcome. *Medicine.* 1997;76(3):192-202.

30. Chung SM, Lee CK, Lee EY, Yoo B, Lee SD, Moon HB. Clinical aspects of pulmonary hypertension in patients with systemic lupus erythematosus and in patients with idiopathic pulmonary arterial hypertension. *Clin Rheumatol.* 2006;25(6):866-872.

31. Kamata Y, Iwamoto M, Minota S. Consecutive use of sildenafil and bosentan for the treatment of pulmonary arterial hypertension associated with collagen vascular disease: sildenafil as reliever and bosentan as controller. *Lupus.* 2007;16(11):901-903.

32. Makol A, Petri M. Pancreatitis in systemic lupus erythematosus: frequency and associated factors – a review of the Hopkins Lupus Cohort. *J Rheumatol.* 2010;37(2):341-345.

33. Serrano Lopez MC, Yebra-Bango M, Lopez Bonet E. Acute pancreatitis and systemic lupus erythematosus: necropsy of a case and review of pancreatic vascular lesions. *Am J Gastroenterol.* 1991;86:764-767.

34. Espinosa G, Santos E, Cervera R, et al. Adrenal involvement in the antiphospholipid syndrome: clinical and immunologic characteristics of 86 patients. *Medicine.* 2003;82(2):106-118.

35. Chen SY, Xu JH, Shuai ZW, et al. A clinical analysis 30 cases of lupus mesenteric vasculitis. *Zhonghua Nei Ke Za Zhi.* 2009;48(2):136-139.

36. Zizic TM, Classen JN, Stevens MB. Acute abdominal complications of systemic lupus erythematosus and polyarteritis nodosa. *Am J Med.* 1982;73:525-531.

37. Ko SF, Lee TY, Cheng TT, et al. CT findings at lupus mesenteric vasculitis. *Acta Radiol.* 1997;38(1):115-120.

38. Birnbaum J, Petri M, Thompson R, Izbudak I, Kerr D. Distinct subtypes of myelitis in systemic lupus erythematosus. *Arthritis Rheum.* 2009;60(11):3378-3387.

Catastrophic Antiphospholipid Syndrome

3

Maria J. Cuadrado, Giovanni Sanna, Maria Laura Bertolaccini,
and Munther A. Khamashta

Abstract Antiphospholipid syndrome (APS) is characterized by the development of arterial and/or venous thrombosis and/or pregnancy morbidity in the presence of antiphospholipid antibodies (aPL) anticardiolipin (aCL), anti-β2-glycoprotein I (anti-β2GPI), and lupus anticoagulant (LA). Catastrophic antiphospholipid syndrome (CAPS) is a very severe variant of the classic APS, with predominant and extensive small-vessels occlusion that causes multiple organs thrombosis. Multiple thrombotic events occur in a short period of time and frequently lead to a life-threatening condition because of multiorgan failure. The mortality rate is high, but an early diagnosis and treatment with anticoagulation, corticosteroids, plasma exchange, and intravenous immunoglobulin (IVIG) may reduce this rate.

Keywords Anticoagulation • Catastrophic • IVIG • Plasmapheresis

3.1
Introduction

In this chapter, we review a life-threatening condition, associated with the presence of antiphospholipid antibodies (aPL) characterized by a different clinical presentation, pathogenesis, and a higher mortality rate than the classical antiphospholipid syndrome (APS). This variant of APS is known as the catastrophic APS (CAPS).

CAPS was defined in 1992.[1] It presents as multiple vascular occlusive events, presenting over a short period of time, in patients who are aPL-positive. It is an uncommon presentation that happens in <1% of APS patients, often after a triggering factor such as anticoagulation withdrawal, minor surgical procedures, or infections. Mortality rate is

M.J. Cuadrado (✉)
Lupus Unit, The Rayne Institute, St. Thomas' Hospital,
Lambeth Palace Road, London SE1 7EH, UK
e-mail: mjcuadrado@yahoo.com

M.A. Khamashta and M. Ramos-Casals (eds.), *Autoimmune Diseases*,
DOI: 10.1007/978-0-85729-358-9_3, © Springer-Verlag London Limited 2011

around 50%, and treatment includes corticosteroids, anticoagulation, intravenous immunoglobulin (IVIG), and plasma exchange.[2]

3.2
Pathogenesis

The pathogenesis of CAPS is not fully understood. It seems that occlusion of multiple vessels occur, beginning at the microvascular level rather than at the macrovascular one. Kitchens et al.[3] have suggested that the vascular occlusions are themselves responsible for the ongoing thrombosis. Clots continue to generate thrombin, fibrinolysis is depressed by an increase in plasminogen activator inhibitor type-1 (PAI-1), and there is consumption of the natural anticoagulant proteins such as protein C and antithrombin. These multiple small-vessel occlusions cause extensive tissue necrosis which results in a systemic inflammatory response syndrome (SIRS), with excessive cytokine release from affected and necrotic tissues.[4] Proinflammatory cytokines, several products of the activated complement system (e.g., C3b, iC3b, and C5a), and aPL themselves have each been demonstrated to activate endothelial cells, provide a stimulatory signal, and upregulate adhesion molecules and tissue factor. These molecules can also act on leukocytes and platelets to increase their adhesion to vascular endothelium and to promote microthrombosis and the local release of toxic mediators, including proteases and oxygen-derived free radicals. The interaction between all these cells in the presence of aPL leads to the diffuse microvasculopathy that characterizes CAPS and leads to multiorgan failure.[4-6]

3.3
Clinical Manifestations

The most common known trigger for CAPS is infection. Trauma, surgery, oral contraceptive, neoplasia, and warfarin withdrawal have also been reported. In almost half of the cases, no obvious precipitating factors have been identified. Frequently, CAPS appears in patients without any previous thrombotic history.[7]

The clinical manifestations of CAPS depend on the organs that are affected by the thrombotic events and the extent of the thrombosis, together with manifestations of the SIRS. Multiple organ dysfunction and failure, as a consequence of thrombotic microangiopathy, are responsible for the majority of the clinical features; however, large venous or arterial thrombosis can also occur in about one fifth of patients. In a review of 220 patients with CAPS,[8] 70% of patients presented with renal involvement (renal insufficiency, proteinuria, hypertension); 66% with pulmonary complications (acute respiratory distress syndrome and pulmonary emboli being the most frequent); 60% with cerebral symptoms (encephalopathy, infarcts, seizures, venous occlusions); 52% with cardiac (myocardial infarction, Libman–Sacks endocarditis, acute valve dysfunction); and 47% with skin necrosis. Hematological manifestations of CAPS include hemolytic anemia, usually

Coombs' positive (32%), thrombocytopenia (63%), and in up to 21% of patients, serological evidence of disseminated intravascular coagulation.[9] Although the initial presentation of CAPS may involve a single organ, in a very short period of time, typically days to weeks, patients develop clinical evidence of multiple organ thrombosis and dysfunction leading to organ failure that requires ICU admission.

CAPS clinical presentation is considerably different from the classical APS with the main difference being the rapid development of multiorgan failure. CAPS is said to affect small vessels primarily, whereas APS predominantly affects large vessels. The involvement of organs, such as bowel, reproductive organs, and bone marrow, is unusual in APS. Disseminated intravascular coagulation, acute respiratory distress syndrome, and severe thrombocytopenia are also common in CAPS patients and not in the classic APS.[2]

3.4
Diagnosis

The diagnosis of CAPS can be challenging because of the acute onset of thrombosis at multiple levels with simultaneous dysfunction of different organs. The survival of the patients is dependent on an early diagnosis and administration of the appropriate treatment.

Preliminary CAPS classification criteria (Table 3.1) was proposed and agreed in Taormina, Sicily during the 10th International Congress on aPL. Although these criteria are accepted for classification purposes, they might be a guide to a more consistent approach to the diagnosis.[10] Therefore, to make the diagnosis, there should be clinical evidence of multiple organ involvement developed over a very short time, histopathologic evidence of multiple small-vessel occlusions, and laboratory confirmation of the presence of aPL, usually in high titer. The positivity of aPL should be confirmed by at least another test when the acute clinical situation has passed. aPL can be also positive in sepsis and other critical situations

Table 3.1 International classification criteria for CAPS

1. Evidence of involvement of 3 organs, systems, and/or tissues
2. Development of manifestations simultaneously or in less than 1 week
3. Confirmation by histopathology of small-vessel occlusion in at least 1 organ/tissue
4. Laboratory confirmation of the presence of aPL (LAC and/or aCL and/or anti-2GPI antibodies)

Definite CAPS:
- All 4 criteria

Probable CAPS:
- All 4 criteria, except for involvement of only 2 organs, system, and/or tissues
- All 4 criteria, except for the absence of laboratory confirmation at least 6 weeks apart attributable to the early death of a patient never tested for aPL before onset of CAPS
- 1, 2, and 4
- 1, 3, and 4, and the development of a third event in >1 week but <1 month, despite anticoagulation treatment

Table 3.2 Differential diagnosis of catastrophic antiphospholipid syndrome

	CAPS	Sepsis	TTP-HUS	DIC
Hemolytic anemia	+/−	+	+	+/−
Schistocytes	+/−	+/−	++	+/−
Thrombocytopenia	+/−	+/−	++	+
Fibrinogen	Normal	Normal/low	Normal	Low
aPL	++	+/−	−	−

which share several clinical features with CAPS. In a large series of patients with CAPS, IgG aCL was positive in 84%, IgM aCL in 41%, and LA in 76% of patients.[8]

The differential diagnosis for sepsis, thrombotic thrombocytopenic purpura (TTP), hemolytic uremic syndrome (HUS), acute disseminated intravascular coagulation (DIC), and HELLP syndrome (hemolysis, elevated liver enzymes, and low platelets) has to be done. Some of the differences between these entities are summarized in Table 3.2.

CAPS resembles severe sepsis in its presentation. Both share the symptoms of SIRS [temperature >38°C, tachycardia, increased respiratory frequency, hypotension, elevated white blood cell count, or with >10% immature forms (band)]. Infection is the most common trigger factor of CAPS and, sometimes, both situations can coexist. An aggressive treatment of the infection can markedly improve the prognosis.

TTP, characterized by thrombocytopenia and microangiopathic hemolytic anemia, also shares with CAPS the presence of renal dysfunction and neurological features. Microangiopathic hemolytic anemia consists of nonimmune hemolysis (direct antiglobulin test negative) together with the presence of red cell fragmentation (schistocytes), in peripheral blood smear. The presence of more than 1% of schistocytes strongly suggests the diagnosis of TTP.[11]

DIC causes multiple thrombosis and hemorrhage. Its features also include renal, liver, lung, and central nervous system involvement. The presence of widespread hemorrhage is not so frequent in CAPS.

3.5
Treatment

The optimal treatment regime in CAPS is unknown. The combination of anticoagulation, corticosteroids, plasma exchange, and intravenous immunoglobulin (IVIG) has been associated with the highest rate of survival.[2]

Intravenous heparin is usually administrated during the critical period. When the patient is stable, oral anticoagulation with an INR target around 3.0 can be initiated. Heparin is discontinued when the target INR is achieved with warfarin. The beneficial effects of heparin are mediated by its capacity to inhibit thrombin, factor Xa, and other activated clotting factors.[12] Heparin also inhibits complement activation.[13] Although this mechanism has not been proven in humans, in the setting of CAPS where there is an important inflammatory component, might be relevant.

Although corticosteroids do not prevent further thrombosis, they are recommended in a situation with SIRS and excessive cytokine release where it also inhibits complement activation. Activation of endothelial cells and monocytes induced by aPL are mediated by NF-kB and the mitogen-activated protein kinase (MPK) mainly p38.[14] Corticosteroids are able to inhibit the proinflammatory status mediated by both the NF-kB and MPK pathway.[15]

When initiated promptly, plasma exchange (PE) can be considered an effective and safe treatment for CAPS. It is useful by removing pathological aPL, cytokines, and complement and also incorporating natural anticoagulants like antithrombin and protein C. The treatment of CAPS with PE is not, however, well defined and has not yet been standardized. The best replacement fluid for PE is still a controversial issue.[16] However, the efficacy of PE has been shown in other thrombotic microangiopathy and since CAPS is a critical situation with a high rate of mortality, it is recommended as part of the CAPS treatment.[17]

The rationale to use IVIG in the treatment of CAPS is based on its capacity to block pathological antibodies, increase its clearance, act on the complement system, and suppress cytokines.[18] IVIG should be specially indicated in situations where there is concomitant infection because of its antibacterial/antiviral activity and its role as immunomodulator rather than immunosuppressor.[19]

Immunosuppressive drugs such as i.v. cyclophosphamide might be helpful in patients with active systemic autoimmune disease mainly SLE and systemic vasculitis, but its use in CAPS is not associated with an improvement in the survival rate.[2]

Some case reports about the use of rituximab – an anti-CD20 monoclonal – in the treatment of CAPS have been published.[20,21] Although more data is necessary to support the use of this drug in the setting of CAPS, current experience seems quite promising, especially in patients with severe thrombocytopenia.

Patients with CAPS have a life-threatening condition and high mortality. They need adequate management in ICU that should include hemodialysis, mechanical ventilation, or cardiovascular support for shock. Other factors like aggressive treatment of infection, debridement or amputation of necrotic tissues/organs, careful management of intravascular instrumentation, especially arterial which can lead to new clots, are extremely important and can substantially improve the rate of survival.

3.6
Prognosis

CAPS is a life-threatening condition with a mortality rate around 50% at the time of the event.[22] However, in a recent article by Bucciarelli et al.,[2] mortality has fallen by some 20%. This is probably due to more awareness of the condition between physicians, early diagnosis, and the use of therapies such as PE, IVIG, full anticoagulation, steroid, and, if necessary, antibiotics.

There is only one study addressing the long-term follow-up of patient with one episode of CAPS.[23] A review including published patients with CAPS showed that 63/136 (46%) died at the time of the event. Seventy three patients survived but information was available only from 58 (79%). Thirty-eight of 58 (66%) patients did not develop any other thrombotic event during a medium follow-up time of 67.2 months. Fifteen of 58 (26%) patients developed further APS-related thrombosis after the initial catastrophic APS event, and the mortality rate of these patients was about 25% (4/15 patients). In summary, 66% of survivors remained thrombosis free and 17% developed further APS-related thrombosis. None of the patients developed further catastrophic APS.

Comparing the demographic, clinical, and immunologic characteristics of patients who survived to those who died, older age, pulmonary and renal involvement, the presence of SLE and high titer of antinuclear antibodies (ANA) were associated with a higher mortality rate.[24]

There is little data regarding CAPS relapse. In the CAPS registry, a total of 18 episodes of relapse in eight patients have been described.[25-30] The precipitating factors in these patients were infection, subtherapeutic anticoagulation level, and anticoagulation withdrawal. The symptoms were very similar to the first CAPS episodes (renal failure followed by cerebral, cardiac, and pulmonary involvement). Thrombocytopenia was present in 17 patients and hemolytic anemia in 13. LA test was the most common aPL positive.[2]

In conclusion, every physician managing patients with multiorgan failure should be aware of the possibility of CAPS. This diagnosis should be strongly suspected in patients previously diagnosed with APS or any underlying systemic autoimmune disease. A prompt diagnosis will enable physicians to take measures to prevent death from this syndrome. An aggressive treatment with steroids, anticoagulation, and IVIG in an ICU setting will help prevent the progression of organ failure or the development of septic shock in the infected patients.

References

1. Asherson RA. The catastrophic antiphospholipid syndrome. *J Rheumatol.* 1992;19:508-512.
2. Bucciarelli S, Espinosa G, Cervera R, et al. Mortality in the catastrophic antiphospholipid syndrome: causes of death and prognostic factors in a series of 250 patients. *Arthritis Rheum.* 2006;54:2568-2576.
3. Kitchens CS. Thrombotic storm: when thrombosis begets thrombosis. *Am J Med.* 1998;104: 381-385.
4. Vora S, Asherson RA, Erkan D. Catastrophic antiphospholipid syndrome. *J Intensive Care Med.* 2006;21:144-159.
5. Bhatia M, Moochhala S. Role of inflammatory mediators in the pathophysiology of acute respiratory distress syndrome. *J Pathol.* 2004;202:145-156.
6. Ortega-Hernandez O, Agmon-Levin N, Blank M, Asherson R, Shoenfeld Y. The physiopathology of the catastrophic antiphospholipid (Asherson's) syndrome: compelling evidence. *J Autoimmun.* 2009;32:1-6.
7. Asherson RA. The catastrophic antiphospholipid (Asherson's) syndrome in 2004 – a review. *Autoimmun Rev.* 2005;4:48-54.
8. Cervera R, Font J, Gomez-Puerta JA, et al. Validation of the preliminary criteria for the classification of catastrophic antiphospholipid syndrome. *Ann Rheum Dis.* 2005;64:1205-1209.
9. Cervera R, Asherson RA. Multiorgan failure due to rapid occlusive vascular disease in antiphospholipid syndrome: the "catastrophic" antiphospholipid syndrome. *APLAR J Rheumatol.* 2004;7:254-262.

10. Asherson RA, Cervera R, de Groot P, et al. Catastrophic antiphospholipid syndrome (CAPS): international consensus statement on classification criteria and treatment guidelines. *Lupus.* 2003;12:530-534.
11. Burns ER, Lou Y, Pathak A. Morphologic diagnosis of thrombotic thrombocytopenic purpura. *Am J Hematol.* 2004;75:18-21.
12. Weitz JI, Hirsh J, Samama MM. New anticoagulant drugs: the seventh ACCP conference on antithrombotic and thrombolytic therapy. *Chest.* 2004;126:265S-286S.
13. Girardi G, Redecha P, Salmon JE. Heparin prevents antiphospholipid antibody-induced fetal loss by inhibiting complement activation. *Nat Med.* 2004;10:1222-1226.
14. Lopez-Pedrera Ch, Buendia P, Cuadrado MJ, et al. Antiphospholipid antibodies from patients with the antiphospholipid syndrome induce monocyte tissue factor expression through the simultaneous activation of NF-kappaB/Rel proteins via the p38 mitogen-activated protein kinase pathway, and of the MEK1/ERK pathway. *Arthritis Rheum.* 2006;54:304-311.
15. Auphan N, DiDonato JA, Rosette C, et al. Immunosuppression by glucocorticoids: inhibition of NF-kB activity through induction of I kappa B synthesis. *Science.* 1995;270:286-290.
16. Marson P, Bagatella P, Bortolati M, et al. Plasma exchange for the management of the catastrophic antiphospholipid syndrome: importance of the type of fluid replacement. *J Intern Med.* 2008;264:201-203.
17. Espinosa G, Bucciarelli S, Cervera R, et al. Thrombotic microangiopathic haemolytic anaemia and antiphospholipid antibodies. *Ann Rheum Dis.* 2004;63:730-736.
18. Lee SJ, Chinen J, Kavanaugh A. Immunomodulator therapy: monoclonal antibodies, fusion proteins, cytokines and immunoglobulins. *J Allergy Clin Immunol.* 2010;125:S314-S323.
19. Hartung HP, Mouthon L, Ahmed R, Jordan S, Laupland KB, Jolles S. Clinical applications of intravenous immnoglobulins (IVIg) – beyond immunodeficiencies and neurology. *Clin Exp Immunol.* 2009;158:23-33.
20. Rubenstein E, Arkfeld DG, Metyas S, Shinada S, Ehresmann S, Liebman HA. Rituximab treatment for resistant antiphospholipid syndrome. *J Rheumatol.* 2006;33:355-357.
21. Iglesias-Jiménez E, Camacho-Lovillo M, Falcón-Neyra D, Lirola-Cruz J, Neth O. Infant with probable catastrophic antiphospholipid syndrome successfully managed with rituximab. *Pediatrics.* 2010;125:1523-1528.
22. Asherson RA, Cervera R, Piette JC, Shoenfeld Y, Espinosa G, Petri MA. Catastrophic antiphospholipid syndrome: clues to the pathogenesis from a series of 80 patients. *Medicine.* 2001;80:355-377.
23. Erkan D, Asherson RA, Espinoza G. Long term outcome of catastrophic antiphospholipid syndrome survivors. *Ann Rheum Dis.* 2003;62:530-533.
24. Bayraktar UD, Erkan D, Bucciarelli S, Espinosa G, Asherson RA, Catastrophic Antiphospholipid Syndrome Project Group. The clinical spectrum of catastrophic antiphospholipid syndrome in the absence and presence of lupus. *J Rheumatol.* 2007;34:346-352.
25. Murphy JJ, Leach IH. Finding at necropsy in the heart of a patient with anticardiolipin syndrome. *Br Heart J.* 1989;62:61-64.
26. Neuwelt CM, Daiki DI, Linfoot JA, et al. Catastrophic Antiphospholipid syndrome. Response to repeated plasmapheresis over three years. *Arthritis Rheum.* 1997;40:1534-1539.
27. Undas A, Swadzba J, Undas R, Musial J. Three episodes of acute multiorgan failure in a woman with secondary antiphospholipid syndrome. *Pol Arch Med Wewn.* 1998;100:556-560.
28. Cerveny K, Sarwitzke AD. Relapsing catastrophic antiphospholipid antibody syndrome: a mimic for thrombotic thrombocytopenic purpura. *Lupus.* 1999;8:477-481.
29. Gordon A, McLean CA, Ryan P, Roberts SK. Steroids responsive catastrophic antiphospholipid syndrome. *J Gastroenterol Hepatol.* 2004;19:479-480.
30. Asherson RA, Espinosa G, Menahen S, et al. Relapsing catastrophic antiphospholipid syndrome: report of three cases. *Semin Arthritis Rheum.* 2008;37:366-372.

Complex Situations in Rheumatoid Arthritis

4

Miriam García-Arias, Gema Bonilla, Luis Gómez-Carreras, and Alejandro Balsa

Abstract Rheumatoid arthritis (RA) is a systemic autoimmune disease involving large and small joints resulting in pain, joint destruction, and disability. The disease course of RA is unpredictable with some patients having only mild symptoms while others may experience persistent and acute synovitis leading to severe joint destruction. However, being a systemic disease, it can affect other tissues and organs, causing a wide range of symptoms and complications that although usually not life threatening are the cause of significant morbidity. Knowledge of articular or extra-articular complications may aid in promoting a high index of suspicion and contribute significantly to an early diagnosis and avoid many potentially dangerous conditions.

Keywords Baker's cyst • Cervical spine • Extra-articular manifestations • Rheumatoid arthritis • Rheumatoid lung • Septic arthritis

4.1
Introduction

Rheumatoid arthritis (RA) is a systemic autoimmune disease affecting 0.5–1% of the population, which is characterized clinically by pain, stiffness, and joint swelling. The chronic inflammation of synovial joints and other synovial structures such as tendon sheets will eventually lead to extensive articular and periarticular destruction, functional decline, and premature death. Being a systemic disease, it can affect other tissues and organs, causing a wide range of different extra-articular disease manifestations in a very heterogeneous way, making clinical features very different between individuals or even within the same individual in different time points. It is usually thought that extra-articular features of RA

A. Balsa (✉)
Rheumatology Unit, Hospital Universitario La Paz,
Paseo de la Castellana, 261, 28046 Madrid, Spain
e-mail: abalsa.hulp@salud.madrid.org

M.A. Khamashta and M. Ramos-Casals (eds.), *Autoimmune Diseases*,
DOI: 10.1007/978-0-85729-358-9_4, © Springer-Verlag London Limited 2011

occur mainly in patients with long-standing or severe disease, but although unusual, can occur in early RA or even can precede the onset of articular symptoms.[1]

Several constitutional symptoms can be a major problem during the course of the disease, such as weight loss, fatigue, muscle weakness, or depression, but although important due to its chronic course, generally are not seen in the emergency room. The ability to manage the patient with RA has improved over the past decades; however, RA is still a significant cause of rheumatological emergencies, either from exacerbation of articular symptoms or complications of extra-articular manifestations, representing one third of all rheumatological emergencies attended in a teaching hospital.[2]

4.2
Rheumatoid Articular Flare

The nature of clinical symptoms in RA differs between individuals. In some patients, the disease may be present with a slow or rapid course of progressive disease while in others, it is characterized by exacerbations and remissions of variable duration and extension.

There are no criteria for a disease flare, but from the patient's perspective, it can be defined as any relevant clinical worsening, that would, if persistent, in most cases lead to initiation or change of therapy.[3] Although the flare of disease activity is usually evident in patients with a well-established RA diagnosis, being a patient perception, not always can be objectively assessed, because pain is always present in a flare but not necessarily is synovitis. Different measures have been used to measure the intensity of a flare, which include the increase in number of tender and swollen joints, patient global assessment and pain, acute phase reactants, fatigue or morning stiffness, systemic complaints or physician's assessments, but patient's perspectives are critical.[3]

Most flares are polyarticular but sometimes are restricted to a smaller number of joints, and physicians should always consider the possibility of concurrent septic arthritis in patients with one or two new inflamed joints. Although infrequent, "pseudoseptic arthritis" is a condition that can mimic an infected joint. The clinical presentation is similar to acute septic arthritis; however, negative cultures and the short course of the flare, which usually resolve in 2–3 days without antibiotics, help to differentiate between the two situations.[4] Even patients with widespread joint destruction may have a worsening of their symptoms that can be referred to as a deterioration of their functional capacity, general health, or an increase of pain or fatigue. This can be attributed to an exacerbation of the underlying disease, to mechanical problems secondary to joint destruction, or to systemic involvement of the disease such as severe anemia or organ failure. Differentiation between these three possibilities may be difficult because of the presence of deformed and swollen joints, and sometimes, hospital admission is necessary to exclude concurrent diseases. The increase in acute phase reactants and the use of modern imaging techniques such as articular Power Doppler ultrasonography can help accurately separate different causes.[5]

The management of a flare of RA is similar to that of an established disease. Local steroid injections into active joints can be very useful when few are affected and can be combined with systemic steroids or used alone in polyarticular symptoms; however, it is important to use them in short courses due to increase in side effects with cumulative doses. Usually, a new second-line drug needs to be started, but it is necessary to know that the response is not immediate, and it may take several weeks for an effect to occur.

4.3
Septic Arthritis

Joint infections are true rheumatologic emergencies because they may cause serious morbidity, permanent disability, or death. The two most significant problems relating to joint infections are early diagnosis and prompt and effective treatment.[6]

The estimated incidence of septic arthritis in RA is 0.3–3% and affects mainly patients with long-standing, erosive, and seropositive disease, and the functional outcomes are worse and the mortality is high.[7] Patients with RA are at high risk for septic arthritis due to a combination of joint damage, immunosuppressive medications, local joint injections, and skin breakdown and delayed diagnosis is not uncommon due to insidious onset, low frequency of fever, and polyarticular joint involvement in up to 20–30% of the patients.[8] *Staphylococcus aureus* has been the microorganism isolated in up to 75% of cases, but other less frequent pathogens include *Streptococci*, gram-negative bacilli, fungi, and mycobacteria[9] and the knee is the most commonly involved joint, followed by the wrist, ankle, and shoulder.

A clinical diagnosis can be difficult to make, even in the hands of experienced doctors, and can be difficult to distinguish from those of an exacerbation of RA, resulting in a delay in the appropriate treatment, but must be suspected in all patients who show a deterioration in their clinical course;[9] however, the "gold standard" for diagnosis of septic arthritis is the level of clinical suspicion of a physician experienced.[10] A definitive diagnosis requires identification of bacteria either by Gram's stain or by culture. Clinical suspicion of joint sepsis should prompt immediate synovial fluid aspiration. If synovial fluid cannot be obtained by closed needle aspiration, the joint should be aspirated again using imaging guidance or it may even be necessary to rely on a surgical arthrotomy. There is limited evidence to suggest that any clinical or laboratory feature is specific for septic arthritis. The absence of fever, elevated blood or synovial white cell counts (WCC), raised erythrocyte sedimentation rate (ESR), or C-reactive protein could reliably exclude the diagnosis of septic arthritis. A high synovial fluid WCC increased the likelihood of a diagnosis of joint sepsis; however, these results should be used in conjunction with clinical and other laboratory findings.[11] Overall, 37% of infectious arthritis cases had a WCC >100,000 mm³, and 67% had counts >50,000 mm³. A majority of these infections were related to *S. aureus*, while 5–7% infections associated with counts <20,000 mm³ were associated with atypical organisms.[12] Levels of CRP and ESR were higher in patients with septic arthritis compared to other rheumatic inflammatory diseases; however, the overlap between the groups was too high to preclude the use of these tests as discriminatory.

Treatment of septic arthritis includes admission to the hospital and daily removal of purulent synovial fluid during the first 5–7 days. It is not necessary to immobilize the infected joint, although weight bearing should be avoided until signs of inflammation and pain have disappeared. There is little evidence on which to base the choice and duration of antibiotic treatment, and there are no randomized clinical trials. The current choice of antibiotics is based on the presence of risk factors and the likelihood of the organism involved, the patient's age, history of sexual activity, and the Gram's stain results. The usual course of therapy lasts 2 weeks for streptococci or gram-negative cocci, 3 weeks for staphylococci, and 4 weeks for pneumococci or gram-negative bacilli.[13]

4.4
Cricoarytenoid Arthritis

Cricoarytenoid arthritis (CA) is a disorder that may present to the emergency room with a number of symptoms and signs referable to the larynx. It is most commonly seen in RA, but it can also be found in other arthropathies like spondyloarthropathies or systemic lupus erythematosus. The overall incidence of CA in RA is about 55%, with radiographic evidence of erosive arthritis in 45% of the patients; however, clinical acute arthritis is rare.[14] The incidence is higher in females and in patients with long-standing and severe RA; however, arthritis of the CA joint was asymptomatic in 58% of cases.[14]

Clinical symptoms of CA involvement frequently appear after laryngeal manipulation or infection and include hoarseness, waking of the voice, sensation of foreign body, fullness or tension in the throat, and inspiratory wheezing that may be confused with asthma or bronchitis.[4] Symptoms tend to run a very slow course and may be present for several years before significant obstruction that can be precipitated by an upper respiratory tract infection that can produce hypoxemia, hypercapnia, and respiratory failure. The preferred method of viewing the vocal cords is by fiber-optic laryngoscope and usually shows edema and reduced vocal cord motility and arytenoid cartilage asymmetry. High-resolution computed tomography may be useful to investigate CA and cervical involvement and to exclude possible causes of laryngeal signs and symptoms or brain stem compression by the odontoid peg. The most frequent findings were CA prominence, density and volume changes, CA subluxation, and soft tissue swelling near the CA joint and narrowing in the piriform sinus.[15]

In nonacute situations, treatment with systemic or locally injected steroids may control symptoms; however, the management of acute airway obstruction can present important technical problems as intubation may be extremely difficult due to involvement of the cervical spine or temporomandibular joints. In patients with cervical spine instability, neck extension may produce fracture and dislocation of the spine resulting in permanent neurological sequelae or death. In the rare situations in which intubation is not possible, an emergency tracheotomy may be necessary.[16]

4.5
Insufficiency Fractures

Stress fractures are divided into two groups: fatigue fractures, which occur in normal bones by abnormal stress and insufficiency fractures, which occur when normal forces are applied to weakened bones with diminished elasticity. RA patients have an increased risk for pelvic or low limb fractures as they can occur in up to 0.8% of patients[17] secondary to generalized osteoporosis related to long-standing active disease, steroid use, previous surgery, and severe functional impairment and can be precipitated by concurrent low-grade trauma or abnormal mechanical stress caused by rheumatoid deformities. Most patients with fractures of the lower tibia or fibula had valgus malalignment of the ankle.

The most frequent fracture sites are in the pelvis and lower limbs (metatarsal bones, tibia, fibula, calcaneus, femur, and tarsal bones) and multiple fractures are relatively uncommon.[18] Diagnosis is usually difficult and is delayed several weeks, and frequently, patients are misdiagnosed as an exacerbation of their RA. Patients may have an acute or gradual onset of symptoms which can be referred to as local pain, which is "different from that of active RA" and not related to a joint, difficulty weigh bearing and local swelling and erythema, but what makes clinicians aware of the possible presence of an insufficiency fracture is an increase of pain at a single site, particularly when the pain is periarticular in origin.[17] On examination, there is a local area of tenderness located over a bone surface, but sometimes, local edema can miss bony edges. Initial radiographs are usually normal, only showing generalized osteoporosis, and other techniques like bone scan or magnetic resonance imaging are needed. Osteomalacia or rarely a pathologic fracture should be excluded.

Osteoporosis prevention in RA patients should be mandatory, including an adequate control of the disease process and calcium and vitamin D intake, avoiding long-term steroid use. The therapy for insufficiency fractures is usually conservative. Prolonged and absolute rest should be avoided, and analgesics to keep patients as active as possible are needed. When healed, antireabsortive or anabolic drugs should be used.

4.6
Baker's Cyst

Baker's cysts is the distension of the gastrocnemius-semimembranosus bursa which is usually found posteriorly in the knee between the tendons of the medial-head of gastrocnemius and semimembranosus muscles.[19] Symptoms are pain at the back of the knee and swelling with bulge and tightness on walking. It is important to diagnose a ruptured cyst early to avoid complications like compartment syndrome or compression of adjacent nerve which may lead to entrapment neuropathies.[19] On examination, the popliteal fossa is explored in full extension and in up to 90° of flexion, as the patient lies flat on the back. The mass is usually found in the medial side of the fossa with an increased tension on extension and may soften or disappear on flexion to 45°.[20]

Patient's symptoms and clinical examination may lead us to suspect the presence of a Baker's cyst; however, imaging techniques need to be used. Plain radiographs are of limited help. They may be useful to identify underlying joint disorders such as osteoarthritis or RA, but a Baker's cyst cannot be seen. Arthrography involves direct injection of the knee joint with iodinated contrast medium, but now, it is seldom used as it is an invasive

Fig. 4.1 (**a**) Ultrasound of a
non-complicated Baker's
cysts. Cysts appear as
fluid-filled structures
extending between the
tendons of semimembranosus
and the medial-head of
gastrocnemius. (**b**) In Baker's
cyst, the inferior pole should
appear smooth with a convex
contour, when irregular,
or forms a thin rat-tail,
the cyst is ruptured

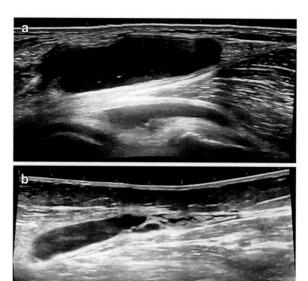

technique with ionizing radiation. Non-contrast computed tomography (CT) can detect
Baker's cyst by their location and their fluid-like attenuation in uncomplicated cases. CT
shows cyst in typical or atypical positions and can separate lipomas, aneurysm, and malignancies from cyst, but hematomas and cyst look alike. Magnetic resonance imaging allows
the precise localization of the cyst and detects associated knee pathology.[19] Ultrasound
(US) is relatively inexpensive, noninvasive, and does not use ionizing radiation, making it
the imaging technique of choice in the initial assessment of Baker's cysts[21] (Fig. 4.1a).
Cysts appear as fluid-filled structures extending between the tendons of semimembranosus
and the medial-head of gastrocnemius along the posteriomedial aspect of the knee and can
be useful in the differential diagnosis which includes popliteal artery aneurysm, venous
thrombosis, lipomas, liposarcoma, popliteal varices, hematoma, ganglionic cysts, synovial
hemangioma, abscess, and malignant fibrous histiocytoma.[21]

The main complication is the rupture of the cyst (Fig. 4.1b) which may be felt as an
acute pain in the back of the knee, sometimes with a decrease in knee swelling, but with
swelling and edema in the calf, which can be clinically indistinguishable from the symptoms of acute deep venous thrombosis.[19] The problem exacerbates when patients are incor-
rectly treated with anticoagulants which may result in the formation of hematoma and
secondary compartment syndrome. US, arthrography, and venography can help in differentiating these two entities.

Treatment is primarily nonsurgical and includes bed rest, elevation of the limb, cold packs,
and nonsteroidal anti-inflammatory drugs. If knee effusion is present, joint aspiration with
corticosteroid injection into the knee joint may be beneficial. Surgical excision is indicated
only for substantial local symptoms or when other conservative treatments are not helpful.[22]

4.7
Instability of the Cervical Spine

Cervical spine is commonly affected in RA, in particular in the atlantoaxial complex of the upper cervical spine. RA can cause degeneration of the ligaments, leading to laxity, instability, and subluxation of the vertebral bodies in 17–85% of cases.[23] This severe destruction of the cervical spine and periodontoid pannus formation may cause compression of the spinal cord or brainstem, which may result in myelopathy or sudden death. Horizontal subluxation is the most common disorder of the cervical spine occurring in 43% of patients with a mean disease duration of 12 years, and vertical subluxation is the most ominous.[4] Other characteristic cervical spine deformities are atlantoaxial impaction and subaxial subluxation, which may result from rheumatoid inflammation of the facet joints below the second cervical vertebra.[24] The rheumatoid disorders of the cervical spine are known to be associated with the extent of erosions in the peripheral joints and the HLA status, as well as with the presence of rheumatoid factor (RF) and rheumatoid nodules.[25] These findings suggest that cervical spine disorders mainly occur in patients with long-standing and severe RA.

The first clinical signs and symptoms that usually describe our patients are neck pain and new occipital pain due to the compression of the greater occipital nerve (Arnold's neuralgia), as well as sensory and eventually motor loss strength in the arms and legs. The vibration sense is lost and the position sense retained in the majority of patients with rheumatoid cervical myelopathy. Neurological examination may be difficult due to joint deformities, muscle wasting, and entrapment neuropathies secondary to RA. It may be impossible to elicit reflexes.[4] Once neurologic deficits occur, progression seems inevitable[23], and it makes essential the establishment of an early diagnosis. Clinical and imagine techniques can be helpful tools in this way. Forward and vertical dislocations of the atlantoaxial joint can be seen on a lateral radiograph of the upper cervical spine in maximal active anterior flexion (Fig. 4.2a, b), but this radiological abnormalities can remain asymptomatic for years. Computed tomography and, especially, magnetic resonance imaging (MRI) are useful whenever plain radiographs leave any doubt about the diagnosis[4] (Fig. 4.2c).

Active conservative treatment includes not only medical treatment, but also patient education, physical training of the deep muscles, and collars. For occipital headache, a collar may be sufficient and, if necessary, analgesics and neck traction. Biologics and combination therapy with traditional DMARDs retarded the early development of atlantoaxial subluxations.[24] Generally accepted indications for surgical intervention include anterior atlantoaxial subluxation with intractable pain and/or neurologic deficits, severe vertical translocation with compromise of the vertebral artery, or evidence of increased signal intensity on T1-weighted MRI sequences.[23] A single horizontal or vertical spinal dislocation without significant neurologic features and no visible dislocation in MRI requires no surgical management. The primary surgical objectives are to relieve neural compression by reduction of subluxation or direct decompression, and/or achieve stabilization of affected segments and reduce pannus formation.[25] A literature review shows that surgery has better neurologic outcomes in symptomatic patientsw, however, in asymptomatic patients surgical and conservative treatment have similar results.

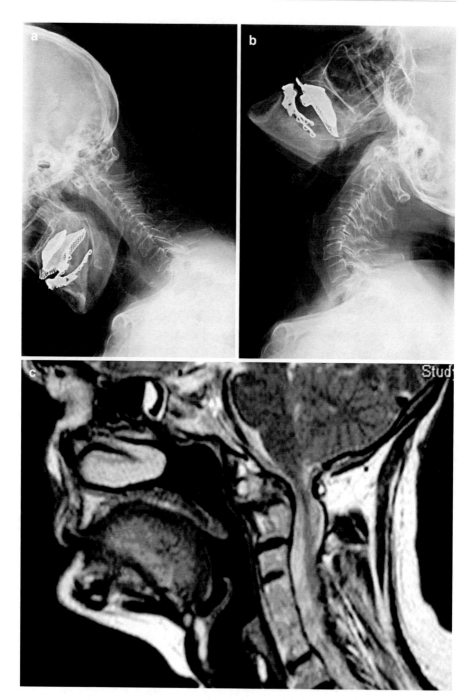

Fig. 4.2 Dynamic radiographs of cervical spine in a patient with rheumatoid arthritis in flexion (**a**) and extension (**b**) Showing a distance between the anterior arch of atlas and the odontoid process greater than 3 mm which characterizes atlantoaxial subluxation. (**c**) T1-weighted sagittal

4.8
Carpal Tunnel Syndrome

Carpal tunnel syndrome (CTS) results from compromise of the median nerve at the wrist caused by an increased pressure in the carpal tunnel, an anatomical compartment bounded by the bones of the carpus and the transverse carpal ligament.[26] The cause of the increased canal pressure must result from either an increase in content, or a decrease in size of the carpal canal, or some combination of the two. There does seem to be an increase in the amount of connective tissue within the carpal canal. However, the mechanism by which this develops remains unclear. The incidence is higher in female gender, obese patients as well as in older age.[27]

The mainstay of diagnosis remains clinical assessment of the patient history, being the most characteristic symptom the nocturnal paresthesia or pain in the median nerve distribution.[28] Some patients will also complain of sensory disturbance in the whole hand or pain radiating up the arm to the shoulder, and they may notice them with particular activities, particularity those that involve holding the arm raised. About 55–65% of cases are bilateral at first presentation, and most patients present first with the dominant hand. Patients may complain of a perception of swelling of the hand or fingers. Sensory loss in median nerve territory and weakness are reliable but late indicators of CTS.[26] The provocative physical test used are *Phalen's sign*: the provocation of median paresthesias by flexion of the wrist to 90° for 60 s, and *Tinel's sign*: the provocation of paresthesias by tapping over the carpal tunnel. Many studies have reported that Phalen's sign has sensitivity from 10% to 73% and a specificity from 55% to 86%. Tinel's sign has a sensitivity from 8% to 100% and a specificity from 55% to 87%.[26]

To confirm the diagnosis and exclude other lesions, nerve conduction studies (NCSs) are the most reliable method. However, false negatives and false positives may occur, even when the most sensitive methods are used.[29] Magnetic resonance imaging (MRI) and high-resolution ultrasonography (US) of the median nerve have been shown to be useful diagnosis tools in CTS, providing information on the median nerve and surrounding structures.[29] Ultrasonography has advantages over MRI in terms of cost and provides dynamic images. It has been shown to produce accurate measurements of carpal tunnel and nerve diameters and is more comfortable than NCSs for patients but will not detect other nerve problems that may be contribute to presentation. Ultrasound (US) is not an alternative diagnostic tool to electrodiagnostic test, but they are complementary. MRI can make similar measurements of median nerve dimensions, but it is more expensive.[26]

The purpose of treatment is to alleviate the symptoms and to prevent any worsening. When symptoms are mild and intermittent, and for those patients who have mild or moderate impairment of median nerve function, we must try conservative management, including splinting and local steroids that are supported by experimental evidence.[26] Splints

image magnetic resonance image of the cervical spine of the same patient showing atlantoaxial subluxation with increased space between the posterior margin of the atlas and the anterior margin of the odontoid, with and abnormal signal between consisting of pannus. A high-grade spinal stenosis most marked at the C1-2 interspace with compression of the cervical cord is shown

should be individually fashioned from lightweight materials for each patient and extend from the upper forearm to include the hand and all of the digits. Splints maintain the wrist in a natural angle without applying direct compression over the carpal tunnel, providing mechanical relief to median nerve. They should be worn at night and as much as possible during the day. CTS has been shown to respond to both systemic and local steroids. The initial response rate to a single injection is about 70%, but relapse is common.[26] No evidence is available about the management after relapse following a successful first injection, though it is common practice to inject a second or even a third more time. Local steroid injection has no discernible systemic effects and very low incidence of local complications. Patients failing such conservative management and those who present at a later stage with objective neurological sings or delayed motor conduction on nerve should be offered the option of surgical treatment. Carpal tunnel decompression is considered the definitive treatment.[26] Endoscopic methods of carpal tunnel decompression have been popular in recent years, but it does not offer any overall benefit compared with traditional open surgery, with the possible exception of quicker recovery after endoscopic surgery.

4.9
Leg Ulcers

Approximately 10% of patients with RA will experience leg ulceration and as many as 10% of leg ulcers can be seen in association with RA.[30] Ulceration is most commonly in females with long-standing disease, and they are usually situated between the ankle and the knee. These patients are seropositive for IgM rheumatoid factor, and they may have rheumatoid nodules. Patients with RA exhibited a multifactorial etiology of leg ulcers[30]: venous stasis and immobility together with factors as trauma, pressure, thinning of the skin due to steroid therapy, and coexistent conditions such as diabetes and atheroma must be considered. Another important cause is systemic vasculitis with occlusion of small vessels. Leg ulcers may contribute to a range of additional problems for patients with RA that include increased pain, restricted choice of footwear, reduced mobility, and the risk of lower limb amputation.[31]

Patients usually consult because a small bruise that has developed after a minor traumatism in a lower limb has been breaking down into an ulcer. Physical examination shows a full-thickness skin defect with a blue and cold distal lower extremity and sometimes small infarcts in some of the nail edges.

Leg ulcers are difficult to treat in patients with RA, often involves long periods of hospitalization, and the recurrence rates are high.[30] Due to these facts, an important part of their management starts with the education of patients on the prevention of ulceration by avoidance of trauma, prolonged sitting, and by active exercises. With established ulceration, the limb must be kept in an elevated position as much as possible. Normal saline must be used for cleaning and hydrocolloid dressing, which are nonadherent and protective, for helping to promote granulation and reepithelialization. If a hard and dry scar has formed, application of a hydrogel dressing can be considered: a thick liquid gel that promotes rapid debridement by facilitating rehydration and autolysis of dead tissue. If swabbing reveals the presence of pathogenic bacteria, a course of systemic antibiotics must be considered. Surgical treatment has demonstrated an improvement in healing rates as compared with conservative treatment.[30] Recent studies have reported the effectiveness of leukocytaphere-sis (LCAP) for refractory ulcers in RA because due to its cellular and molecular mecha-nisms, it may accelerate the healing process of inflammatory skin ulcers.[32] If the ulceration is part of a diffuse vasculitic syndrome, this should receive appropriate drug medication.

4.10
Rheumatoid Pachymeningitis

Rheumatoid pachymeningitis is a rare manifestation. It is more frequently in elderly popu-lation with long-standing, erosive, and seropositive RA, and it can be present even in the absence of active systemic disease. Its prognosis is ominous, with a high mortality rate (70%) despite intensive treatment.[33] Although patients with pachymeningitis may remain asymptomatic (up to 26% in some series), the majority of patients experience neurological symptoms like seizure, cranial nerve dysfunction, headaches, mental status change, altered level of consciousness, and hemiparesis or paraparesis.[34]

A definite diagnosis of rheumatoid meningitis is in general difficult without positive histopathology as there are few clinical markers specific for this disease. Rheumatoid fac-tor (RF) in cerebrospinal fluid (CSF) is often used as a diagnostic marker because the strongly positive results specifically indicate this disease.[35] Analysis of CSF usually shows an elevated protein level with occasional pleocytosis and hypoglycorrhachia. MRI is the imaging method of choice for diagnosing pachymeningitis[36] (Fig. 4.3). It shows increased T2 signal in the hemispheric subarachnoid space and leptomeningeal enhancement after gadolinium administration, but these findings are nonspecific and can result from various etiologies including infectious, inflammatory, and neoplastic ones. The biopsy specimen

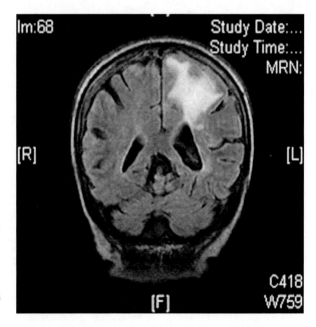

Fig. 4.3 Rheumatoid meningitis seen on magnetic resonance image showing an increased signal in the left hemispheric subarachnoid space and leptomeningeal enhancement after gadolinium administration in a flair sequence

reveals infiltration of inflammatory cells, fibrosis and, rarely, typical rheumatoid nodules. The presence of epithelioid granulomas typically in the cranial meninges or choroid plexus confirms the diagnosis of rheumatoid meningitis but is not a specific finding.[37] Differential diagnosis of pachymeningitis includes meningeal carcinomatosis, lymphoma, neurofibromatosis, Sturge–Weber angiomatosis, infective disorders such as tuberculosis and syphilis and granulomatous disease like sarcoidosis and Wegener disease.

An early diagnosis and immediate initiation of treatment is fundamental to avoid neurological sequelae.[34] There are no clear guidelines for the treatment of rheumatoid cranial pachymeningitis. This entity can respond to steroids, but there is some evidence that steroids alone may not be sufficient[35] and other immunosuppressant agents such as cyclophosphamide and azathioprine must be added to treatment. The use of methotrexate in rheumatoid vasculitic is controversial as some reports have described accelerated nodulosis and vasculitis during methotrexate treatment.[33]

4.11
Interstitial Lung Disease

Interstitial lung disease (ILD) is the most common manifestation of rheumatoid lung disease that is clinically detected in less than 5% of patients, although studies using high-resolution computer tomography (HRCT) have shown a much higher prevalence.[38] In general, ILD is seen more frequently in men, between 50–60 years, with a smoking history and in erosive and rheumatoid factor positive disease.[39] The onset of symptoms is usually slow and includes dyspnea on exertion and a nonproductive cough. Physical signs may be absent in early disease, but later, bibasilar crackles and clubbing may appear and finally signs of pulmonary hypertension. ILD has poor prognosis, but there is some evidence that the natural history is better than in cryptogenic fibrosis. The diagnosis is based on clinical symptoms, respiratory function tests, and HRCT. In some cases, bronchoscopy with bronchoalveolar lavage and biopsy may be needed. Chest radiographs can be normal in early phases, but in established disease, chest radiographs are indistinguishable from those seen in idiopathic pulmonary fibrosis or ILD associated with other connective tissue disease. Only 2–9% of patients have abnormalities in the chest radiograph, which is characterized by a reticular pattern or reticulonodular pattern with predominant involvement of lower lobes (Fig. 4.4a). In later stages, it shows the typical honeycomb pattern changes and reveals findings associated with the coexistence of pulmonary hypertension. HRCT has an increased sensitivity and specificity for analysis of the pulmonary parenchyma and provides an excellent diagnostic tool for determining the presence and type of pulmonary abnormality. HRCT has great ability to discriminate different stages of the disease and can differentiate between the presence of predominantly ground glass pattern from reticular changes and honeycombing (Fig. 4.4b). In this clinical setting, ground glass opacification suggests inflammation consistent with nonspecific interstitial pneumonia (NSIP) and reticular changes and honeycombing reflect fibrosis, and are more typical of usual interstitial pneumonia (UIP). Restrictive abnormalities on pulmonary function tests are common even in the absence of symptoms. Up to 40–50% of patients in some series have alterations in

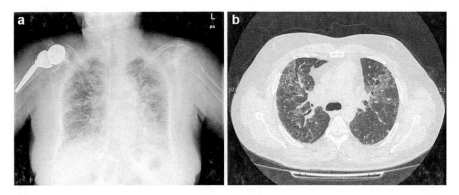

Fig. 4.4 (a) Chest radiograph showing subpleural interstitial pattern in bases, most evident in left hemithorax. (b) High-resolution computer tomography showing subpleural reticular interstitial pattern with ground glass areas

respiratory function tests suggestive of interstitial disease. The first change observed is the desaturation during exercise and decreased diffusion capacity, measured using single-breath carbon monoxide diffusion capacities and appears in 40% of patients even in cases with normal chest radiograph. In later stages, a restrictive pattern in spirometry with reductions in lung volume measure by pletismography is shown. Bronchio-alveolar lavage (BAL) is frequently abnormal with an increase in the number of white cells with neutrophilia and occasionally eosinophils. An increase of lymphocytes in BAL is usually an indicator of response to treatment and good prognosis, but the predominance of neutrophils or eosinophils is not always correlated with the severity of the disease. Bronchoscopy and bronchoalveolar lavage is a useful technique for the differential diagnosis of infection, bleeding, tumors, and other systemic diseases such as sarcoidosis. Although, HRCT has replaced lung biopsy, when atypical features are present in HRCT, pathological diagnosis may be required. The most common pathologic findings are those of UIP and NSIP, while the nonspecific interstitial pneumonia (NSIP) pattern predominates in most forms of collagen vascular disease (CVD)–associated ILD. Studies in patients with RA-associated ILD (RA-ILD) suggest that the usual interstitial pneumonia (UIP) pattern is the most common.[40] The decision to treat depends on patient's age, severity, and rate of progression and the presence of coexisting diseases. Deterioration of lung function over a period of 1–3 months strengthens the case for intervention. More aggressive treatment is justified in patients with evidence of inflammation on HRCT, lymphocytes on BAL or no-UIP pattern on biopsy. Treatment is based primarily on high-dose steroids, a dose of 0.5–1.0 mg/kg per day as a single morning doses. If a response is going to occur, it is usually seen within 1–3 months. The prednisolone dose should be slowly reduced to a maintenance dose of 10 mg/day once a response occurs; pulmonary function test is used to monitor disease activity. If patient fails to respond or deteriorates during the initial treatment, addition of an immunosuppresive agent like cyclophosphamide or azathioprine is recommended. In severe disease, therapy with intravenous methylprednisolone should be considered during the first week, while oral prednisolone and immunosuppressive agent are introduced later.

4.12
Rheumatoid Nodules

Pulmonary nodulosis is an unusual extra-articular manifestation of rheumatoid disease but the only pulmonary manifestation specific for RA. The prevalence of pulmonary rheumatoid nodules is not clearly established. An open lung biopsies study including 40 patients with suspected lung disease found that rheumatoid nodules were the most common abnormality, being present in 13 subjects (32%) and in 8 out of 13, there were multiple nodules.[41] Lung nodules may appear singly or in clusters that coalesce and are more frequently seen in long-term disease, but in some cases, may precede RA diagnosis. They are more frequent in men, with subcutaneous nodules and high titers of rheumatoid factor and are usually an incidental radiographic finding. In some cases, rheumatoid nodules are associated with pneumoconiosis (Caplan syndrome). Although pulmonary rheumatoid nodules are generally asymptomatic, they may lead to complications like pleural effusion, pneumothorax, pyopneumothorax, bronchopleural fistula, hemoptysis, and infection, but prognosis is generally good, with occasional spontaneous resolution and rare complications. The first step in their diagnosis is plain chest radiography (Fig. 4.5a). Upper lobes are the most frequent localization, generally located in subpleural areas or in association with interlobular septa, well delimitated and their size varies between 1 and 7 cm. CT is a more sensible imaging technique to discriminate nodule characteristics and allows to diagnose other findings in lung or mediastinum (Fig. 4.5b). It is recommended that asymptomatic nodules be followed with a repeat CT. Depending upon the clinical circumstances, fine needle aspiration may be performed to exclude the possibility of malignancy. In several cases, solitary pulmonary nodules in RA patients have proved to be a rheumatoid nodule and a coexistent bronchogenic carcinoma. Differential diagnosis includes primary lung cancer or lung metastasis, mycosis, histiocytosis, and vasculitis. Histologically nodules are similar to that at other sites, with central necrosis, palisading epithelioid cells, a mononuclear

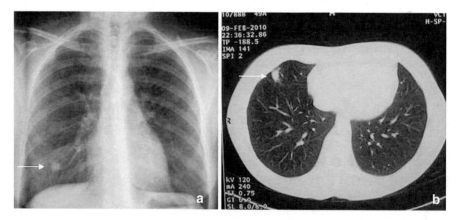

Fig. 4.5 (**a**) Chest radiograph of a rheumatoid nodule (*arrow*). (**b**) High-resolution computer tomography of the same patient showing the subpleural rheumatoid nodule (*arrow*)

cell infiltrate, and associated vasculitis. Although occasionally revert spontaneously and evolved separately to joint involvement. The nodules do not usually respond to drug treatment. Surgery is indicated in cases where there is a secondary bronchopleural fistula.

4.13
Bronchiectasis

Although Bronchiectasis (BR) is not usually included in the category of extra-articular manifestation, it has been recognized in the setting of RA for many years, especially in patients with more severe disease[42] and occurs in up to 10% of RA patients. In a HRCT study, 30% of RA patients were noted to have BR without evidence of ILD. BR is usually characterized by chronic cough and purulent sputum production with a variable clinical course with periods of stability punctuated by exacerbations that may include respiratory distress or hemoptysis.[43] Pulmonary infectious complications are common with the most common bacteria found being *Haemophilus influenzae* and in more severe stages *Pseudomonas aeruginosa*. Most patients complain of chronic symptoms with worsening sputum volume and dyspnea. Destruction or weakening of the bronchial cartilage with airway dilation and acute and chronic inflammation are the most common pathologic findings. HRCT is a more sensitive image technique for detecting BR that bronchography. Although the presence of ILD with honeycombing may confound the diagnosis of BR on HRCT, the clinical history will often help clarify the situation. In those patients that require therapy, treatment should be similar to that used for other forms of BR, including some combination of oral or intravenous antibiotics in case of exacerbation, if it is possible in function of the results of sputum culture. Chronic colonization by *Pseudomonas aeruginosa* must be treated with inhaled antibiotics. Other concomitant therapies include bronchodilator treatment, vaccination, chest physiotherapy, and possibly anti-inflammatory drugs.

4.14
Pleural Disease

Pleural disease in RA is usually subclinical and appears in 40–75% of autopsies. Is most common in patients with long-standing RA, but can precede joint disease. In about 20% of patients, pleuritis develops concurrently with the onset of the arthritis, is more common in men, and coexists with rheumatoid nodules, high rheumatoid factor titers, and ILD in up to 30% of patients.[44] The most common symptoms are chest pain and fever, and some patients with significant pleural effusions may report dyspnea. Physical examination may reveal a pleural rub and there may be unilateral or bilateral effusions, being more frequent in the right chest. Thoracentesis should be performed in patients who have RA and a pleural effusion. The purpose of pleural fluid analysis is to confirm that the pleural fluid is an exudate with pH less than 7.3, glucose 10–50 mg/dL, pleural fluid glucose-to-serum glucose ratio less than 0.5, protein concentration higher than 4 g/dL, white cells

100–3,500/mm^3 (<5,000/mm^3), high lactate dehydrogenase, and low CH50. Pleural effusions are rarely pseudoquilosum, owing to the accumulation of cholesterol in chronic spills. These may occur in patients with secondary amyloidosis, although the most common cause is tuberculosis. The presence of bloody fluid requires ruling out other causes of pleural effusion such as tuberculosis and malignancy. The cellularity of the fluid in early stages is of predominantly polymorphonuclear while in the more chronic phases are lymphocytes. The presence of multinucleated cells and histiocytosis is more specific of subpleural rheumatoid nodules. Other pleural abnormalities include empyema, bronchopleural fistula, or pyopneumothorax. Empyema due to infection should be excluded by Gram stain and culture. A pleural biopsy may be helpful in excluding other disorders, such as tuberculosis or malignancy. Pleural effusion can be caused by necrosis and cavitations of a nodule into the pleural space.

The resolution of the pleural effusion is usually slow and residual pleurisy may persist for years. Rheumatoid pleuritis and pleural effusion usually do not require specific treatment as they commonly resolve spontaneously. Several therapies have been reported to be useful including nonsteroidal anti-inflammatory drugs, glucocorticoids, pleurodesis, and decortication. The pleural effusion will resolve with treatment of rheumatoid joint disease. If the pleural effusion is refractory, a dose of oral glucocorticoids may be beneficial.

References

1. Young A, Koduri G. Extra-articular manifestations and complications of rheumatoid arthritis. *Best Pract Res Clin Rheumatol*. 2007;2:907-927.
2. Smith EC, Berry H, Scott DL. The clinical need for an acute rheumatology referral service. *Br J Rheumatol*. 1996;35:389-391.
3. Bingham CO III, Pohl C, Woodworth TG, et al. Developing a standardized definition for disease "flare" in rheumatoid arthritis (OMERACT 9 special interest group). *J Rheumatol*. 2009;36:2335-2341.
4. Slobodin G, Hussein A, Rozenbaum M, Rosner I. The emergency room in systemic rheumatic diseases. *Emerg Med J*. 2006;23:667-671.
5. Wakefield RJ, Brown AK, O'Connor PJ, Emery P. Power Doppler sonography: improving disease activity assessment in inflammatory musculoskeletal disease. *Arthritis Rheum*. 2003;48:285-288.
6. Goldenberg DL. Septic arthritis. *Lancet*. 1998;351:197-202.
7. Goldenberg DL. Infectious arthritis complicating rheumatoid arthritis and other chronic rheumatic disorders. *Arthritis Rheum*. 1989;32:496-502.
8. Nolla JM, Gomez-Vaquero C, Fiter J, et al. Pyarthrosis in patients with rheumatoid arthritis: a detailed analysis of 10 cases and literature review. *Semin Arthritis Rheum*. 2000;30:121-126.
9. Mateo SL, Miquel Nolla SJ, Rozadilla SA, Valverde GJ, Roig ED. Infectious arthritis in patients with rheumatoid arthritis. *Ann Rheum Dis*. 1992;51:402-403.
10. Mathews CJ, Kingsley G, Field M, et al. Management of septic arthritis: a systematic review. *Ann Rheum Dis*. 2007;66:440-445.
11. Margaretten ME, Kohlwes J, Moore D, Bent S. Does this adult patient have septic arthritis? *JAMA*. 2007;297:1478-1488.
12. Coutlakis PJ, Roberts WN, Wise CM. Another look at synovial fluid leukocytosis and infection. *J Clin Rheumatol*. 2002;8:67-71.

13. Smith JW, Chalupa P, Shabaz HM. Infectious arthritis: clinical features, laboratory findings and treatment. *Clin Microbiol Infect.* 2006;12:309-314.
14. Jurik AG, Pedersen U. Rheumatoid arthritis of the crico-arytenoid and crico-thyroid joints: a radiological and clinical study. *Clin Radiol.* 1984;35:233-236.
15. Bayar N, Kara SA, Keles I, Koc C, Altinok D, Orkun S. Cricoarytenoiditis in rheumatoid arthritis: radiologic and clinical study. *J Otolaryngol.* 2003;32:373-378.
16. McGeehan DF, Crinnion JN, Strachan DR. Life-threatening stridor presenting in a patient with rheumatoid involvement of the larynx. *Arch Emerg Med.* 1989;6:274-276.
17. Kay LJ, Holland TM, Platt PN. Stress fractures in rheumatoid arthritis: a case series and case-control study. *Ann Rheum Dis.* 2004;63:1690-1692.
18. Peris P. Stress fractures in rheumatological practice: clinical significance and localizations. *Rheumatol Int.* 2002;22:77-79.
19. Torreggiani WC, Al-Ismail K, Munk PL, et al. The imaging spectrum of Baker's (Popliteal) cysts. *Clin Radiol.* 2002;57:681-691.
20. Canoso JJ, Goldsmith MR, Gerzof SG, Wohlgethan JR. Foucher's sign of the Baker's cyst. *Ann Rheum Dis.* 1987;46:228-232.
21. Handy JR. Popliteal cysts in adults: a review. *Semin Arthritis Rheum.* 2001;31:108-118.
22. Burger C, Monig SP, Prokop A, Rehm KE. Baker's cyst – current surgical status. Overview and personal results. *Chirurg.* 1998;69:1224-1229.
23. Wolfs JF, Kloppenburg M, Fehlings MG, van Tulder MW, Boers M, Peul WC. Neurologic outcome of surgical and conservative treatment of rheumatoid cervical spine subluxation: a systematic review. *Arthritis Rheum.* 2009;61:1743-1752.
24. Kauppi MJ, Neva MH, Laiho K, et al. Rheumatoid atlantoaxial subluxation can be prevented by intensive use of traditional disease modifying antirheumatic drugs. *J Rheumatol.* 2009;36:273-278.
25. Rasker JJ, Cosh JA. Radiological study of cervical spine and hand in patients with rheumatoid arthritis of 15 years' duration: an assessment of the effects of corticosteroid treatment. *Ann Rheum Dis.* 1978;37:529-535.
26. Bland JD. Carpal tunnel syndrome. *BMJ.* 2007;335:343-346.
27. Day CS, Makhni EC, Mejia E, Lage DE, Rozental TD. Carpal and cubital tunnel syndrome: who gets surgery? *Clin Orthop Relat Res.* 2010;468(7):1796-1803. Epub ahead of print.
28. Bland JD. Carpal tunnel syndrome. *Curr Opin Neurol.* 2005;18:581-585.
29. Mondelli M, Filippou G, Gallo A, Frediani B. Diagnostic utility of ultrasonography versus nerve conduction studies in mild carpal tunnel syndrome. *Arthritis Rheum.* 2008;59:357-366.
30. Hafner J, Schneider E, Burg G, Cassina PC. Management of leg ulcers in patients with rheumatoid arthritis or systemic sclerosis: the importance of concomitant arterial and venous disease. *J Vasc Surg.* 2000;32:322-329.
31. Firth J, Hale C, Helliwell P, Hill J, Nelson EA. The prevalence of foot ulceration in patients with rheumatoid arthritis. *Arthritis Rheum.* 2008;59:200-205.
32. Sato T, Hagiwara K, Kobayashi S, Inokuma S, Akiyama O. Effectiveness of leukocytapheresis for refractory foot ulceration in rheumatoid arthritis. *Intern Med.* 2008;47:1763-1764.
33. Inan AS, Masatlioglu S, Ozyurek SC, Engin D, Erdem I. Unusual central nervous system involvement of rheumatoid arthritis: successful treatment with steroid and azathioprine. Rheumatol Int. 2009; Dec 15, PMID 20012963, doi: 10.1007/s00296-009-1266-z.
34. Koide R, Isoo A, Ishii K, Uruha A, Bandoh M. Rheumatoid leptomeningitis: rare complication of rheumatoid arthritis. *Clin Rheumatol.* 2009;28:1117-1119.
35. Kato T, Hoshi K, Sekijima Y, et al. Rheumatoid meningitis: an autopsy report and review of the literature. *Clin Rheumatol.* 2003;22:475-480.
36. Yucel AE, Kart H, Aydin P, et al. Pachymeningitis and optic neuritis in rheumatoid arthritis: successful treatment with cyclophosphamide. *Clin Rheumatol.* 2001;20:136-139.

37. Jones SE, Belsley NA, McLoud TC, Mullins ME. Rheumatoid meningitis: radiologic and pathologic correlation. *AJR Am J Roentgenol.* 2006;186:1181-1183.
38. Rajasekaran A, Shovlin D, Saravanan V, Lord P, Kelly C. Interstitial lung disease in patients with rheumatoid arthritis: comparison with cryptogenic fibrosing alveolitis over 5 years. *J Rheumatol.* 2006;33:1250-1253.
39. Gochuico BR, Avila NA, Chow CK, et al. Progressive preclinical interstitial lung disease in rheumatoid arthritis. *Arch Intern Med.* 2008;168:159-166.
40. Kim EJ, Collard HR, King TE Jr. Rheumatoid arthritis-associated interstitial lung disease: the relevance of histopathologic and radiographic pattern. *Chest.* 2009;136:1397-1405.
41. Yousem SA, Colby TV, Carrington CB. Lung biopsy in rheumatoid arthritis. *Am Rev Respir Dis.* 1985;131:770-777.
42. Shadick NA, Fanta CH, Weinblatt ME, O'Donnell W, Coblyn JS. Bronchiectasis. A late feature of severe rheumatoid arthritis. *Medicine.* 1994;73:161-170.
43. Lieberman-Maran L, Orzano IM, Passero MA, Lally EV. Bronchiectasis in rheumatoid arthritis: report of four cases and a review of the literature – implications for management with biologic response modifiers. *Semin Arthritis Rheum.* 2006;35:379-387.
44. Anaya JM, Diethelm L, Ortiz LA, et al. Pulmonary involvement in rheumatoid arthritis. *Semin Arthritis Rheum.* 1995;24:242-254.

Sjögren's Syndrome: Beyond Sicca Involvement

5

Manuel Ramos-Casals, Pilar Brito-Zerón, Albert Bové Boada, and Antoni Sisó-Almirall

Abstract Sjögren syndrome (SS) is a systemic autoimmune disease that presents with sicca symptomatology of the major mucosal surfaces. The clinical spectrum of this condition often extends to systemic involvement (extraglandular manifestations) and may be complicated by the development of lymphoma. SS is one of the most prevalent autoimmune diseases (with an estimated 0.5–3 million sufferers in the United States), and primarily affects perimenopausal women. When sicca symptoms appear in a previously healthy person, the syndrome is classified as primary SS. This chapter summarizes recent work focused on extending and characterizing the acute and/or complex clinical presentations of patients with primary SS, including a wide variety of symptoms and the involvement of internal organs. As a general rule, the management of extraglandular features in primary SS should be targeted to the specific organ involved. The mainstays of such treatment regimens remain glucocorticoids and immunosuppressive agents. Such therapies are more likely to affect favorably the extraglandular manifestations of SS, even though the patients' most intense complaints often pertain to sicca features. Severe, life-threatening involvement has rarely been reported in primary SS. There are now substantially more data on the outcome of patients with primary SS, which indicate that patients with a predominantly extraepithelial expression (often associated with cryoglobulinemia) should be monitored and managed differently from patients with a predominantly periepithelial or sicca-limited disease.

Keywords Cryoglobulinemia • Interstitial nephritis • Lymphoma • Myelitis • Neuropathy • Primary biliary cirrhosis • Pulmonary fibrosis • Sjögren syndrome • Vasculitis

Sjögren syndrome (SS) is a systemic autoimmune disease that presents with sicca symptomatology of the major mucosal surfaces.[1] The clinical spectrum of this condition often extends to systemic involvement (extraglandular manifestations) and may be complicated

M. Ramos-Casals (✉)
Department of Autoimmune Diseases, Laboratory of Autoimmune Diseases
Josep Font, Institut d'Investigacions Biomèdiques August Pi i Sunyer
(IDIBAPS), Hospital Clinic, Barcelona, Spain
e-mail: mramos@clinic.ub.es

M.A. Khamashta and M. Ramos-Casals (eds.), *Autoimmune Diseases*,
DOI: 10.1007/978-0-85729-358-9_5, © Springer-Verlag London Limited 2011

by the development of lymphoma.[2] SS is one of the most prevalent autoimmune diseases (with an estimated 0.5–3 million sufferers in the United States)[3] and primarily affects perimenopausal women. When sicca symptoms appear in a previously healthy person, the syndrome is classified as primary SS.[4] The standard management approach is centered on the control of sicca features using substitutive agents, while extraglandular features are managed with glucocorticoids and broad-spectrum immunosuppressive agents.[5]

The increasing amount of SS-related publications in the last 5 years has contributed to a better understanding of the systemic involvement and the outcome of the disease. Advances in the treatment of extraglandular features are especially noteworthy. This chapter summarizes recent work focused on extending and characterizing the acute and/or complex clinical presentations of patients with primary SS (Table 5.1) and evaluating new therapeutic approaches.

Table 5.1 Complex and acute clinical presentations in patients with primary Sjögren syndrome

- Parotid and submandibular gland enlargement
- Cutaneous and vascular involvement
  - Ro-associated cutaneous lesions
  - Raynaud phenomenon
  - Life-threatening vasculitis
- Liver involvement
  - Coexistence with hepatitis C virus infection
  - Primary biliary cirrhosis
- Nephrourological involvement
  - Interstitial nephritis
  - Glomerulonephritis
  - Interstitial cystitis
- Peripheral neuropathy
  - Axonal polineuropathy
  - Ataxic neuronopathy
  - Small-fiber neuropathy
- Central nervous system involvement
  - Cerebral white matter lesions
  - Neuromyelitis optica
  - Myelitis
- Sensorineural hearing loss
- Hematological involvement
  - Neutropenia
  - Agranulocytosis
  - Hemolytic anemia
  - Severe thrombocytopenia
  - Monoclonal gammopathy
  - Lymphoma

5.1
Parotid and Submandibular Involvement

Patients with primary SS have a range of major salivary gland involvement, mainly parotid enlargement, but also isolated submandibular gland enlargement.[6] The course of glandular enlargement in SS varies from patient to patient. Some develop parotid enlargement that persists largely unchanged for years (Fig. 5.1). In others, the glandular involvement waxes and wanes over periods of several weeks or months. This is often asymmetric. Nearly 90% of patients with primary SS present inflammatory, benign parotid enlargement. However, B-cell lymphoma should be always suspected, especially in patients with persistent enlargement. A more recently recognized cause of salivary gland enlargement is IgG4-associated systemic disease, a disorder in which IgG4-producing plasma cells infiltrate certain exocrine glands, for example, the salivary glands, pancreas, and biliary tract.[7]

5.2
Ro-Associated Cutaneous Lesions

Although SS-associated annular erythema (AE) has been considered as the Asian counterpart of subacute cutaneous lupus erythematosus (SCLE) in Caucasians, a growing number of cases have been reported in white SS patients. In a recent study,[8] polycyclic, photosensitive, erythematosus maculopapulae lesions, clinically identical to AE or SCLE, were reported in patients with primary SS, all of whom had positive anti-Ro/SS-A antibodies (Fig. 5.2). McCauliffe et al.[9] could not identify disease-specific Ro autoantibodies in sera from patients with SS-AE and SCLE, and suggested that the two diseases might have a

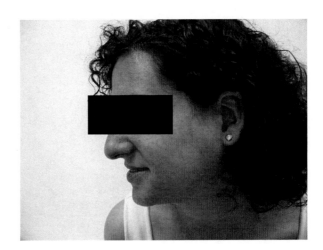

Fig. 5.1 Unilateral parotid enlargement

Fig. 5.2 Polycyclic, photosensitive, erythematosus maculopapulae lesions, clinically identical to AE or SCLE, in a 62-year-old woman with primary SS, with positive anti-Ro/SS-A antibodies

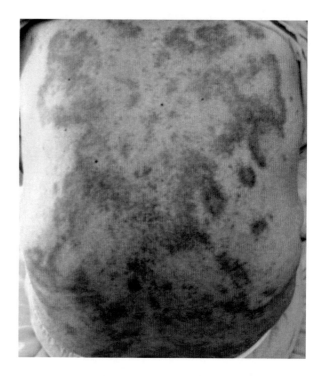

common pathogenic origin. Thus, polycyclic, photosensitive cutaneous lesions (clinically identical to Asian AE or Caucasian SCLE) may occur in a specific subset of patients with primary SS and positive anti-Ro/SS-A antibodies. This cutaneous manifestation of primary SS may be considered the counterpart of the SCLE lesions observed in SLE patients with positive anti-Ro/SS-A antibodies. Some patients diagnosed with isolated SCLE (without additional clinical or immunological data of systemic lupus) may have an underlying primary SS. Nevertheless, SS patients with these photosensitive lesions should always be followed up in order to discard a possible evolution to SLE.

5.3
Raynaud Phenomenon

Raynaud phenomenon (RP) is the most frequent vascular feature observed in primary SS (Fig. 5.3). We have reported[10] a prevalence of 13% in 320 patients with primary SS, with RP being the first autoimmune symptom in almost 50% of cases. Patients with RP have a higher frequency of some extraglandular features and positive immunological markers. The clinical course of RP in primary SS is milder than in other systemic autoimmune diseases such as systemic sclerosis, with no vascular complications and with pharmacological treatment needed in only 40% of patients. In patients with primary SS presenting with severe local

Fig. 5.3 Raynaud's phenomenon

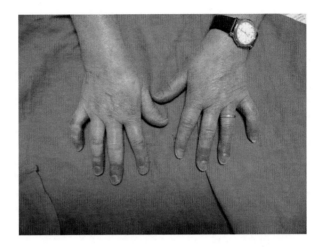

sequelae such as digital ulcers or gangrene, a specific search for anticentromere antibodies (ACA) should be performed, especially when high titers of ANA and negative anti-Ro/La antibodies are present.[11,12] SS patients with severe RP need a closer follow-up paying special attention to the possible development of clinical features of limited systemic sclerosis, mainly dermatological and pulmonary manifestations, and treatment with endothelin antagonists may be considered.

5.4
Life-Threatening Vasculitis

In primary SS, vasculitis can range from a benign, restricted process (e.g., cutaneous leucocytoclastic angiitis) to a life-threatening systemic vasculitis. All types of vessels from any organ may be affected, with a wide variety of signs and symptoms. Tsokos et al.[13] pointed out that the severity of vasculitis in SS depends on the histological type (necrotizing vasculitis being more severe than leukocytoclastic) and the site (internal more severe than external) of the vasculitic lesions. We have differentiated between vasculitis confined to the skin, observed in 56% of patients, from systemic vasculitis, observed in the remaining 44%.[8] This suggests that cutaneous vasculitis expresses systemically in almost half of patients. The main systemic vasculitic involvement was neuropathic, pulmonary and renal, associated with cryoglobulinemia in more than half the cases, with severe cutaneous involvement, intestinal and pancreatic vasculitis being infrequent. Although most of the severe cases of vasculitis reported in SS patients were due to necrotizing vasculitis, there are some reports of life-threatening leukocytoclastic vasculitis, with intestinal involvement in four patients and cutaneous involvement in two.[8]

Necrotizing vasculitis of the medium arteries is a very infrequent SS-associated vasculitic process, occurring in less than 5% of SS patients with vasculitis, and the coexistence of SS with a true primary medium vessel vasculitis is an exceptional situation. Acute necrotizing vasculitis in patients with primary SS manifesting as a PAN-like vasculitis was first described by Tsokos et al. in 1987.[13] We have identified nearly 20 reports of additional SS cases[8] with necrotizing vasculitis involving muscle (10 cases), gastrointestinal tract (7 cases), peripheral nerve (4 cases), kidney (3 cases), CNS (2 cases), and pancreas, gallbladder, spleen, parotid gland and spinal cord (1 case each). Finally, the coexistence of small- and medium-sized vessel vasculitis in the same SS patient has also been described.[8,13]

Although infrequent, systemic vasculitis is one of the main autoimmune causes of death in patients with primary SS. In our patients with cutaneous vasculitis, 6/52 (12%) died due to multisystemic vasculitic involvement[8]; Molina et al.[14] described a similar percentage (10%) in 50 patients with cutaneous vasculitis. Of the 19 reporting deaths of SS patients with vasculitis, the main causes were CNS involvement in 6, gastrointestinal perforation in 5, hematological neoplasia in 3, sepsis in 2, renal failure in 1, and hemolytic anemia in 1. Cryoglobulins were determined in 12 of these patients and were positive in 10 (83%) cases.

5.5
Coexistence with HCV

Patients with chronic hepatitis C virus (HCV) infection present some extrahepatic manifestations that may mimic the clinical, immunologic, and histological manifestations of primary Sjögren's syndrome (SS). However, various demographic, clinical, and immunologic features may aid differentiation between the two processes.[15] Immunologically, SS-HCV patients present a higher frequency of cryoglobulinemia and hypocomplementemia and a lower prevalence of anti-Ro/SS-A and anti-La/SS-B antibodies in comparison with patients with primary SS. Chronic HCV infection should be considered an exclusion criterion for the classification of primary SS, not because it mimics primary SS, but because the virus may be implicated in the development of SS in a specific subset of patients.[16]

5.6
Primary Biliary Cirrhosis

After discarding HCV infection, primary biliary cirrhosis (PBC) is the main cause of liver disease in patients with primary SS.[17-19] Studies in non-SS patients have shown that AMA-M2 patients with any clinical or analytical sign of liver involvement have a high risk of developing symptomatic PBC,[20] underlining the key role of AMA-M2 as an early immunological marker of PBC.[21] Nearly 10% of patients with primary SS have positive AMA-M2+ pattern.[22] Primary SS patients with AMA-M2 showed a broad spectrum of abnormalities in the analytical liver profile, including patients with no clinical or analytical data suggestive of liver disease.[17-19] For these reasons, we recommend the inclusion of AMA in the routine immunologic follow-up of SS patients, independently of whether the analytical liver profile is altered or not, due to the strong association between AMA and the development of PBC. Although historically these patients have been considered as having a "secondary" SS, it seems more rational to use the term "SS associated with PBC," due to the clinical-based evidence that SS is associated with (and not secondary to) other autoimmune diseases. Although there are no therapeutic guidelines for these asymptomatic patients, early use of ursodeoxycholic acid may be considered, since some studies in non-SS patients with mild analytical abnormalities have suggested that treatment with ursodeoxycholic acid might prevent a possible evolution to liver cirrhosis.[23]

5.7
Interstitial Nephritis

Tubulointerstitial disease is usually found in younger patients and is characterized by an indolent course in which renal dysfunction is often subclinical.[6] IgM and complement proteins comprise the primary deposits in the glomerulonephritis of SS. This contrasts with the immunopathologic lesion of lupus nephritis, in which a "full house" of immunoreactant deposition (immunoglobulin and complement) is observed. Interstitial nephritis can be an early manifestation of SS.[24] This condition is usually manifested by a low urine specific gravity (hyposthenuria) and an alkaline urine pH. Elevated serum creatinine as a complication of interstitial nephritis is uncommon. Nephrocalcinosis that presents with renal colic is a common clinical expression of distal renal tubular dysfunction in these patients. The classic renal manifestation of SS is a distal renal tubular acidosis (RTA) caused by interstitial nephritis. Hypokalemia can also result from the mechanism of a distal RTA. Patients who develop distal RTAs may require spironolactone to control hypokalemia, and the use of loop diuretics should be discouraged. Proximal RTAs, which can lead to osteomalacia and the Fanconi syndrome, are rare in SS.[24]

5.8
Glomerulonephritis

Although tubulointerstitial disease is regarded widely as the most common form of renal dysfunction in primary SS, some patients may present with glomerulonephritis. In fact, among 27 SS patients with documented renal biopsy reported in the literature,[24] 15 had tubulointerstitial nephritis, 11 had glomerulonephritis, and one had both tubulointerstitial disease and glomerulonephritis. Among the patients with glomerulonephritis, the most common glomerular lesions were membranoproliferative (7 patients), mesangial proliferative (6 patients), and membranous (2 patients). Cryoglobulinemia was detected in half of the patients with glomerulonephritis. Only two patients ultimately developed end-stage renal disease. SS-glomerulonephritis usually responds to glucocorticoids at a starting dose of 0.5–1.0 mg/kg of body weight per day.

5.9
Peripheral Neuropathy

A wide range of peripheral neuropathies can complicate primary SS. Early attention to peripheral neuropathies is extremely important. Sensory neuropathies and ganglionic neuropathies are the most common forms that afflict SS patients.[25] Pathology in cases of sensory ganglioneuronopathy consists of loss of neuronal cell bodies and infiltration of T cells. Peripheral motor neuropathies can include mononeuritis multiplex (which stems from vasculitis) or CIDP (chronic idiopathic demyelinating polyneuropathy), the latter of which is linked in some cases to anti-myelin-associated glycoprotein. SS patients can also suffer from trigeminal and other cranial neuropathies, autonomic neuropathy, and mixed patterns of neuropathy.

Sural nerve biopsy may show vascular or perivascular inflammation of small epineurial vessels (both arterioles and venules) and in some cases necrotizing vasculitis. The loss of myelinated nerve fibers is common and loss of small-diameter nerve fibers occurs. The histopathology of sensory ganglioneuronopathy consists of the loss of neuronal cell bodies and T cell infiltration. Peripheral neuropathy in primary SS often is refractory to treatment with currently available agents.

5.10
Ataxic Neuronopathy

Pure sensory neuropathy (PSN) is recognized as a characteristic neurological complication of primary SS caused by damage of the sensory neurons of the dorsal root and gasserian ganglia. The differential diagnosis of PSN includes paraneoplastic syndrome, *tabes dorsalis*, vitamin B12 or E deficiency, paraproteinemias, and acute idiopathic cases. PSN is a neuropathy that affects nearly 5% of patients with primary SS, who often have a high prevalence of positive immunological markers (ANA and anti-Ro/SS-A). Clinically, PSN may be the first manifestation of a latent primary SS, and is characterized by asymmetrical sensory involvement, usually starting in the upper limbs and predominantly affecting kinesthesic and vibratory sensations. Some patients also have associated Adie's pupil or trigeminal sensory involvement. The diagnosis of PSN is important because, although it may precede that of primary SS, it is not associated with systemic vasculitis, and treatment with corticosteroids may be ineffective. We have reported three differentiated clinical courses[26]: subacute progression of PSN in less than 1 month (7%); late acceleration of PSN some years after an initial indolent onset (20%); and a very long-term insidious, chronic evolution (73%). This study also demonstrated a poor response to treatment with corticosteroids or immunosuppressive agents, although stabilization of symptomatology (spontaneously or after treatment) during very long periods was often observed. First-line therapy consisted of intravenous immunoglobulins.[27] In refractory cases, some authors have obtained a good treatment response using plasma exchanges[28] or rituximab.[29]

5.11
Small-Fiber Neuropathy

Some patients with primary SS present with a painful sensory neuropathy but normal nerve conduction studies.[6] Small-fiber neuropathy occurs in patients with primary SS.[30,31] These patients often present with burning pain in the feet. Small-fiber neuropathy can develop either in isolation as the sole neurologic manifestation of disease, or in combination with larger sensory fiber involvement. The diagnosis often relies on quantitative sensory testing and sural nerve biopsy, but skin biopsy is an increasingly useful technique for demonstrating small-fiber neuropathy.[32] The pathological finding on skin biopsy is a decrease in the density of epidermal nerve fibers.[33] Patients with small-fiber neuropathy have normal nerve conduction studies, because the size of nerve fibers involved is below the resolution of conventional electrodiagnostic studies.

5.12
Central Nervous System Involvement: Differential Diagnosis

The clinical approach to primary SS patients with suspected CNS involvement requires not only the diagnostic procedures to define the type of neurological involvement, but also consideration of processes not directly related to primary SS that also cause neurological involvement. These include the coexistence of other systemic autoimmune diseases (antiphospholipid syndrome, systemic lupus erythematosus, and systemic vasculitis), the differential diagnosis with primary CNS disorders (multiple sclerosis, Devic disease), and the role played by non-autoimmune processes that frequently provoke CNS involvement in patients aged >50 years (cardiovascular disease, neurodegenerative processes).

5.13
Cerebral White Matter Lesions

In primary SS patients with suspected neurological involvement, MRI often discloses the presence of hyperintense white matter lesions (WML). These lesions are associated with a wide variety of processes, including vasculitic, inflammatory, infectious, metabolic, and neoplasic causes. Multiple sclerosis (MS) is probably the disease most often considered in the differential diagnosis of these lesions, and one of the most difficult diagnostic issues is dealing with a patient with sicca syndrome and WML in whom two different clinical scenarios may be hypothesized:

5.13.1
Coexistence of MS and SS

Several studies have investigated the prevalence of SS-related features in MS patients. Seze et al. found a prevalence of SS of 17% in patients with MS, a higher prevalence than that observed in the general population[34] but not confirmed by other studies: Miro et al.[35] found a prevalence of 3% of SS in 64 MS patients and three studies including a total of 270 patients with MS found any case.[36-38] The majority of these studies suggest that SS is rarely associated with MS, although some patients may have the two diseases. This may be considered an additional example of the frequent association of primary SS with organ-specific autoimmune diseases as occurs with thyroiditis or primary biliary cirrhosis.

5.13.2
MS-Like Lesions in Primary SS

Diagnosis of WML in a patient with primary SS leads to a difficult differential diagnosis between MS- and SS-related CNS involvement (Fig. 5.4). In the study by Delalande et al.,[39] these authors found that 40% of patients with primary SS and neurological involvement had WML suggestive of MS. There are some clinical, analytical, and imaging features that may help in differentiating both situations. The clinical course is probably a key factor that may allow to differentiate MS and the CNS involvement associated to primary SS. In patients with primary SS, WML are often diagnosed in asymptomatic patients or in those with nonspecific neurological symptoms (migraine, psychiatric involvement, depression). In contrast, a diagnosis of MS requires neurological symptoms suggesting a MS flare together with the appearance of new WML lesions during follow-up (the so-called dissemination in time and space). In patients with primary SS presenting with nonspecific symptoms, a close clinical follow-up should be carried out by neurologists and specialists in autoimmune diseases. Cerebrospinal fluid (CSF) analysis may help in the differential diagnosis, although both diseases may have an elevated index of IgG and oligoclonal bands. A greater percentage of CSF lymphocytes and elevated proteins is more frequently seen in SS patients, although this is not an always-valid feature. CSF immunoelectrophoresis seems to play a more useful role,

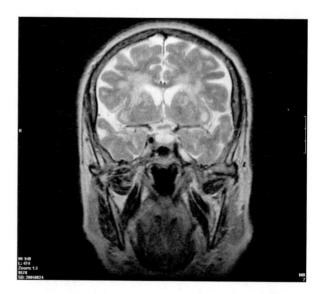

Fig. 5.4 Multiple sclerosis-like white matter lesions in a 45-year-old woman with primary SS

since there is a lower number of oligoclonal bands in primary SS (less than 5 with respect to more than 10 in MS patients).[40] Finally, MRI should be a clue diagnostic tool to differentiate both entities. The application of the Barkhof criteria may help in diagnosing MS, especially if the size and location of the lesions are carefully evaluated.

5.14
Neuromyelitis Optica

Devic disease or neuromyelitis optica (NMO) is an inflammatory demyelinating disease that affects selectively the optic nerve and the spinal cord. The recent identification of a highly specific biomarker for NMO (NMO-IgG/aquaporin-4-water-channel specific antibody)[41] has extended the clinical spectrum of NMO to other neurological diseases such as recurrent longitudinally extensive transverse myelitis (LETM) and recurrent optic neuritis (ON).[42] A new set of diagnostic criteria of the disease[43] has been recently proposed which not only incorporates the new biomarker, but also eliminates the mandatory criteria of having no demyelinating disease beyond optic nerve and spinal cord.[44]

Recent studies have suggested a close association between NMO and primary SS, since aquaporin has also been described as a potential autoantigen involved in primary SS etiopathogenesis.[45] A recent study has found anti-Ro/SS-A antibodies in 11% of the so-called NMO idiopathic cases, with a higher prevalence in patients with positive IgG-NMO antibodies. Javed et al.[46] have found salivary gland infiltration in 80% of patients with NMO or LETM, while Wandinger et al.[47] found that 7 out of 8 primary SS patients with myelitis fulfilled the diagnostic criteria of NMO. These studies suggest that NMO and primary SS may coexist more frequently than previously supposed.[48] IgG-NMO antibodies should be tested and visual evoked potentials carried out in primary SS patients with suspected CNS involvement, especially in those presenting with optic neuritis or myelitis. Thus, Delalande et al.[39] showed alteration of visual evoked potentials in 61% of patients with CNS involvement, confirming the diagnosis of optical neuritis in 13 patients who presented visual involvement and detecting subclinical manifestations in other 12. The majority of these patients probably may be currently diagnosed as NMO according to the new proposed criteria.

5.15
Myelitis

Spinal cord involvement has been reported in nearly 50 patients with primary SS, most of which are included in the two major studies on neurological involvement in primary SS.[39,49] The clinical presentation is normally acute or chronic myelitis, although spinal subarachnoid hemorrhage, Brown-Sequard syndrome, and a motor neurone disease resembling lateral amyotrophic sclerosis have been also reported.[39,50] Symptoms include sensitive and motor involvement, loss of sphincter control, and optic neuritis in 10–20% of cases. Chronic myelitis may have a clinical course similar to MS.[39] Spinal MRI shows vertebral

Fig. 5.5 Spinal MRI showing multiple vertebral methameric involvement in a patient with cervical myelitis

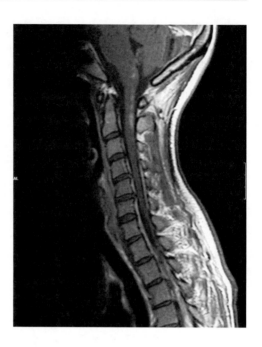

methameric involvement (65%), predominantly cervical (82%) (Fig. 5.5), thoracic (47%), and less frequently, lumbar (12%); there is centromedullary involvement in 40%.[39] Visual evoked potentials may be altered in more than 50% of cases in the absence of overt optical neuritis. The differential diagnosis includes ataxic neuronopathy, progressive forms of MS, Devic disease, and CNS retroviral infections (HIV, HTLV-1, JVC).[51,52]

5.16
Interstitial Cystitis

Two studies have analyzed lower urinary tract symptoms in patients with primary SS. Walker et al. found severe urological symptoms (increased frequency, urgency, and nicturia) in 61% of patients, some of them with autonomic neuropathy and positive anti-M3R antibodies, with a biopsy-proven interstitial cystitis being found in some cases.[53] Lepilahti et al.[54] have recently studied interstitial cystitis–like urinary symptoms in a population-based study of Finnish SS patients, and found that 45 (5%) fulfilled the criteria for probable interstitial cystitis.

5.17
Sensorineural Hearing Loss

Ear, nose, and throat involvement in patients with primary SS has been little studied. Some studies have described sensorineural hearing loss in a substantial percentage of SS patients. Of the 140 patients included in these studies,[55-58] 38 (27%) showed sensorineural loss.

Some of these studies suggested an association with immunologic parameters such as aPL,[55] ANA, Ro, or La.[55,56] Boki et al.[56] found that primary SS is associated with sensorineural hearing loss affecting preferentially the high frequencies, although clinically significant defects are not common, with no evidence of retrocochlear disease or increased vestibular involvement.

5.18
Neutropenia and Agranulocytosis

Nearly 30% of patients with primary SS may present autoimmune neutropenia,[59] a percentage much higher than that of other cytopenias such as leukopenia or thrombocytopenia. In a recent study,[59] neutrophil counts oscillate between normal and low values in the majority of patients during the follow-up, with minimum values of between $1.5-2.5 \times 10^9/L$ in 60% of cases. In this study, 7 (2%) out of 300 patients presented agranulocytosis, mainly related to neoplasia (5 cases). No apparent cause was identified in the remaining two patients, who were classified as having an SS-related agranulocytosis, although their neutrophil counts varied widely during the follow-up. Two recent studies have reported a total of 20 patients with primary SS and agranulocytosis.[60,61] One of our 90 patients with SS-related neutropenia developed large granular lymphocyte lymphoma (LGL) a T-cell leukemia closely associated with agranulocytosis. A recent study found that around 25% of patients with LGL have an associated, underlying primary SS, suggesting a closer relationship than previously suspected.[62]

More than 80% of our SS patients with neutropenia had other cytopenias and a high frequency of altered immunological markers including autoantibodies and low complement levels, especially those with lower neutrophil counts ($<1.5 \times 10^9/L$), who presented a twofold higher prevalence of RF and a threefold higher prevalence of anti-Ro/La antibodies in comparison with patients without neutropenia.[59] This association with positive anti-Ro/La antibodies has been previously described for other cytopenias such as leukopenia, lymphopenia, and thrombocytopenia.[59]

A significant finding in our study[59] was the higher rate of hospital admission due to infection in our patients with primary SS and neutropenia. The clinically significant findings of our study are that, on the one hand, patients with primary SS and neutropenia should be followed closely due to the high risk of presenting infections and that, on the other hand, some therapeutic agents such as immunosuppressive (cyclophosphamide and mycophenolate) and biological agents (anti-TNF and rituximab) should be used carefully in these patients. In patients with primary SS presenting severe systemic involvement who may require treatment with these agents, routine neutrophil count should be made, previous to and during treatment.

Probably, the majority of SS patients with autoimmune neutropenia do not require specific therapy, with standard antibiotic therapy often being sufficient to deal with infections. In patients with severe infections or those requiring surgery, specific treatment with corticosteroids, intravenous immunoglobulins, and granulocyte colony–stimulating factor (G-CSF) has been suggested,[63-65] although Vivancos et al.[66] have reported the failure of G-CSF therapy in a patient with primary SS and neutropenia.

5.19
Hemolytic Anemia

Clinically significant hemolysis is very rare in primary SS, with less than 30 cases of hemolytic anemia reported.[67] These patients present with symptoms related to acute anemia (weakness, pallor, dyspnea) with a significant decrease of hemoglobin values. All reported cases but one received initial treatment with corticosteroids and, as maintenance therapy, danazol in two patients, azathioprine in two, and oral cyclophosphamide in other one. The outcome of these patients was excellent, with improvement of hemoglobin values in most. Nevertheless, due to the rarity of hemolytic anemia in patients with primary SS, we consider that hemolytic assays (haptoglobin, Coombs test) should only be performed in those SS patients with clinical evidence of acute anemia and/or laboratory evidence of hemolysis (raised LDH and bilirubin). In these patients, high-dose corticosteroid therapy is recommended.

5.20
Severe Thrombocytopenia

Severe thrombocytopenia ($<50,000/mm^3$) is very infrequent in primary SS.[67] Patients often present with cutaneous purpura, bruises, and oral mucosal bleeding. All reported cases were treated with corticosteroids, although associated with immunosuppressive agents in two and danazol as maintenance therapy in three. A good response was observed in most patients, although one was refractory to corticosteroids, danazol, and vincristine and partially responded to cyclosporin A.

5.21
Monoclonal Gammopathy

Monoclonal gammopathies (MG) are a heterogeneous group of disorders characterized by the clonal proliferation of plasma cells that produce a homogenous monoclonal protein. In the absence of a malignant disorder, patients with MG are classified as having monoclonal gammopathy of undetermined significance (MGUS).[68] However, this asymptomatic disorder requires routine clinical and analytical surveillance, since some patients with MGUS may develop an overt hematological neoplasia, mainly multiple myeloma (MM).[69] Studies performed in the 1980s described the presence of monoclonal immunoglobulins in urine of SS patients[70,71] and its association with extraglandular manifestations and lymphoproliferative disorders. More recently, the clinical significance of serum monoclonal immunoglobulins has been studied in a large series of patients with SS,[72] with circulating monoclonal immunoglobulins (mIg) being detected in nearly 20% of patients with primary SS. The most frequent type of circulating mIg is mIgG (57%), and the type of light chain predominantly found is "κ" (60%). The main features associated with the presence of circulating mIgs were hypergammaglobulinemia, cryoglobulinemia, and hematologi-cal neoplasia, which is reported in 6–8% of primary SS patients with monoclonal gam-mopathy.[72-74] In primary SS patients with circulating mIgs associated with hematological neoplasia, IgMκ is the most common type of circulating mIg associated with B-cell lym-phoma and IgGκ the monoclonal band most frequently associated with multiple myeloma. A change in the monoclonal component has been observed previous to the development of neoplasia.[72] This suggests that sequential determinations of serum mIgs are useful to detecting possible changes in the monoclonal components, with these changes or switches of mIgs being a possible marker of an emergent hematological neoplasia. Thus, we rec-ommend the inclusion of serum IE in the routine immunological tests performed during the follow-up of patients with primary SS.

5.22
Lymphoma

Primary SS patients are at higher risk of lymphoma than are healthy individuals and patients with other autoimmune diseases. Different studies have estimated the relative risk of lymphoma in patients with primary SS compared with the general population to range from 10- to 44-fold. A meta-analysis of five studies in four different countries that included a combined total of 1,200 primary SS patients confirmed the high risk of non-Hodgkin's lymphoma and calculated a standardized incidence rate (SIR) of 18.8.[75] This SIR contrasts with those for SLE and RA of 7.4 and 3.9, respectively, from the same study.

The incidence of malignant lymphoproliferation in SS is the highest among all autoim-mune diseases, and primary SS is often considered to be a link between autoimmune and lymphoproliferative disease. Interestingly, most lymphomas observed in patients with SS are of B-cell origin, despite the fact that the vast majority of cells infiltrating the salivary glands are T cells. Cross-sectional studies have reported that only 98 (4%) of 2,311 patients with primary SS developed lymphoma.[76] The main clinical characteristics of B-cell lym-phoma in primary SS are lymphadenopathy, skin vasculitis, peripheral nerve involvement, fever, anemia, and lymphopenia. B-cell lymphoma was primarily located in the marginal zone, with a predominantly extranodal involvement, mainly in the salivary glands.

There are two main types of clinical presentation of lymphoma in patients with SS. Some patients present with a predominant nodal involvement with fever, general malaise, splenom-egaly, and peripheral adenopathies, more commonly in the cervical or supraclavicular regions. However, the most frequent type of lymphoma in primary SS affects the salivary glands or major parenchymal organs such as the lungs, kidneys, or gastrointestinal tract. Gastrointestinal symptoms are nonspecific with vague abdominal pain as the most common presenting symp-tom in intestinal lymphoma. With respect to pulmonary involvement, Hansen et al.[77] described pulmonary involvement in 10 out of 50 patients with SS and lymphoma. Pulmonary involve-ment by lymphoma is more likely to occur in those patients with systemic lymphoma, although in some cases, the lungs were the only organs involved. Unusual metabolic presentations include hyperuricemic renal failure[78] and hypercalcemia. Neurologic symptoms and signs, including headache or cranial nerve palsies, may be the presenting features, and they are more

Fig. 5.6 MALT lymphoma of
the ocular adnexa

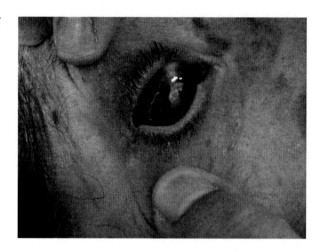

commonly associated with high-grade lymphomas. Genitourinary presentations include renal mass, ureteral obstruction, testicular mass, ovarian mass, and vaginal bleeding. Other unusual sites of lymphoma involvement are thymus, skin, and ocular adnexa (Fig. 5.6).[76]

The main clinical characteristics of B-cell lymphoma in primary SS were well described in a multicenter European study, including 33 patients followed up in nine centers.[79] Lymphadenopathy, skin vasculitis, peripheral nerve involvement, fever, anemia, and lymphopenia were observed significantly more frequently than in the general SS population. B-cell lymphoma was primarily located in the marginal zone (49%), with a predominantly extranodal involvement (79%), mainly in the salivary glands (55%). Patients with lymphoma had significantly worse survival rate, with high-to-intermediate grade lymphoma, B symptoms (fever, night sweats, and weight loss) and a large tumor diameter (>7 cm) being independent risk factors for death.[79] Recent reports have used rituximab in SS patients with lymphoma.[80] The results provide preliminary evidence that rituximab may be a worthwhile therapeutic option for indolent B-cell lymphoma in patients with HCV-related SS, and could be an alternative to aggressive chemotherapy options currently available. Rituximab may be considered as a safe and effective therapy for indolent B-cell lymphoma in elderly patients with SS, either in its primary or HCV-associated form.

Lymphoma tends to occur in a subgroup of SS patients who express special risk factors from early on in their disease course. These risk factors include palpable purpura and C4 hypocomplementemia. This patient subgroup has increased mortality.[81-83] The long-term risk of lymphoma for patients with primary SS is often estimated to be in the order of 5%.

5.23
Conclusion

The spectrum of SS extends from sicca syndrome to systemic involvement. Few studies have prospectively analyzed the outcome of patients with primary SS, a disease characterized by a chronic, insidious evolution. However, some patients with primary SS may present a complicated evolution of the disease due to the development of vasculitic involvement and the high incidence of lymphoma, which are closely related to a higher risk of death. The identification of markers prospectively associated with a poor prognosis could play a significant role in identifying those patients requiring a closer follow-up.

The increasing amount of published data on primary SS has contributed to a better understanding of the extraglandular expression of the disease and has changed the therapeutic management of these patients.[84] A wide spectrum of extraglandular features has been studied in the last 5 years, with understanding of the involvement of some organs and systems being expanded. There are now substantially more data on the outcome of patients with primary SS, which indicate that patients with a predominantly extraepithelial expression (often associated with cryoglobulinemia) should be monitored and managed differently from patients with a predominantly periepithelial or sicca-limited disease.

References

1. Sjögren H. Zur kenntnis der keratoconjunctivitis sicca (keratitis filiformis bei hypofunktion der tränendrüsen). *Acta Ophthalmol.* 1933;11(suppl 2):1-151.
2. Kassan SS, Moutsopoulos HM. Clinical manifestations and early diagnosis of Sjögren syndrome. *Arch Intern Med.* 2004;164:1275-1284.
3. Helmick CG, Felson DT, Lawrence RC, National Arthritis Data Workgroup, et al. Estimates of the prevalence of arthritis and other rheumatic conditions in the United States. Part I. *Arthritis Rheum.* 2008;58:15-25.
4. Ramos-Casals M, Tzioufas AG, Font J. Primary Sjögren's syndrome: new clinical and therapeutic concepts. *Ann Rheum Dis.* 2005;64:347-354.
5. Ramos-Casals M, Font J. Primary Sjögren syndrome. In: Imboden J, Hellman D, Stone JH, eds. *Current Diagnosis & Treatment in Rheumatology.* New York: McGraw-Hill; 2007:237-245.
6. Ramos-Casals M, Daniels TE, Fox RI, et al. Sjögren's syndrome. In: Stone JH, ed. *A Clinician's Pearls and Myths in Rheumatology.* London: Springer; 2009:107-130.
7. Kamisawa T, Nakajima H, Egawa N, Funata N, Tsuruta K, Okamoto A. IgG4-related sclerosing disease incorporating sclerosing pancreatitis, cholangitis, sialadenitis and retroperitoneal fibrosis with lymphadenopathy. *Pancreatology.* 2006;6:132-137.
8. Ramos-Casals M, Anaya JM, García-Carrasco M, et al. Cutaneous vasculitis in primary Sjögren syndrome: classification and clinical significance of 52 patients. *Medicine.* 2004;83: 96-106.
9. McCauliffe DP, Faircloth E, Wang L, Hashimoto T, Hoshino Y, Nishikawa T. Similar Ro/SS-A autoantibody epitope and titer responses in annular erythema of Sjögren's syndrome and subacute cutaneous lupus erythematosus. *Arch Dermatol.* 1996;132:528-531.
10. García-Carrasco M, Sisó A, Ramos-Casals M, et al. Raynaud's phenomenon in primary Sjögren's syndrome. Prevalence and clinical characteristics in a series of 320 patients. *J Rheumatol.* 2002;29:726-730.
11. Nakamura H, Kawakami A, Hayashi T, et al. Anti-centromere antibody-seropositive Sjögren's syndrome differs from conventional subgroup in clinical and pathological study. *BMC Musculoskelet Disord.* 2010;11:140.
12. Salliot C, Gottenberg JE, Bengoufa D, Desmoulins F, Miceli-Richard C, Mariette X. Anticentromere antibodies identify patients with Sjögren's syndrome and autoimmune overlap syndrome. *J Rheumatol.* 2007;34:2253-2258.
13. Tsokos M, Lazarou SA, Moutsopoulos HM. Vasculitis in primary Sjögren's syndrome. Histologic classification and clinical presentation. *Am J Clin Pathol.* 1987;88:26-31.

14. Molina R, Provost TT, Alexander EL. Two types of inflammatory vascular disease in Sjögren's syndrome. Differential association with seroreactivity to rheumatoid factor and antibodies to Ro (SS-A) and with hypocomplementemia. *Arthritis Rheum*. 1985;28:1251-1258.

15. Ramos-Casals M, Loustaud-Ratti V, De Vita S, SS-HCV Study Group, et al. Sjögren syndrome associated with hepatitis C virus: a multicenter analysis of 137 cases. *Medicine*. 2005;84:81-89.

16. Ramos-Casals M, De Vita S, Tzioufas AG. Hepatitis C virus, Sjögren's syndrome and B-cell lymphoma: linking infection, autoimmunity and cancer. *Autoimmun Rev*. 2005;4:8-15.

17. Ramos-Casals M, Sánchez-Tapias JM, Parés A, et al. Characterization and differentiation of autoimmune versus viral liver involvement in patients with Sjögren's syndrome. *J Rheumatol*. 2006;33:1593-1599.

18. Lindgren S, Manthorpe R, Eriksson S. Autoimmune liver disease in patients with primary Sjögren's syndrome. *J Hepatol*. 1994;20:354-358.

19. Skopouli FN, Barbatis C, Moutsopoulos HM. Liver involvement in primary Sjögren's syndrome. *Br J Rheumatol*. 1994;33:745-748.

20. Prince MI, Chetwynd A, Craig WL, Metcalf JV, James OF. Asymptomatic primary biliary cirrhosis: clinical features, prognosis, and symptom progression in a large population based cohort. *Gut*. 2004;53:865-870.

21. Abraham S, Begum S, Isenberg D. Hepatic manifestations of autoimmune rheumatic diseases. *Ann Rheum Dis*. 2004;63:123-129.

22. Ramos-Casals M, Nardi N, Brito-Zerón P, et al. Atypical autoantibodies in patients with primary Sjögren syndrome: clinical characteristics and follow-up of 82 cases. *Semin Arthritis Rheum*. 2006;35:312-321.

23. Beswick DR, Klatskin G, Boyer JL. Asymptomatic primary biliary cirrhosis. A progress report on long-term follow-up and natural history. *Gastroenterology*. 1985;89:267-271.

24. Goules A, Masouridi S, Tzioufas AG, Ioannidis JP, Skopouli FN, Moutsopoulos HM. Clinically significant and biopsy-documented renal involvement in primary Sjögren syndrome. *Medicine*. 2000;79:241-249.

25. Mellgren SI, Conn DL, Stevens JC, Dyck PJ. Peripheral neuropathy in primary Sjögren's syndrome. *Neurology*. 1989;39:390-394.

26. Font J, Ramos-Casals M, de la Red G, et al. Pure sensory neuropathy in primary Sjögren's syndrome. Longterm prospective followup and review of the literature. *J Rheumatol*. 2003;30:1552-1557.

27. Morozumi S, Kawagashira Y, Iijima M, et al. Intravenous immunoglobulin treatment for painful sensory neuropathy associated with Sjögren's syndrome. *J Neurol Sci*. 2009;279:57-61.

28. Chen WH, Yeh JH, Chiu HC. Plasmapheresis in the treatment of ataxic sensory neuropathy associated with Sjögren's syndrome. *Eur Neurol*. 2001;45:270-274.

29. Gorson KC, Natarajan N, Ropper AH, Weinstein R. Rituximab treatment in patients with IVIg-dependent immune polyneuropathy: a prospective pilot trial. *Muscle Nerve*. 2007;35:66-69.

30. Mori K, Iijima M, Sugiura M, et al. Sjögren's syndrome associated painful sensory neuropathy without sensory ataxia. *J Neurol Neurosurg Psychiatry*. 2003;74:1320-1322.

31. Gorson KC, Ropper AH. Positive salivary gland biopsy, Sjögren syndrome, and neuropathy: clinical implications. *Muscle Nerve*. 2003;28:553-560.

32. Chai J, Herrmann DN, Stanton M, Barbano RL, Logigian EL. Painful small-fiber neuropathy in Sjögren syndrome. *Neurology*. 2005;65:925-927.

33. Gøransson LG, Herigstad A, Tjensvoll AB, Harboe E, Mellgren SI, Omdal R. Peripheral neuropathy in primary Sjögren syndrome: a population-based study. *Arch Neurol*. 2006;63:1612-1615.

34. de Seze J, Devos D, Castelnovo G, et al. The prevalence of Sjögren syndrome in patients with primary progressive multiple sclerosis. *Neurology*. 2001;57:1359-1363.

35. Miro J, Pena-Sagredo JL, Berciano J, Insua S, Leno C, Velarde R. Prevalence of primary Sjögren's syndrome in patients with multiple sclerosis. *Ann Neurol*. 1990;27:582-584.

36. Montecucco C, Franciotta DM, Caporali R, DeGennaro F, Citterio A, Melzi d'Eril GV. Sicca syndrome and anti-SSA/Ro antibodies in patients with suspected or definite multiple sclerosis. *Scand J Rheumatol.* 1989;18:407-412.
37. Metz LM, Seland TP, Fritzler MJ. An analysis of the frequency of Sjögren's syndrome in a population of multiple sclerosis patients. *J Clin Lab Immunol.* 1989;30:121-125.
38. Noseworthy JH, Bass BH, Vandervoort MK, et al. The prevalence of primary Sjögren's syndrome in a multiple sclerosis population. *Ann Neurol.* 1989;25:95-98.
39. Delalande S, de Seze J, Fauchais AL, et al. Neurologic manifestations in primary Sjögren syndrome: a study of 82 patients. *Medicine.* 2004;83:280-291.
40. Vrethem M, Ernerudh J, Lindström F, Skogh T. Immunoglobulins within the central nervous system in primary Sjögren's syndrome. *J Neurol Sci.* 1990;100:186-192.
41. Saikali P, Cayrol R, Vincent T. Anti-aquaporin-4 auto-antibodies orchestrate the pathogenesis in neuromyelitis optica. *Autoimmun Rev.* 2009;9:132-135.
42. Nandhagopal R, Al-Asmi A, Gujjar AR. Neuromyelitis optica: an overview. *Postgrad Med J.* 2010;86:153-159.
43. Saiz A, Zuliani L, Blanco Y, et al. Revised diagnostic criteria for neuromyelitis optica (NMO). Application in a series of suspected patients. *J Neurol.* 2007;254:1233-1237.
44. Wingerchuck DM, Hogancamp WF, O'Brien PC, Weinshenker BG. The clinical course of neuromyelitis optica (Devic's syndrome). *Neurology.* 1999;53:1107-1114.
45. Ramos-Casals M, Font J. Primary Sjögren's syndrome: current and emergent aetiopathogenic concepts. *Rheumatology.* 2005;44:1354-1367.
46. Javed A, Balabanov R, Arnason BG, et al. Minor salivary gland inflammation in Devic's disease and longitudinally extensive myelitis. *Mult Scler.* 2008;14:809-814.
47. Wandinger KP, Stangel M, Witte T, et al. Autoantibodies against aquaporin-4 in patients with neuropsychiatric systemic lupus erythematosus and primary Sjögren's syndrome. *Arthritis Rheum.* 2010;62:1198-1200.
48. Pittock SJ, Lennon VA, de Seze J, et al. Neuromyeltis optica and non-organ-specific autoimmunity. *Arch Neurol.* 2008;65:78-83.
49. de Seze J, Delalande S, Fauchais AL, et al. Myelopathies secondary to Sjögren's syndrome: treatment with monthly intravenous cyclophosphamide associated with corticosteroids. *J Rheumatol.* 2006;33:709-711.
50. Alexander EL, Craft C, Dorsch C, Moser RL, Provost TT, Alexander GE. Necrotizing arteritis and spinal subarachnoid hemorrhage in Sjögren syndrome. *Ann Neurol.* 1982;11: 632-635.
51. Sá MJ. Acute transverse myelitis: a practical reappraisal. *Autoimmun Rev.* 2009;9:128-131.
52. Ramírez M, Ramos-Casals M, Graus F. Central nervous system involvement in primary Sjögren syndrome. *Med Clín.* 2009;133:349-359.
53. Shibata S, Ubara Y, Sawa N, et al. Severe interstitial cistitis associated with Sjögren's syndrome. *Intern Med.* 2004;43:248-252.
54. Leppilahti M, Tammela TL, Huhtala H, Kiilholma P, Leppilahti K, Auvinen A. Interstitial cystitis-like urinary symptoms among patients with Sjögren's syndrome: a population-based study in Finland. *Am J Med.* 2003;115:62-65.
55. Tumiati B, Casoli P, Parmeggiani A. Hearing loss in the Sjögren's syndrome. *Ann Intern Med.* 1997;126:450.
56. Ziavra N, Politi EN, Kastanioudakis I, Shevas A, Drosos AA. Hearing loss in Sjögren's syndrome patients: a comparative study. *Clin Exp Rheumatol.* 2000;18:725-728.
57. Boki KA, Ioannidis JP, Segas JV, et al. How significant is sensorineural hearing loss in primary Sjögren's syndrome? *J Rheumatol.* 2001;28:798-801.
58. Hatzopoulos S, Amoroso C, Aimoni C, Lo Monaco A, Govoni M, Martini A. Hearing loss evaluation of Sjogren's syndrome using distortion product otoacoustic emissions. *Acta Otolaryngol Suppl.* 2002;54:20-25.

59. Brito-Zerón P, Soria N, Muñoz S, et al. Prevalence and clinical relevance of autoimmune neutropenia in patients with primary Sjögren's syndrome. *Semin Arthritis Rheum.* 2009;38: 389-395.

60. Coppo P, Sibilia J, Maloisel F, et al. Primary Sjögren's syndrome associated agranulocytosis: a benign disorder? *Ann Rheum Dis.* 2003;62:476-478.

61. Friedman J, Klepfish A, Miller EB, Ognenovski V, Ike RW, Schattner A. Agranulocytosis in Sjogren's syndrome: two case reports and analysis of 11 additional reported cases. *Semin Arthritis Rheum.* 2002;31:338-345.

62. Friedman J, Schattner A, Shvidel L, Berrebi A. Characterization of T-cell large granular lymphocyte leukemia associated with Sjogren's syndrome – an important but under-recognized association. *Semin Arthritis Rheum.* 2006;35:306-311.

63. Maheshwari A, Christensen RD, Calhoun DA. Immune-mediated neutropenia in the neonate. *Acta Pediatr Suppl.* 2002;438:98-103.

64. Shastri KA, Logue GL. Autoimmune neutropenia. *Blood.* 1993;81:1984-1995.

65. Bux J, Behrens G, Jaeger G, Welte K. Diagnosis and clinical course of autoimmune neutropenia in infancy: analysis of 240 cases. *Blood.* 1998;91:181-186.

66. Vivancos J, Vila M, Serra A, Loscos J, Anguita A. Failure of G-CSF therapy in neutropenia associated with Sjögren's syndrome. *Rheumatology.* 2002;41:471-473.

67. Ramos-Casals M, Font J, Garcia-Carrasco M, et al. Primary Sjögren syndrome: hematologic patterns of disease expression. *Medicine.* 2002;81:281-292.

68. Kyle RA, Rajkumar SV. Monoclonal gammopathies of undetermined significance. *Rev Clin Exp Hematol.* 2002;6:225-252.

69. Zandecki M, Genevieve F, Jego P, Grosbois B. Monoclonal gammopathies of undetermined significance. *Rev Méd Interne.* 2000;21:1060-1074.

70. Sugai S, Shimizu S, Konda S. Lymphoproliferative disorders in Japanese patients with Sjögren's syndrome. *Scand J Rheumatol Suppl.* 1986;61:118-122.

71. Walters MT, Stevenson FK, Herbert A, Cawley MI, Smith JL. Lymphoma in Sjögren's syndrome: urinary monoclonal free light chains as a diagnostic aid and a means of tumour monitoring. *Scand J Rheumatol Suppl.* 1986;61:114-117.

72. Brito-Zerón P, Ramos-Casals M, Nardi N, et al. Circulating monoclonal immunoglobulins in Sjögren syndrome: prevalence and clinical significance in 237 patients. *Medicine.* 2005;84: 90-97.

73. Moutsopoulos HM, Steinberg AD, Fauci AS, Lane HC, Papadopoulos NM. High incidence of free monoclonal lambda light chains in the sera of patients with Sjögren's syndrome. *J Immunol.* 1983;130:2663-2665.

74. Sibilia J, Cohen-Solal J. Prevalence of monoclonal gammopathy and myeloma in a cohort of primary Sjögren's syndrome. *Arthritis Rheum.* 1999;42(suppl 9):S140.

75. Zintzaras E, Voulgarelis M, Moutsopoulos HM. The risk of lymphoma development in autoimmune diseases: a meta-analysis. *Arch Intern Med.* 2005;165:2337-2344.

76. García-Carrasco M, Ramos-Casals M, Cervera R, Font J. Primary Sjögren's syndrome and lymphatic proliferation. *Med Clín.* 2000;114:740-746.

77. Hansen LA, Prakash UB, Colby TV. Pulmonary lymphoma in Sjögren's syndrome. *Mayo Clin Proc.* 1989;64:920-931.

78. Gentric A, Hervé JP, Cledes J, Pennec Y, Leroy JP. Renal insufficiency as a manifestation of lymphoma with acquired hypocomplementemia and Gougerot-Sjögren syndrome. Apropos of a case. *Ann Méd Interne.* 1987;138:668-669.

79. Voulgarelis M, Dafni UG, Isenberg DA, Moutsopoulos HM. Malignant lymphoma in primary Sjögren's syndrome: a multicenter, retrospective, clinical study by the European Concerted Action on Sjögren's syndrome. *Arthritis Rheum.* 1999;42:1765-1772.

80. Ramos-Casals M, Brito-Zerón P. Emerging biological therapies in primary Sjögren's syndrome. *Rheumatology.* 2007;46:1389-1396.

81. Ioannidis JP, Vassiliou VA, Moutsopoulos HM. Long-term risk of mortality and lymphoprolif-erative disease and predictive classification of primary Sjögren's syndrome. *Arthritis Rheum.* 2002;46:741-747.
82. Theander E, Manthorpe R, Jacobsson LT. Mortality and causes of death in primary Sjögren's syndrome: a prospective cohort study. *Arthritis Rheum.* 2004;50:1262-1269.
83. Brito-Zerón P, Ramos-Casals M, Bove A, Sentis J, Font J. Predicting adverse outcomes in primary Sjögren's syndrome: identification of prognostic factors. *Rheumatology.* 2007;46: 1359-1362.
84. Ramos-Casals M, Tzioufas AG, Stone JH, Sisó A, Bosch X. Treatment of primary Sjögren syndrome: a systematic review. *JAMA.* 2010;304:452-460.

Systemic Sclerosis: Severe Involvement of Internal Organs

6

Niamh P. Quillinan and Christopher P. Denton

Abstract Systemic sclerosis (SSc) is a multisystem autoimmune rheumatic disease characterized by inflammation, fibrosis, and vasculopathy. SSc has very high morbidity and the highest case-specific mortality of any rheumatic disorder with 50% of patients dying or developing major internal organ complications within 3 years of diagnosis. The most frequent causes of death are pulmonary and cardiac diseases although severe gastrointestinal involvement and renal disease can also develop. In this chapter, we review the clinical features, outcome, and management of the major internal organ complications of systemic sclerosis.

Keywords Complications • Management • Pulmonary fibrosis • Pulmonary hypertension • Renal crisis • Screening • Systemic sclerosis

6.1
Introduction

Systemic sclerosis (SSc) is a multisystem disease that is associated with inflammation, fibrosis, and vasculopathy. It is clinically heterogeneous although certain clinical and investigational features are common to the majority of cases. Although some cases are relatively mild, there is overall a high frequency of internal organ manifestations, and these are responsible for substantial morbidity and mortality. SSc has the highest case-specific mortality of any of the autoimmune rheumatic diseases. The most frequent causes of death are pulmonary and cardiac diseases although severe gastrointestinal involvement and renal disease can also develop. The latter was previously the most common cause for SSc-associated death, but outcomes have improved over the past 30 years.[1]

N.P. Quillinan (✉)
Centre for Rheumatology, Royal Free Campus, University College
Medical School, Rowland Hill Street, Hampstead, London, NW3 2PF, UK
e-mail: n.quillinan@medsch.ucl.ac.uk

M.A. Khamashta and M. Ramos-Casals (eds.), *Autoimmune Diseases*,
DOI: 10.1007/978-0-85729-358-9_6, © Springer-Verlag London Limited 2011

Table 6.1 Key features of the two major subsets of systemic sclerosis

Disease subset	
Limited cutaneous systemic sclerosis (lcSSc)	Diffuse cutaneous systemic sclerosis (dcSSc)
Distal skin involvement ± face	Proximal skin involvement including trunk
Anti-centromere antibody most common antibody	Anti-topoisomerase or anti-RNA polymerase III most common
Long history of Raynaud's, can be severe	Short history of Raynaud's
Maximum skin score < 18	Maximum skin score > 18, plateaus/improves after 2–3 years
Pulmonary arterial hypertension and pulmonary fibrosis associated	Pulmonary fibrosis and renal crisis associated
	Other organ involvement more common

lcSSc Limited cutaneous systemic sclerosis, *dcSSc* diffuse cutaneous systemic sclerosis

Systemic sclerosis is clinically heterogeneous. All cases manifest Raynaud's phenomenon and most have features of gastroesophageal reflux. There is a variable extent of skin involvement, and this forms the basis for classification of SSc cases into one of the two major subsets, namely, limited or diffuse disease.[2] The key features of each subset are indicated in Table 6.1. Prevalence estimates vary depending on the population studied; however, it is generally accepted to be 1 per 10,000 individuals. Systemic sclerosis is more common in Afro-Caribbeans and in females.

Approximately one fifth of cases of SSc also manifest features of another autoimmune rheumatic disease. These are designated as SSc overlap syndromes. The commonest overlap feature is myositis, but other cases manifest arthritis, Sjogrens, vasculitis, or inflammatory arthritis. Clinical or serological features of SLE may also be present. These overlap features are important because they may be amenable to treatment independent of the SSc and also their management may need to be modified to take account of the coexistent SSc.

Immunosuppressive treatments for SSc have often been borrowed from treatment strategies used in other autoimmune diseases such as rheumatoid arthritis and systemic lupus erythematosus. Currently, no treatment is proven to be effective in preventing progression of disease, reversing fibrosis, or improving long-term outcome. The EULAR Scleroderma Trials and Research group (EUSTAR) recently published a set of core recommendations for treatment of SSc.[3] Cyclophosphamide is recommended for skin disease in diffuse cutaneous systemic sclerosis (dcSSc) and for lung fibrosis. Methotrexate can be used in skin disease or in patients with features of overlap inflammatory arthritis. Mycophenolate mofetil is increasingly being used in skin and lung disease with azathioprine as an alternative option.[4] Other therapies are prescribed for symptom control and will be discussed separately with each organ system below (Fig. 6.1).

The benefit of regular screening should not be underestimated. A recent report has demonstrated that regular screening has led to better ascertainment of organ-based complications, with earlier diagnosis and treatment of these complications, contributing to increased survival in these patients.[5] It is therefore recommended to perform noninvasive screening for organ-based complications on an annual basis.

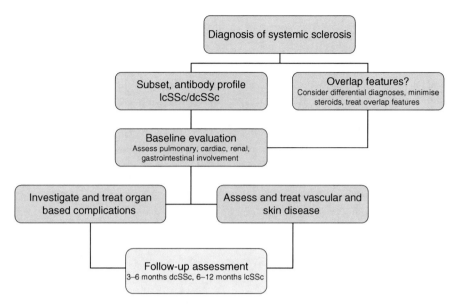

Fig. 6.1 Management of systemic sclerosis

Although the frequency of each of the major internal organ involvements in SSc may differ between subsets, any one of the major features can occur in any subset. Despite the absence of effective disease-modifying therapy, there has been an improvement in overall outcome in SSc and overall survival is now in excess of 85% at 5 years. However, the outcome is much poorer if there is severe involvement of internal organs. The purpose of this chapter is to review the clinical features, outcome, and management of the major internal organ complications of systemic sclerosis.

6.2
Renal Involvement

6.2.1
Scleroderma Renal Crisis (SRC)

6.2.1.1
Frequency

Scleroderma renal crisis affects 5–10% of all scleroderma patients, and is more common in females with dcSSc.[6] Other renal complications can occur including chronic kidney disease and overlap renal vasculitis disorders; however, SRC is the most prominent and is discussed below.

6.2.1.2
Clinical Features and Risk Factors

Typical features of SRC are new-onset accelerated phase systemic hypertension (>150/85 mmHg) and progressive renal impairment with ≥30% reduction of estimated glomerular filtration rate (eGFR). Other features are headaches, encephalopathy, seizures, visual disturbances associated with hypertensive retinopathy, pulmonary edema, pyrexia, and general malaise. SRC can occur in the setting of a normal blood pressure, but the blood pressure is usually relatively elevated from baseline for that patient. This is uncommon, however, and indicates a poorer prognosis. Other factors that indicate poor prognosis are intervening pericarditis, myocarditis, and arrhythmias. Renal failure is usual, but occurs over days to weeks. Oliguria or anuria is worrying and rare in patients diagnosed and treated appropriately.[7]

DcSSc patients especially in early disease are at greatest risk, with two-thirds of patients developing SRC within the first year of diagnosis. LcSSc patients usually develop SRC later in the disease process.[7,8] Rapidly progressive skin disease is also another risk factor. SRC has been linked to steroid therapy especially high-dose steroids, although patients are at higher risk even with low-dose steroids compared to controls in some studies.[9] Anemia, cardiac abnormalities, hormone replacement therapy, and the presence of antibodies to RNA polymerase III are also risk factors.[10]

An important differential diagnosis is renal vasculitis or glomerulonephritis as the treatment for these conditions are different than for SRC. Patients can have overlap features of vasculitis or lupus as well as established SSc. Other important differential diagnoses to consider are interstitial and tubular nephritis, thrombotic thrombocytopenia purpura, prerenal causes, and acute kidney injury secondary to drugs.

6.2.1.3
Investigation

Renal function tests show high creatinine and hyper-reninemia, and urinalysis frequently demonstrates non-nephrotic proteinuria and hematuria, with granular casts on microscopy. Microangiopathic hemolytic anemia (MAHA) and thrombocytopenia are common, but severe coagulopathy is rare. Renal biopsy can be helpful, especially if the diagnosis is unclear and other differential diagnoses are possible. Cardinal features of SRC on renal biopsy are intimal and medial proliferation with luminal narrowing especially in the arcuate arteries, fibrinoid necrosis, and thrombosis. Vascular changes are associated with a poorer outcome.[7]

6.2.1.4
Management

Early and aggressive management of hypertension is essential to prevent end-organ damage. ACE inhibitors are essential and have dramatically improved outcome in SRC.[11] The aim of treatment is to gradually reduce blood pressure to a normal level, avoiding episodes of prolonged hypotension which will reduce renal perfusion and cause further acute tubular necrosis, compounding the problem. Continuous intravenous prostacyclin may also be helpful for controlling hypertension and also increasing renal perfusion in the acute hypertensive phase. This should be discontinued when blood pressure is controlled or on initiation of dialysis.

Other antihypertensive agents may be required for adequate blood pressure control. Calcium channel blockers and alpha-blockers can be particularly useful in this setting, and angiotensin receptor blockers can be added to ACE inhibitors but are usually not sufficient when used on their own. Nitrate infusions or labetalol may be required if there is associated pulmonary edema and plasma exchange can be helpful in the setting of MAHA.

6.2.1.5
Outcome

Approximately 66% patients with SRC require renal replacement therapy, but 50% of these patients will recover sufficient renal function to discontinue dialysis, with median time to recovery ~1 year. Renal recovery can occur out to 2 years but is unlikely after 3 years. Renal transplantation may be considered if dialysis is still required after 2 years, but should not be considered before this. Transplant survival is similar in SSc patients to those undergoing renal transplant for other reasons.[12]

In patients requiring dialysis, those with higher blood pressures and serum creatinine are most likely to recover sufficient renal function to discontinue dialysis and those presenting with a normotensive SRC, or older age at presentation of SRC are at greatest risk of requiring long-term renal replacement therapy.

The routine use of ACE inhibitors has dramatically improved survival in patients with SRC. Prior to ACE inhibitors, mortality from SRC was >80% at 1 year; however, mortality is estimated in recent cohorts at 24%.[11] In spite of this, long-term survival remains poor, especially in those patients requiring ongoing renal replacement therapy.

6.2.1.6
Screening and Prevention

Newly diagnosed SSc patients, those with a history of corticosteroid therapy and those with the presence of anti-RNA polymerase III, should be carefully monitored, as these are known risk factors for SRC. In these patients, blood pressure should be monitored at monthly intervals, with daily self-monitoring introduced if the patient becomes hypertensive and measures taken to improve blood pressure control.

Urinalysis should be routinely performed at clinic visits and significant proteinuria should be investigated. Serum creatinine, protein–creatinine ratio, and calculated eGFR are helpful to identify patients with impaired renal function, who may need to be more carefully monitored.

Prophylactic use of ACE inhibitors has not been proven to prevent SRC and may potentially be associated with a worse outcome, therefore is not advised at present.

6.2.1.7
Future Developments and Challenges

Recent studies have reported an association between the endothelin receptor signaling system and pathogenesis of SRC, making this an attractive area for future research and possibility for new therapies such as endothelin receptor antagonism for SRC.[13]

6.3
Lung Involvement

Pulmonary involvement is very common in SSc, with the two major patterns of disease being pulmonary fibrosis (PF) and pulmonary vasculopathy leading to pulmonary arterial hypertension (PAH). Pulmonary arterial hypertension can also develop as a consequence of long-standing pulmonary fibrosis. Pulmonary complications are now the leading cause of mortality in systemic sclerosis. Causes of breathlessness in SSc are summarized in Table 6.2.

6.3.1
Pulmonary Fibrosis

6.3.1.1
Frequency

Pulmonary fibrosis is a major cause of death in systemic sclerosis, occurring in 19% patients with systemic sclerosis (35% of deaths attributable to systemic sclerosis).[14] Around 40% of dcSSc patients and 16% lcSSc patients develop clinically significant pulmonary fibrosis within 5 years of diagnosis.[5] However, mild pulmonary fibrosis is detectable in

Table 6.2 Causes of dyspnea in systemic sclerosis

- Pulmonary fibrosis (PF)
- Pulmonary hypertension (PAH or PH), right heart failure
- Anemia (GAVE, medications)
- Intercurrent infection
- Bronchiectasis
- Pleural/pericardial effusion
- Pulmonary embolism
- Concomitant ischemic heart disease, congestive cardiac failure
- Other (pneumothorax, neoplasm etc.)
- Deconditioning

PF pulmonary fibrosis, *PAH* pulmonary arterial hypertension, *PH* pulmonary hypertension, *GAVE* gastric antral vascular ectasia

many more SSc patients on HRCT chest. Pulmonary function test abnormalities are also extremely common in SSc, even in patients who are asymptomatic and have a normal chest radiograph.

6.3.1.2
Clinical Features and Differential Diagnosis

Early pulmonary fibrosis is often asymptomatic. Clinical features of pulmonary fibrosis include dyspnea (initially on exertion, then at rest in later stages), cough, usually non-productive, chest discomfort/tightness, and fatigue. Clinical signs include crackles on auscultation of the chest, usually at the lung bases and signs of pulmonary hypertension (if associated) as detailed below. It can often be challenging to identify the cause of breathlessness in scleroderma patients as the differential diagnosis can be wide (Table 6.2).

6.3.1.3
Investigation

Pulmonary function tests are an extremely valuable tool in the investigation of breathlessness in systemic sclerosis. Reduction in diffusion capacity for carbon monoxide (DLco) is an early marker of lung involvement, both PF and PAH. Lung fibrosis causes a restrictive pattern on lung function tests; therefore, forced vital capacity (FVC) and total lung capacity are reduced. A pattern of normal lung volumes with a reduced DLco is more suggestive of pulmonary vascular disease.

Plain chest radiographs may pick up more severe lung fibrosis but are often normal even in symptomatic patients. The introduction of high-resolution CT (HRCT) scanning of the chest has improved identification of early lung fibrosis and is very useful for following progression of disease. Features of pulmonary fibrosis on HRCT include ill-defined sub-pleural increased opacification in the posterior lower lobes, more defined ground glass shadowing, reticular patterns, traction bronchiectasis, and, occasionally, evidence of honeycombing. HRCT should be performed in both prone and supine positions to exclude congestion of fluid in the dependant areas, which can have the same appearance as early fibrosis (Fig. 6.2).

Bronchoscopy with bronchoalveolar lavage is not generally useful for diagnosis or prognosis unless it is being performed to rule out other causes of dyspnea, such as active tuberculosis or neoplastic disease. Histologically, SSc-related lung fibrosis is classified as nonspecific interstitial pneumonia or occasionally usual interstitial pneumonia. However, lung biopsy is an invasive procedure and not generally helpful for diagnosis and management of SSc-related lung fibrosis. Goh et al. have developed a simple staging system using a combination of lung function tests and HRCT to separate cases into prognostic groups.[15] This has been very helpful to identify patients at risk of deterioration, who would benefit from immunosuppression.

Fig. 6.2 HRCT showing basolateral parenchymal fibrosis including areas of amorphous shadowing likely to represent fine fibrosis as well as more established reticular change. CT pattern cannot be used to reliably define inflammation and extent of disease is emerging as the most robust predictor of future progression

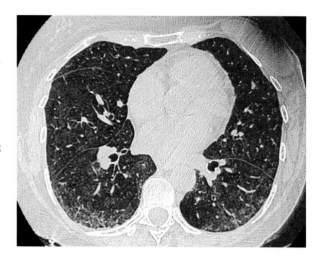

6.3.1.4
Management

Early detection of pulmonary fibrosis is paramount as the goal of treatment is to treat reversible interstitial lung disease as well as prevent progression of disease. Patients with newly diagnosed disease, more severe or progressive disease, tend to respond better to treatment.

Mild cases of pulmonary fibrosis, that is, those with <20% lung involvement on HRCT and normal pulmonary function tests can be monitored routinely with annual review and lung function tests. If there is deterioration in symptoms and/or lung function, a repeat HRCT should be performed and treatment initiated if there is worsening of fibrosis.

For moderate or severe lung fibrosis, extent is determined by: >20% involvement on HRCT and/or FVC <70% if extent on HRCT cannot be determined.[15] There is now evidence from a number of trials that cyclophosphamide has limited benefit in the treatment of lung fibrosis. However, the efficacy of treatment should be carefully balanced with known side effects and toxicities. Cyclophosphamide is usually given in pulses monthly in a dose of 0.6 mg/m² intravenously for 6 months as induction treatment and then followed by an oral immunosuppressive agent such as mycophenolate mofetil or azathioprine for maintenance. Cyclophosphamide can also be given orally, but the toxicity profile is a concern. Other options for moderate lung fibrosis are mycophenolate mofetil and azathioprine alone, which have better toxicity profiles and moderate efficacy in small case series; however, there are little published data on these treatments, but further studies are in the pipeline.[4,16,17]

Low-dose oral steroids are often used in combination with immunosuppressive regimes. However, high-dose steroids are not recommended especially in patients carrying the RNA polymerase III antibody in view of the potential to trigger a renal crisis.

Lung transplantation may be an option in selected patients with end-stage lung fibrosis as the posttransplant outcome in patients with systemic sclerosis is similar to other patients undergoing lung transplantation.[18]

6.3.1.5
Screening and Prevention

The benefits of immunosuppressive treatment are greatest in those with early or less severe pulmonary fibrosis, underlining the importance of early diagnosis and treatment. Screening with annual review and pulmonary function testing is therefore highly recommended in all patients with systemic sclerosis.

6.3.1.6
Future Developments and Challenges

Other pathways are now being investigated in pulmonary fibrosis associated with SSc with a view to identifying new therapeutic targets. Imatinib mesylate, other tyrosine kinase inhibitors, and pirfenidone have potent anti-fibrotic effects in vitro; they are also currently under investigation.

Lessons learned in idiopathic pulmonary fibrosis (IPF) may also be translatable to SSc-related pulmonary fibrosis. N-acetylcysteine has been found to be beneficial in patients with IPF, but there is no published evidence at present in systemic sclerosis–related pulmonary fibrosis.[19] A clinical trial involving bosentan, an endothelin receptor antagonist, showed a trend to efficacy of this medication in IPF,[20] but did not show significant efficacy in patients with SSc-related PF.[21] Bosentan may still be helpful in patients with progressive disease and requires further investigation.

6.3.2
Pulmonary Hypertension

6.3.2.1
Types of PH in SSc

Pulmonary hypertension (PH) is defined as mean pulmonary arterial pressure (mPAP) ≥ 25 mmHg at rest assessed by right heart catheterization (RHC). Pulmonary arterial hypertension (PAH) is the presence of precapillary PH not due to other causes of precapillary PH (lung diseases etc.) and is defined as mPAP ≥ 25 mmHg at rest with pulmonary capillary wedge pressure ≤ 15 mmHg.

Although PAH is the most common type of PH in SSc, PH due to lung fibrosis and also due to systolic or diastolic dysfunction or valve disease is not uncommon. Chronic thromboembolic PH can also occur, especially in patients with overlap features such as SLE.

6.3.2.2
Brief Review of Classification and Diagnosis

Initial classification criteria for PH provided only two categories: primary or secondary PH. However, due to further understanding of the pathophysiology of PH, the most recent classification groups together diseases that share similarities in pathophysiological mechanisms and clinical presentations (Table 6.3).[22,23]

Table 6.3 Clinical classification of pulmonary hypertension

Class		
1	Pulmonary arterial hypertension (PAH)	Idiopathic PAH
		Heritable
		BMPR2, ALK1, endoglin, unknown
		Drug and Toxin induced PAH
		Associated PAH
		Connective tissue diseases
		HIV infection
		Portal hypertension
		Congenital heart diseases
		Schistosomiasis
		Chronic hemolytic anemia
		Persistent pulmonary hypertension of the newborn
1'	Pulmonary veno-occlusive disease (PVOD) and/or pulmonary capillary hemangiomatosis (PCH)	
2	Pulmonary hypertension due to left heart disease	Systolic dysfunction
		Diastolic dysfunction
		Valvular disease
3	Pulmonary hypertension due to lung disease and/or hypoxia	Chronic obstructive pulmonary disease
		Interstitial lung disease
		Other lung diseases with mixed restrictive/obstructive pattern
		Sleep disorders
		Alveolar hypoventilation disorders
		Chronic exposure to high altitude
		Developmental abnormalities
4	Chronic thromboembolic pulmonary hypertension (CTEPH)	
5	Pulmonary hypertension with unclear multifactorial mechanisms	Hematological disorders
		Myeloproliferative disorders
		Systemic disorders
		Sarcoidosis, vasculitis, etc.
		Metabolic disorders
		Thyroid disease, Gaucher's, etc.
		Others
		Renal failure on dialysis, etc.

PAH Pulmonary arterial hypertension, *PVOD* Pulmonary veno-occlusive disease, *PCH* pulmonary capillary hemangiomatosis, *CTEPH* Chronic thromboembolic pulmonary hypertension

6.3.2.3
Frequency

The prevalence of PAH in SSc is estimated to be 10–15%, more common in the lcSSc subtype. PAH is a leading cause of mortality and is responsible for 14% of deaths overall (26% deaths attributable to SSc).[14]

6.3.2.4
Clinical Features and Differential Diagnosis

Many patients are asymptomatic until late into the course. The commonest symptom is dyspnea on exertion and fatigue, with chest pain and syncope occurring less often. Cough, if present, is suggestive of associated pulmonary fibrosis. Clinical signs include right ventricular heave, loud second heart sound, and raised jugular venous pressure. Bibasilar crackles, hepatomegaly, or peripheral edema may be present if there is associated pulmonary fibrosis or congestive heart failure. The differential diagnosis is similar to that mentioned for pulmonary fibrosis above (Table 6.2).

6.3.2.5
Investigation

The 6-minute walking distance (6MWD) is a useful noninvasive test that gives an idea of exercise tolerance and can be measured serially to monitor progression of disease. The World Health Organisation/ New York Heart Association Functional Class (WHO/NYHA FC) is a grading system from I to IV indicating worsening grades of exercise tolerance which is also helpful for evaluating disease progression and prognosis. Advanced PAH is correlated to NYHA FC III and IV.

Electrocardiography (ECG) may show right ventricular hypertrophy and strain, right axis deviation, and right atrial enlargement. Some patients may have arrhythmias, such as atrial flutter or fibrillation. Chest radiograph may demonstrate right atrial or ventricular enlargement, signs of associated lung fibrosis or pulmonary edema but in early stages, is often normal. NT-pro-BNP is a blood test available in many centers and is a measure of right atrial strain. In studies, elevated levels correlate with hemodynamic measures of PAH on RHC and higher levels are associated with a poorer prognosis.[24] NT-pro-BNP can also be used to follow response to treatment.

Patients with PAH typically have reduced DLco with preserved lung volumes on lung function testing. This can be the earliest indicator that the patient may be developing PAH. Arterial blood gases may show reduced carbon dioxide due to hyperventilation. If there is hypoxia, there may be associated Chronic obstructive pulmonary disease (COPD) or asthma. Hypoxia can also occur in late stages of disease. If pulmonary fibrosis is suspected, a HRCT should be performed. A ventilation/ perfusion scan (V/Q) or CT pulmonary angiogram (CTPA) may also be required to exclude pulmonary emboli, which is also associated with PAH and amenable to treatment. The V/Q has higher sensitivity and specificity than CTPA.

Doppler echocardiography is helpful in identifying patients who may be developing PAH. The systolic PAP is estimated using the peak velocity jet of tricuspid regurgitation. If there is little/no tricuspid regurgitation, it is not possible to measure systolic PAP; however, contrast echocardiography with agitated saline (if available) may be used in this instance. Echocardiography is operator and patient dependant and unfortunately overestimation or underestimation of PAP is common. Other echocardiographic findings may also aid in diagnosis, such as increased right atrial or right ventricular dimensions, increased right ventricular wall thickness, and dilated main pulmonary artery.

Cardiac magnetic resonance imaging (MRI) is helpful for providing further structural and functional information about the right ventricle, in addition to identifying myocardial fibrosis. It can also be used for hemodynamics especially in follow-up.

Right heart catheterization (RHC) is essential for diagnosis and invaluable for follow-up of patients with PAH. Although an invasive test, it has low morbidity and mortality when performed in specialist centers. Hemodynamic variables that must be measured include PAP (systolic, diastolic, and mean), pulmonary capillary wedge pressure, right atrial and right ventricular pressures, cardiac output and oxygen saturations (to calculate peripheral vascular resistance). Left heart catheterization and coronary angiography may also be required if there is a suspicion of left heart disease. The vasoreactivity test is not recommended for SSc patients.

6.3.2.6
Management

With major advances in the understanding of pathophysiological mechanisms behind PAH in the past 10 years, there are now a number of therapeutic approaches based on these mechanisms (Table 6.4). However, despite advances in treatment, PAH associated with SSc has a worse prognosis compared to idiopathic PAH. For this reason, the treatment of SSc-associated PAH remains a major unmet medical need.

Treatment options for PAH include phosphodiesterase type 5(PDE-5) inhibitors, endothelin receptor antagonists (ERA), and prostacyclin derivatives. PDE-5 inhibitor or ERA monotherapy is the treatment of choice initially, followed by switching treatments or combination therapy. Other options include the prostacyclin analogues, either inhaled, subcutaneous, or by continuous intravenous infusion if there is further progression. Combination therapy is an attractive option considering that the available medications target different pathways. However, supportive evidence for the use of combination therapy is, as yet, lacking. All of the available medications are best prescribed and monitored in specialist centers. Recently, Barst et al. have published evidence-based guidelines for treatment of PAH.[25]

Oxygen therapy may be helpful in patients with hypoxia. Other supportive therapies are often used if there are no contraindications, such as diuretics, oral anticoagulation, and digoxin. Treatment of concurrent lung fibrosis with immunosuppression may be very helpful especially in the setting of overlap connective tissue diseases.

Table 6.4 Therapeutic options for PAH (current licensed treatments)

Class of drug	Drug	Dose and route of administration	Main side effects	Comments
Prostacyclin analogues	Epoprostenol	Continuous intravenous infusion. Starting dose 2 ng/kg/min then uptitrated	Headaches, muscle cramps, diarrhea. Severe worsening if infusion interrupted. Sepsis and other risks form intravenous administration	Only drug specifically tested in SSc-PAH in placebo-controlled trial. Reserved for advanced disease
	Treprostinil	Subcutaneous or Intravenous infusion starting at 1.25 ng/kg/min then uptitrated. Nebulized inhaled dose 18–54 mcg 4 times daily	Headaches, muscle cramps, diarrhea. Worsening if infusion interrupted (less immediate than epoprostenol). Sepsis and other risks form intravenous administration. Severe local site pain from subcutaneous infusion	Available for intravenous use and being evaluated by inhaled and oral routes in PAH in clinical trials
	Iloprost	Nebulized inhaled dose 2.5–5.0 mcg given 6–9 times daily	Headaches, muscle cramps, diarrhea	Intravenous formulation not licensed for PAH
	Beraprost	Oral dose 60 mcg daily	Headaches, muscle cramps, diarrhea	Licensed in Japan
PDE-5 inhibitors	Sildenafil	Oral dose 20 mg tds licensed	Headache, visual disturbance, epistaxis. Generally well tolerated	Different formulation licensed for erectile dysfunction
	Tadalfil	Oral dose 40 mg once daily	Headache, visual disturbance, epistaxis. Generally well tolerated	Longer duration of action than sildenafil
Endothelin receptor antagonists	Bosentan	Oral dose 62.5 mg bd for 1 month then 125 mg bd	Liver function test abnormalities up to 10% and so needs monthly monitoring. Potentially teratogenic. Fluid retention and anemia. Reduces oral anticoagulant efficacy	Nonselective ETA and ETB receptor blockade
	Sitaxentan	Oral dose 100 mg once daily	Liver function test abnormalities up to 10%. Needs monthly monitoring. Potentially teratogenic. Fluid retention and anemia. Increases oral anticoagulant efficacy – needs dose reduction of warfarin	Highly selective for ETA receptor. In use in EU but not licensed in USA. Recently taken off the market due to concern about fulminant hepatic failure
	Ambrisentan	Oral dose 5 or 10 mg daily	Low risk of liver function test abnormalities. Fluid retention common. Anemia occurs. No interaction with oral anticoagulants	Partially selective ERA with specificity for ETA

SSc Systemic sclerosis, *PAH* Pulmonary arterial hypertension, *PDE 5* Phosphodiesterase type 5, *ETA* Endothelin receptor A, *ETB* Endothelin receptor B, *EU* European Union, *USA* United States of America

6.3.2.7
Screening and Prevention

As PAH is usually asymptomatic until late into the course of disease, the aim of screening is to identify and treat patients as early as possible, to improve quality of life and prognosis. Annual review with electrocardiogram, echocardiogram, and pulmonary function testing is therefore recommended, with early referral to a specialist center for RHC in those patients suspected to have PAH. Additionally, 6-min walking distance and NT-pro-BNP can be helpful in monitoring patients with established PAH.

6.3.2.8
Future Developments and Challenges

Clinical trials on combination therapy and long-term follow-up of early PAH patients are currently underway. These will provide further information on the impact of combination treatment and early monotherapy on morbidity and mortality. As with pulmonary fibrosis, imatinib mesylate is also currently in trials for PAH. Standardization of screening programs is also paramount to identify PAH as early as possible.

6.4
Gastrointestinal Involvement

The gastrointestinal (GI) tract is the organ system most commonly involved and often the first system to be involved in SSc. The same pathophysiology of inflammation, fibrosis, and vascular dysfunction typical of SSc can occur in any part of the GI tract.[26,27]

6.4.1
Clinical Features and Differential Diagnosis

Symptoms of GI involvement are nonspecific, and other causes should be considered and excluded. Malignancy should be excluded in patients with unexplained anemia or weight loss, and abdominal pain should be thoroughly investigated in the absence of an obvious cause. In a recent study, 97% patients reported symptoms at least once a week, while 15% patients reported daily symptoms and only 3% patients had no symptoms at all. Distension and reflux were the most common symptoms.[28]

6.4.1.1
Gastroesophageal Reflux and Stricture

Gastroesophageal reflux disease is extremely common, with up to 90% SSc patients reporting some degree of reflux. Some patients may have asymptomatic reflux. In extreme cases, there may be associated esophageal erosion, esophagitis, Barrett's esophagus, bleeding, or stricture. Associated symptoms include heartburn especially in supine position, dysphagia, anorexia, nausea, regurgitation, vomiting, and weight loss. Significant reflux can also cause chemical pneumonitis, worsening pulmonary fibrosis, and is a relative contraindication to lung transplantation.

6.4.1.2
GAVE, GI Bleeding and Other Gastric Problems

Gastric antral vascular ectasia (GAVE) or watermelon stomach (named for the endoscopic appearance) is an important cause of chronic iron deficiency anemia and sometimes frank hemorrhage. Telangiectasia in other parts of the bowel is common and may bleed leading to anemia. SSc patients may also have comorbid peptic ulcer disease or hiatus hernia. Delayed gastric emptying can cause early satiety, food intolerance, bloating, severe nausea, vomiting, and may worsen reflux (Fig. 6.3).

6.4.1.3
Pseudo-Obstruction

Hypomotility of the small intestine may cause intestinal dilatation, ileus, and pseudo-obstruction. Clinical features include abdominal discomfort or pain, distension, food intolerance, nausea, and vomiting. These episodes can be recurrent and difficult to treat. Complete bowel obstruction is rare. Electrolyte disturbances such as low magnesium,

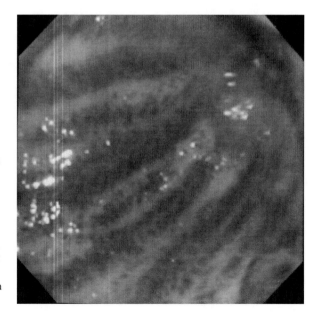

Fig. 6.3 Gastric antral vascular ectasia (GAVE) is a common finding in systemic sclerosis and most often associates with the active stage of the diffuse cutaneous subset. Recurrent anemia is the typical clinical manifestation, and treatment using YAG laser or Argon plasma photocoagulation can be effective

potassium, or calcium can contribute to episodes of pseudo-obstruction. Ileus is also often prolonged after laparotomy, and intestinal stasis may be a problem after contrast studies of the bowel using barium contrast agents.

6.4.1.4
Diarrhea/Malabsorption/Pancreatic Insufficiency

Diarrhea is seen in about 50% of patients and is usually a consequence of bowel hypomotility causing stagnation of intestinal contents and small bowel bacterial overgrowth. It can also be associated with bloating, flatulence, vomiting, and abdominal discomfort and distension. Bacterial overgrowth can lead to malabsorption and weight loss. Malabsorption can be compounded by relative pancreatic insufficiency. Other important differential diagnoses or comorbidities, such as celiac disease and primary biliary cirrhosis, should be excluded. Both of these diseases are autoimmune and more common in patients with SSc.

6.4.1.5
Constipation/Volvulus

Colonic hypomotility can lead to constipation, seen in up to 50% of patients. Many patients have alternating bowel habit, which can be extremely difficult to treat or find a balance between diarrhea and constipation. Chronic constipation may lead to sigmoid volvulus and acute bowel obstruction.

6.4.1.6
Anorectal Disease

Anorectal disease is common and very distressing for the patient. Symptoms include loss of anal sensation, rectal prolapse, and fecal incontinence. Incontinence has a huge impact on the social and emotional well-being of the patient. These symptoms can also be compounded with diarrhea from bacterial overgrowth causing stress or urge incontinence.

6.4.2
Investigation

Routine blood tests should be performed especially in patients with profuse diarrhea or vomiting, to ensure electrolytes are within normal limits and to rule out severe anemia in GAVE. Celiac screen and autoantibody profile including anti-mitochondrial and anti-smooth muscle antibody should be performed to exclude celiac disease and primary biliary cirrhosis.

Upper GI symptoms should be investigated with upper GI endoscopy and barium swallow. Esophageal manometry and pH monitoring may also be helpful if available. Barium follow-through may show characteristic changes such as "stack of coins" sign. Hydrogen breath testing can be helpful to identify patients who have bacterial overgrowth.

Colonoscopy/sigmoidoscopy or CT colonoscopy can be helpful to identify colonic or anorectal disease and to exclude other causes of symptoms such as malignancy and diverticulosis. Anorectal disease can be investigated using anorectal manometry and ultrasound to document sphincter pressure and identify anatomical tears that may be amenable to surgical repair.

6.4.3
Management

Proton pump inhibitors are the mainstay of treatment for reflux symptoms. Increased doses may be required for symptomatic relief. In severe cases, the addition of a H2 blocker at night such as ranitidine may be helpful. Dietary modification is also important with avoidance of spicy foods and late eating patterns. Prokinetic agents such as domperidone, erythromycin, and metoclopramide are the treatment of choice for dysphagia, and esophageal candidiasis should be identified and treated with antifungal agents. Endoscopic balloon dilatation is useful for esophageal strictures.

Bleeding from GAVE is often amenable to laser photocoagulation therapy, but may need to be performed at regular intervals with screening endoscopies to monitor progress. Blood transfusions and oral iron supplementation may be needed. Prokinetic agents may be helpful for delayed gastric emptying to increase transit time.

Pseudo-obstruction should be managed conservatively by avoiding oral feeding and letting the bowel rest, nasogastric tube suction, and intravenous fluids. Surgery should be avoided as outcome is usually very poor.

Cyclical antibiotics are helpful for bacterial overgrowth; however, resistance to the antibiotics can occur. Pancreatic enzyme supplementation is used if pancreatic insufficiency is suspected. Dietary modification to include a low residue diet and exclude complex carbohydrates is recommended in some patients. In severe malabsorption, it may be necessary to consider nasogastric or percutaneous endoscopic gastrostomy/jejunostomy feeding or even in extreme cases, total parenteral nutrition. Some patients may require percutaneous gastrostomy for bowel decompression if there is recurrent pseudo-obstruction.

Constipation is treated primarily with stool bulking agents and stool softeners although prolonged use of laxatives should be avoided. Loperamide can be used in patients with diarrhea in combination with antibiotics if bacterial overgrowth is suspected. Probiotics can also be helpful in some cases. Pelvic floor exercises and biofeedback are used for anorectal disease. In severe cases, sacral nerve stimulation may be beneficial. Defunctioning colostomy is a last resort.

6.4.4
Outcome

GI disease is a leading cause of morbidity and mortality in SSc patients. Several case series have linked severe GI disease to cardiac disease in SSc, possibly from electrolyte abnormalities. Severe GI disease with malnutrition can be very difficult to treat and is often progressive.

6.4.5
Screening and Prevention

New SSc patients should be screened for the presence of GI symptoms, with barium swallow and/or endoscopy for further evaluation if needed. The management of patients with established SSc should include regular monitoring for development and progression of GI symptoms with early referral for specialist treatment.

6.4.6
Future Developments and Challenges

Patients with recurrent intestinal pseudo-obstruction may benefit from octreotide therapy; however, studies are presently lacking.[29] Octreotide is expensive and can be associated with major adverse effects such as bowel perforation; therefore, cautious use is advised.

6.5
Cardiac Involvement

SSc can affect all structures of the heart causing pericardial effusion, valve abnormalities, arrhythmias, conduction defects, myocardial fibrosis, myocarditis, hypertrophy or ischemia and heart failure.[30]

6.5.1
Frequency

Cardiac abnormalities are very common (up to 75% patients with SSc) and often asymptomatic. Hemodynamically insignificant pericardial effusion is found in up to 35% of patients. Fourteen percent of all deaths in a recent study were attributable to myocardial causes with almost half of these due to arrhythmia.[14]

6.5.2
Clinical Features and Differential Diagnosis

Symptoms include dyspnea on exertion, paroxysmal nocturnal dyspnea, orthopnea, pedal edema, ascites, chest pain, and palpitation. One symptom or a combination of symptoms may be present, depending on the underlying cause. Syncope and sudden cardiac death can occur in patients with pulmonary arterial hypertension or left heart disease. Myocardial fibrosis is a hallmark feature of systemic sclerosis. It tends to occur later in the course of disease and can lead to systolic or diastolic dysfunction. It can remain subclinical for a long time before presenting with some of the symptoms mentioned above.

6.5.3
Investigation

Acute phase proteins, creatinine kinase, and troponin levels are often elevated in inflammatory cardiac disease but may be normal. N terminal pro-BNP can be elevated in cardiac congestion. Electrolyte abnormalities need to be identified and corrected. Electrocardiography identifies patients with conduction abnormalities or arrhythmia while a 24-hour electrocardiographic monitor may be required to pick up paroxysmal arrhythmias.

Chest radiographs may demonstrate cardiomegaly, right or left ventricular enlargement, signs of pulmonary edema (upper lobe diversion, basal shadowing), pulmonary hypertension (vascular pruning), or globular heart indicating a pericardial effusion. Echocardiography is useful for identifying valvular heart disease and ventricular wall hypokinesis, estimating systolic function and pulmonary arterial pressure and demonstrating pericardial effusion with or without tamponade.

Cardiac MRI and myocardial perfusion scans are helpful imaging modalities to identify myocardial fibrosis and hypoperfusion. Right and left heart catheterization is the gold standard test to identify pulmonary hypertension and ischemic heart disease, respectively.[31]

6.5.4
Management

There are no studies on specific treatments for systemic sclerosis–related cardiac disease. Early identification and management of pulmonary hypertension has already been discussed above. Tight control of blood pressure to prevent further damage is important. Current standard management of left heart disease is advised with ACE inhibition and beta-blockade if tolerated and diuretics for diastolic dysfunction as appropriate. Acute cardiac myositis is treated with immunosuppression such as cyclophosphamide or if less severe, MMF or azathioprine may be appropriate alternatives.[4] Implantable defibrillators may be necessary especially in ventricular arrhythmias or in patients with poor systolic function.

6.5.5
Screening and Prevention

Full history, examination, and ECG should be performed at baseline and at annual review. New symptoms should be investigated and referral to a cardiologist if cardiac involvement is suspected.

6.6
Severe Skin Disease

Skin disease is a hallmark feature of SSc. Although major internal organ involvement in SSc is a major cause of morbidity and mortality, skin involvement can also be associated with severe disability. The severity and extent of skin involvement correlates to internal

Fig. 6.4 Ischemic digital vasculopathy is common in both subsets of SSc and underlies important complications including fingertip digital ulceration (**a**), critical ischemia and gangrene (**b**). Auto-amputation of nonviable tissue often leads to a better cosmetic and functional outcome than surgical intervention

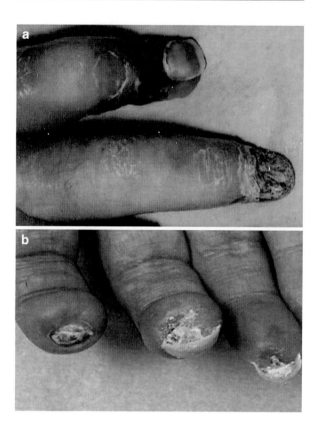

organ involvement.[32] Skin inflammation causes edema, pruritis, hypo-/hyper-pigmentation, and shiny inflamed skin resulting in skin thickening and fibrosis. Skin sclerosis can lead to joint contractures and loss of function. Localized ischemia of finger tips and across joint contractures results in ulcers. These ulcers are slowly healing and may be complicated by bacterial infection. Severe vasculopathy can lead to digital gangrene with sepsis and auto-amputation (Fig. 6.4).

Calcinosis can occur on weight-bearing areas or on the hands or other essential areas which interfere with function and activities of daily living. Calcinotic deposits can also be complicated by bacterial infection necessitating recurrent courses of antibiotics. Debridement can be difficult, and deposits tend to recur.

6.7
Conclusions

Although the major internal organ complications of SSc have been discussed separately, it is important to remember that they most often occur in combination and that the treatment of one manifestation may have to take account of other complications. Some general problems such as medication absorption or tolerability are important. In addition, some discrete complications may impact the outcome of each other (PH and PF). There are clinical and functional links – gut and heart, electrolyte disturbances. Steroids may precipitate renal crisis. Some therapeutic approaches may benefit multiple systems. Finally, there is often interplay and undercurrent illness may be poorly tolerated – infection, fluid shifts, and acidosis with cardiac and other disease.

Some therapies, such as stem cell transplantation, are not feasible if there is major internal organ disease and this is a challenge despite emerging evidence of benefit for skin, function and possible other manifestations of SSc.

References

1. Denton CP, Black CM. Targeted therapy comes of age in scleroderma. *Trends Immunol.* 2005;26:596-602.
2. LeRoy EC, Black C, Fleischmajer R, et al. Scleroderma (systemic sclerosis): classification, subsets and pathogenesis. *J Rheumatol.* 1988;15:202-205.
3. Kowal-Bielecka O, Landewe R, Avouac J, et al. EULAR recommendations for the treatment of systemic sclerosis: a report from the EULAR Scleroderma Trials and Research group (EUSTAR). *Ann Rheum Dis.* 2009;68(5):620-628.
4. Quillinan NP, Denton CP. Disease modifying treatment in systemic sclerosis: current status. *Curr Opin Rheumatol.* 2009;21(6):636-641.
5. Nihtyanova SI, Tang EC, Coghlan JG, Wells AU, Black CM, Denton CP. Improved survival in systemic sclerosis is associated with better ascertainment of internal organ disease: a retrospective cohort study. *QJM.* 2010;103(2):109-115.
6. Denton CP, Black CM. Scleroderma – clinical and pathological advances. *Best Pract Res Clin Rheumatol.* 2004;18:271-290.
7. Penn H, Howie AJ, Kingdon EJ, et al. Scleroderma renal crisis: patient characteristics and long-term outcomes. *QJM.* 2007;100(8):485-494.
8. Teixeira L, Mouthon L, Mahr A, et al. Mortality and risk factors of scleroderma renal crisis: a French retrospective study of 50 patients. *Ann Rheum Dis.* 2008;67:110-116.
9. Steen VD, Medsger TA Jr. Case-control study of corticosteroids and other drugs that either precipitate or protect from the development of scleroderma renal crisis. *Arthritis Rheum.* 1998;41(9):1613-1619.
10. Tormey VJ, Bunn CC, Denton CP, Black CM. Antifibrillarin antibodies in systemic sclerosis. *Rheumatology (Oxford).* 2001;40:1157-1162.
11. Steen VD, Costantino JP, Shapiro AP, Medsger TA Jr. Outcome of renal crisis in systemic sclerosis: relation to availability of angiotensin converting enzyme (ACE) inhibitors. *Ann Intern Med.* 1990;113:352-357.
12. Gibney EM, Pairkh CR, Jani A, et al. Kidney transplantation for systemic sclerosis improves survival and may modulate disease activity. *Am J Transplant.* 2004;4:2027-2031.
13. Müller-Ladner U, Distler O, Ibba-Manneschi L, Neumann E, Gay S. Mechanisms of vascular damage in systemic sclerosis. *Autoimmunity.* 2009;42(7):587-595.
14. Tyndall AJ, Bannert B, Vonk M, et al. Causes and risk factors for death in systemic sclerosis: a study from the EULAR Scleroderma Trials and Research (EUSTAR) database. *Ann Rheum Dis.* 2010;69(10):1809-1815. Epub 2010 Jun 15.
15. Goh NS, Desai SR, Veeraraghavan S, et al. Interstitial lung disease in systemic sclerosis: a simple staging system. *Am J Respir Crit Care Med.* 2008;177(11):1248-1254.

16. Tashkin DP, Elashoff R, Clements PJ, et al. Scleroderma Lung Study Research Group. Effects of 1-year treatment with cyclophosphamide on outcomes at 2 years in scleroderma lung disease. *Am J Respir Crit Care Med.* 2007;176(10):1026-1034.

17. Hoyles RK, Ellis RW, Wellsbury J, et al. A multicenter, prospective, randomized, double-blind, placebo-controlled trial of corticosteroids and intravenous cyclophosphamide followed by oral azathioprine for the treatment of pulmonary fibrosis in scleroderma. *Arthritis Rheum.* 2006;54(12):3962-3970.

18. Schachna L, Medsger TA, Dauber JH, et al. Lung transplantation in scleroderma compared with idiopathic pulmonary fibrosis and idiopathic pulmonary arterial hypertension. *Arthritis Rheum.* 2006;54:3954-3961.

19. Demedts M, Behr J, Buhl R, et al. High-dose acetylcysteine in idiopathic pulmonary fibrosis. *N Engl J Med.* 2005;353(21):2229-2242.

20. King TE Jr, Behr J, Brown KK, et al. BUILD-1: a randomized placebo-controlled trial of bosentan in idiopathic pulmonary fibrosis. *Am J Respir Crit Care Med.* 2008;177(1):75-81.

21. Seibold JR, Black CM, Denton CP, et al. *Bosentan Versus Placebo in Interstitial Lung Disease Secondary to Systemic Sclerosis: The BUILD-2 Trial.* San Diego: American Thoracic Society Poster; 2006.

22. Simonneau G, Robbins IM, Beghetti M, et al. Updated clinical classification of pulmonary hypertension. *J Am Coll Cardiol.* 2009;54(1 suppl):S43-S54.

23. Galiè N, Hoeper MM, Humbert M, et al. Task force for diagnosis and treatment of pulmonary hypertension of European Society of Cardiology (ESC); European Respiratory Society (ERS); International Society of Heart and Lung Transplantation (ISHLT). Guidelines for the diagnosis and treatment of pulmonary hypertension. *Eur Respir J.* 2009;34(6):1219-1263.

24. Mukerjee D, Yap LB, Holmes AM, et al. Significance of plasma N-terminal pro-brain naturetic peptide in patients with systemic sclerosis-related pulmonary arterial hypertension. *Respir Med.* 2003;97:1230-1236.

25. Barst RJ, Gibbs JS, Ghofrani HA, et al. Updated evidence-based treatment algorithm in pulmonary arterial hypertension. *J Am Coll Cardiol.* 2009;54(1 suppl):S78-S84.

26. ClementsPJ B, Becvar R, Drosos AA, et al. Assessment of gastrointestinal involvement. *Clin Exp Rheumatol.* 2003;21(3 suppl 29):S15-S18.

27. Denton CP, Black CM, Abraham DJ. Mechanisms and consequences of fibrosis in systemic sclerosis. *Nat Clin Pract Rheumatol.* 2006;2:134-144.

28. Thoua NM, Bunce C, Brough G, et al. Assessment of gastrointestinal symptoms in patients with systemic sclerosis in a UK tertiary referral centre. *Rheumatology (Oxford).* 2010;49(9):1770-1775.

29. Nikou GC, Toumpanakis C, Katsiari C, et al. Treatment of small intestinal disease in systemic sclerosis with octreotide: a prospective study in seven patients. *J Clin Rheumatol.* 2007;13(3):119-123.

30. Champion HC. The heart in scleroderma. *Rheum Dis Clin North Am.* 2008;34(1):181-190, viii.

31. Boueiz A, Mathai SC, Hummers LK, et al. Cardiac complications of systemic sclerosis: recent progress in diagnosis. *Curr Opin Rheumatol.* 2010;22(6):696-703.

32. Shand L, Lunt M, Nihtyanova S, et al. Relationship between change in skin score and disease outcome in diffuse cutaneous systemic sclerosis: application of a latent linear trajectory model. *Arthritis Rheum.* 2007;56(7):2422-2431.

Vasculitic Emergencies in Patients with Large-Vessel Vasculitis

7

Kathleen Maksimowicz-McKinnon and Gary S. Hoffman

Abstract Takayasu arteritis (TAK) and giant cell arteritis (GCA) are chronic, idiopathic inflammatory diseases preferentially affecting the large arteries. Both TAK and GCA can lead to organ- or life-threatening manifestations at any point during the disease course. Awareness of the potentially serious complications of these disorders is the first step toward prevention, early detection, and successful treatment of these conditions.

Keywords Giant cell arteritis • Large-vessel vasculitis • Takayasu arteritis • Temporal arteritis

7.1
Introduction

The primary large-vessel vasculitides, Takayasu arteritis (TAK) and giant cell arteritis (GCA), are chronic, idiopathic inflammatory diseases preferentially affecting the large arteries. Although there is significant overlap in the signs, symptoms, and vascular manifestations of these disorders, they have traditionally been distinguished by age and the presence or absence of cranial symptoms. Both TAK and GCA can lead to organ- or life-threatening manifestations at any point during the disease course. Awareness of the potentially serious complications of these disorders is the first step toward prevention, early detection, and successful treatment of these conditions.

K. Maksimowicz-McKinnon (✉)
Division of Rheumatology and Clinical Immunology, University of Pittsburgh,
3500 Terrace Street, BST S718, Pittsburgh, PA 15213, USA
e-mail: mckinnonk@dom.pitt.edu

M.A. Khamashta and M. Ramos-Casals (eds.), *Autoimmune Diseases*,
DOI: 10.1007/978-0-85729-358-9_7, © Springer-Verlag London Limited 2011

7.2
Takayasu Arteritis

Takayasu arteritis (TAK) is a rare form of vasculitis, with a reported incidence in the United States (Olmsted County, Minnesota) of 2.6 cases/million/year.[1] Although initially thought to be a disease primarily of young women from the Far East, TAK has been identified in both men (10–20%) and women worldwide. The mean age of affected persons in most reports is approximately 25 years. Over 85% of large-vessel lesions in TAK are stenotic, resulting in organ and tissue ischemia, which leads to the majority of disease-associated morbidity.[2-4] About 15–27% of lesions are aneurysms. The diagnosis of TAK is frequently delayed. This is most striking in children compared to adults, given the rarity of serious vascular diseases in youth.[3,4] Patients may not be symptomatic at disease onset, or only have nonspecific constitutional symptoms (<50%). Because the majority of patients lack systemic inflammatory symptoms at initial presentation, TAK should be included in the differential diagnosis of any young individual with vascular symptoms. The appropriate diagnostic evaluation often does not occur until a clinician becomes inclined to check symmetry of pulses or blood pressure or listen for bruits in a patient with regional ischemic symptoms.

Any tissue or organ is vulnerable to ischemic injury in TAK. Vascular stenosis is frequently slow and progressive, which can allow for enhancement of collateral circulation. Hence, not all stenotic lesions lead to end-organ damage or symptoms. If asymptomatic inflammatory stenotic lesions are compromised further by other factors, such as thrombosis, or focal atheromatous change as may occur in sites of turbulent flow, critical ischemia and subsequent damage may occur.

Hypertension (HTN) frequently contributes to emergent complications. In the USA, about 20–30% of patients present with HTN, but outside of the USA, 50–75% may present with HTN.[2] In many patients, HTN results from stenotic disease of the suprarenal abdominal aorta and/or renal arteries, causing reduction in renal blood flow and a high renin state (Fig. 7.1).

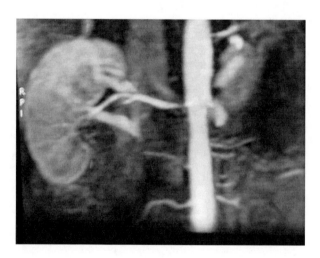

Fig. 7.1 Renal artery stenosis in a patient with Takayasu arteritis

Fig. 7.2 Bilateral subclavian stenosis in a patient with Takayasu arteritis

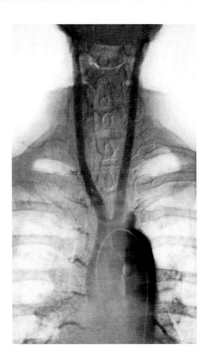

Upper extremity artery stenoses (subclavian and or innominate) are very common (>90% unilateral and >40% bilateral in some series). It is critical for the physician to recognize that this usually leads to inaccurate peripheral cuff blood pressure measurements. The dampening of aortic pressure traveling through large-vessel stenoses may cause central HTN to remain undiagnosed and untreated. The resultant presenting event may be congestive heart failure (CHF), renal failure, or stroke. In patients with bilateral upper extremity disease, lower extremity blood pressures may more accurately reflect true central aortic arch pressures if flow from the arch to the legs is not interrupted (Fig. 7.2). In patients with bilateral upper extremity disease who also have stenotic aortic or bilateral lower extremity arterial stenoses, central arterial pressure measurements should be obtained directly using intravascular pressure transducer catheters to determine whether cuff peripheral blood pressure measurements are an accurate surrogate of central aortic pressure. In the setting of severe central hypertension and no available accurate peripheral site for BP monitoring, consideration should be given to bypass procedures to enable effective monitoring and treatment of this life-threatening complication.

7.2.1
Cerebrovascular Emergencies in Takayasu's Arteritis

Ischemic cerebrovascular disease, such as transient ischemic attack (TIA) or stroke (CVA), occurs in patients with TAK. The reported incidence of TIA in TAK is about 3–7%, and that for CVA is 5–15%.[2-5] Hemorrhagic stroke can also occur in the setting of uncontrolled HTN. Signs and symptoms of cerebrovascular disease are variable, based on anatomic regions affected. The most commonly affected vessels associated with CVA are the carotid arteries. Confirmation of suspected vascular lesions is achieved by brain imaging, including angiographic modalities (catheter-directed/invasive MR or CT).

Patients who require intervention for arterial occlusion with thrombolysis, stenting, or endarterectomy are at risk for cerebral reperfusion syndrome. This is characterized by the onset of headache (usually ipsilateral), seizure (focal or generalized), and neurologic defects (generally contralateral, may be worsening of previous defect) and may occur immediately following revascularization but as late as 1 month following intervention.[6,7] The most common factor contributing to cerebral reperfusion syndrome is hypertension, which should be vigilantly monitored for, even in patients who are initially normotensive, and treated when identified.

7.2.2
Cardiac Emergencies in Takayasu's Arteritis

Only about 5% report angina at first presentation and about 10% of patients with TAK have ischemic heart disease during the course of their illness.[2,3,8] This is important for both patients and providers to be aware of, especially in this young, predominantly female patient population who would otherwise be felt to have minimal cardiovascular disease risk. Signs and symptoms and evaluation of ischemic heart disease in TAK are the same as in the general population.

Congestive heart failure (CHF) has been documented in up to 20% of TAK patients, and may occur from either obstructive coronary artery disease, but more often results from uncontrolled hypertension or aortic insufficiency.[2,3,5] Determining whether one or more of these factors is involved is critical to identifying treatment options. This evaluation usually includes vascular imaging and if there is any question about the reliability of peripheral cuff pressures, would favor invasive angiography with intravascular pressure recordings. Coronary imaging would be included if ischemia was thought to be a factor in CHF.

7.2.3
Abdominal Emergencies in Takayasu's Arteritis

Although mesenteric artery involvement is common in TAK, occurring in up to 40% of patients, the rich collateral flow within the mesentery makes visceral ischemia much less common than the frequency of involved sites.[9] In fact, lesions of just one and sometimes even two vessels may be clinically silent.[9] Patients with critical narrowing of the mesenteric arteries may present with insidious or acute abdominal pain, nausea, vomiting, gastrointestinal bleeding, or postprandial pain. The definition of anatomic etiology of mesenteric ischemia requires vascular imaging studies.

7.2.4
Treating Emergent Conditions in TAK

The conditions detailed above are treated the same way in TAK patients as they would be in the general population, with a few additional considerations. Although it is preferable that TAK patients requiring vascular flow restoration interventions receive them in the setting of quiescent disease, in emergent situations, interventions often cannot be delayed. If vascular interventions are required, it has been demonstrated that arterial bypass, especially with autologous donor vessels (e.g., saphenous vein if size-match is appropriate), is more likely to lead to sustained vessel patency than angioplasty with or without stenting. Patients who are determined to have active disease should be treated with immunosuppressive (corticosteroid with or without a second agent) therapy in addition to having vascular reconstitution. Patients who had been receiving chronic corticosteroid therapy may experience adrenal insufficiency during acute illness. If it occurs, administration of "stress-dose" steroids (i.e., hydrocortisone 50–100 mg IV every 8 h) would be required.

7.3
Giant Cell Arteritis

In contrast to the rarity of TAK, GCA is the most common form of vasculitis in European and North American persons over 50 years of age. The incidence and prevalence varies based on geography. In general, GCA is more common in the most Northern latitudes. Incidence has been reported in the range of <1 (Israel)-56 (Norway)/100,000/year and prevalence as high as 223/100,000.[10-14]

GCA is characterized by granulomatous inflammation of the aorta and its primary branches, most frequently affecting the extracranial branches of the carotid artery. However, with the advent of less invasive, more frequently utilized vascular imaging studies, the prevalence of other large-artery involvement in GCA is becoming better appreciated. In one US cohort, 62% of GCA patients undergoing vascular imaging studies were found to have anatomic changes in large arteries, most frequently of the aorta (65%) and subclavian arteries (37%).[2] This data is an indirect confirmation of the postmortem studies of Ostberg, which revealed 100% of patients having histopathologic features of large-vessel disease.[15] It is likely, given the age of affected patients with GCA, that signs and symptoms of vascular claudication associated with large-vessel involvement are often presumed to be secondary to atherosclerotic vascular disease and hence underdiagnosed. As with TAK, GCA may be a challenging diagnosis, given the many symptoms that patients can present. Patients may demonstrate acute onset of "classic" symptoms, such as headache (60–90%), limb girdle myalgias (polymyalgia rheumatica, 30–50%), jaw claudication (30–70%), and scalp tenderness (40–70%). Others may present with only nonspecific constitutional symptoms (20–50%). In the course of illness, the most feared complications are blindness (5–40%) and stroke (0–10%). The variations in range of reported complications no doubt reflect subspecialty referral bias. Ophthalmologists are most likely to have patients with GCA referred because of visual symptoms, whereas generalists and rheumatologists will see a broader range of presentations. In addition to symptoms from ischemia, aneurysm formation, especially of the thoracic aorta (15–25% of large series), can be associated with rupture or dissection, a dreaded complication that occurs in about half of this subset. This urges careful repeated examination for aortic regurgitant murmurs and thoracic bruits.

7.3.1
Visual Loss: An Ophthalmologic Emergency in GCA

One of the most feared complications of GCA is visual loss, which occurs in 5–58% of patients.[6,10,16,17] The effects of corticosteroids have been striking. Most modern series report only 5–15% frequency of blindness. When initially used, corticosteroids reversed visual symptoms in 35% of patients in whom treatment was provided shortly after the onset of symptoms. Once chronic corticosteroid therapy has been started, blindness is an infrequent complication of GCA (<10%) and may be more related to critical fixed stenoses than active disease.[18] Acute visual loss most frequently results from anterior ischemic optic neuropathy (AION), and can manifest as an initial presenting symptom of GCA, or more insidiously, with blurred vision that gradually progresses to blindness. In addition to AION, visual loss may occur from central retinal artery occlusion or occipital CVA. Other visual manifestations of GCA include scotoma, diplopia, and amaurosis fugax. Patients may have unilateral or bilateral symptoms, which may be transient or permanent. The strongest predictive factors for visual loss are prior transient visual loss and stroke (relative risk 6.35 and 7.65, respectively).[19] Treatment of visual symptoms within 24 h markedly enhanced likelihood of visual improvement compared to patients not treated promptly. Treatment more than 48 h after onset of visual symptoms was not associated with any improvement.[20] Consequently, most authorities would advise to err on the side of overtreatment in elderly patients for whom the cause of acute visual loss is uncertain, but suspected to possibly be due to GCA. Other cohort studies examining risk factors for visual loss in GCA have found that the absence of systemic symptoms and lower sedimentation rates and C-reactive protein levels are associated with increased risk of blindness and other ischemic complications.[16,19] However, not all investigators have reproduced these observations.

Ophthalmologic examination is an essential part of the evaluation of all patients with GCA. This can help establish the etiology of visual symptoms, but also may identify other causes of visual disturbances that may not be related to vasculitis, e.g., glucocorticoid-induced or -aggravated glaucoma, central serous retinopathy, and cataracts. Imaging of the brain and vessels can identify stroke associated with visual loss.

Patients presenting with visual loss are treated with high-dose corticosteroid therapy, usually intravenous pulse therapy with the equivalent of 1 g of methylprednisolone daily for about 3 days, followed by 1 mg/kg of prednisone (or equivalent) daily.

7.3.2
Cerebrovascular Emergencies in GCA

TIA and CVA are relatively uncommon complication of GCA, occurring in about 0–10% of patients.[21-26] CVA is most frequent in patients with active disease, and may occur as the initial presentation of GCA. The majority of CVAs involve the stenosis or occlusion of the carotid and less often vertebral arteries. Vertebrobasilar CVA occurs more frequently in patients with GCA than in an age-matched non-GCA population. Less often, CVA is caused by thromboembolism or thrombus extension from a damaged artery. A study of 287 patients with GCA who presented with CVA at the time of disease diagnosis found that patients with hypertension, smoking history, and those with permanent visual loss had an increased risk of CVA.[27]

If active disease is identified, high-dose glucocorticoid therapy should be initiated. In patients who present with CVA in whom there is a moderate to high suspicion for GCA, glucocorticoid therapy should be initiated and a temporal artery biopsy obtained as soon as possible. The likelihood of a diagnostic biopsy diminishes the longer patients are treated with steroids.

7.3.3
Aortic Aneurysm and Dissection in GCA

With increasing use of large-vessel imaging (especially MRA and MRI) in GCA, there has been greater appreciation for the risk of aortic aneurysm (thoracic >>> abdominal).[28-31] An inception cohort of GCA patients from the Mayo Clinic demonstrated a marked increase in mortality in patients with thoracic aortic dissection, with a median survival after diagnosis of only 1.1 years; this speaks about the serious nature of this comorbidity.[29]

GCA patients with thoracic aortic aneurysm often are asymptomatic, but may manifest with chest or back pain, usually from impingement on surrounding structures. In patients with ascending or arch aneurysm with mediastinal invasion, hoarseness from laryngeal or vagal nerve compression can occur, as can dyspnea, dysphagia, or superior vena cava syndrome from local structural compromise. Signs and symptoms of aortic dissection include severe pain in the chest or back, frequently described as "tearing," hypotension, CHF, acute CVA, or MI. Pericardial tamponade may occur with rupture into the pericardial space, and pleural effusion or hemothorax with rupture into the pleural space. Patients may demonstrate pulse and/or blood pressure inequality between upper extremities, or the murmur of aortic insufficiency. Reported risk factors for aortic aneurysm and/or dissection in GCA include hyperlipidemia, history of coronary artery disease, and hypertension.[29-31]

Aortic aneurysm or dissection is diagnosed by imaging studies. Computed tomography scanning of the chest is frequently used, because of both availability and rapidity. Multiplane transesophageal echocardiography and MR imaging also are utilized in the evaluation of suspected aortic aneurysm or dissection, albeit less frequently, because of the lack of availability of the technology or trained personnel for interpretation of the study. Chest radiography may demonstrate widening of the mediastinum, displaced aortic calcification, or pleural effusion, but has inadequate sensitivity to be used alone for diagnosis.

Acute aortic dissection involving the ascending aorta in GCA, as in the general population, is a surgical emergency. Patients with descending aortic dissections are treated medically if stable, or surgically if there is continued hemorrhage or progression of the dissection. Patients found to have active GCA (based on clinical evaluation or tissue pathology from aortic surgery) should be treated with glucocorticoid therapy, with the timing of institution of therapy dependent on the patient's clinical status and perioperative considerations.

7.3.4
Mesenteric Ischemia in GCA

Because this is a very rare event in GCA, it is often not considered to be part of the illness, even when active GCA is otherwise apparent.[32] It may manifest in the absence of cranial symptoms (40% cases), becoming recognized from either postoperative or postmortem pathology. Mortality rates from GCA-related mesenteric ischemia are about 50%.

7.4
Urgent Complications of Immunosuppressive Therapy

Corticosteroid therapy is the cornerstone of medical treatment for patients with large-vessel vasculitis. For GCA, no adjunctive therapy has been shown to be of proven value. In TAK, second agents have been evaluated in open-labeled trials. Some appear to be promising, but require proof of utility in controlled studies. All of the therapies utilized in the treatment of these disorders can cause a host of adverse effects ranging from mild to life-threatening. It is important to be aware of the more common serious adverse effects in order to provide timely identification and treatment to minimize associated morbidity and mortality.

7.4.1
Infectious Complications of Therapy

Patients with large-vessel vasculitis receiving any immunosuppressive therapy, including corticosteroids and other immunosuppressive agents, are at increased risk of infection. Although common community-acquired bacterial and viral infections are often found in these patients, they are also at risk for infection with uncommon opportunistic pathogens. Patients with large-vessel vasculitis receiving immunosuppressive therapy are also at risk for reactivation of dormant or latent infection, such as herpes simplex virus, varicella zoster virus, or tuberculosis.

A high level of vigilance must be maintained for infectious complications of immunosuppressive therapy, given that "usual" signs and symptoms of infection may be muted or absent in this setting. A focused evaluation is appropriate in nontoxic patients presenting with localized signs or symptoms suggestive of infection. In patients with nonspecific, generalized symptoms, or in those who are systemically ill, a broad initial investigation, usually in-hospital, is warranted, with considerations given to both common and opportunistic pathogens. In critically ill patients, stress-dose steroids may be required to prevent acute adrenal insufficiency. In patients with more aggressive or chronic infections, decreasing corticosteroid doses to the lowest effective dose is required to control vasculitis to facilitate clearing infection.

7.4.2
Cardiovascular Complications of Therapy

Perhaps one of the most underappreciated side effects of glucocorticoid therapy is the potential adverse effects on the cardiovascular system. Increased rates of MI, CVA, and congestive heart failure have been reported in patients without prior hospitalization for cardiovascular disease who have been receiving corticosteroid therapy. Increase in risk has been documented in patients receiving as little as the equivalent of prednisone 7.5 mg/day.[33]

7.4.3
Gastrointestinal Complications of Therapy

Corticosteroid therapy increases the risk of gastrointestinal events, including ulcer disease, gastritis, and bleeding. Although the reported increase in relative risk when corticosteroids are used as single agents is relatively low, in combination with nonsteroidal anti-inflammatory agents, this risk increases to about four times that of a patient using neither agent.[34] Treatment for these conditions is similar to that in the general population. In addition, elimination or minimizing the dose of culprit medications, when possible, is an important facet of therapy.

7.4.4
Central Nervous System Complications of Therapy

Central nervous system side effects are not uncommon in patients receiving corticosteroids. In the majority of patients, these side effects are mild and manageable. However, a small number of patients can develop acute psychiatric symptoms, e.g., psychosis, hypomania, or severe depression. These severe adverse effects may occur within a few days of beginning therapy, and are most frequently seen in patients receiving higher doses of corticosteroids, generally greater than the equivalent of 20 mg/day of prednisone. In some patients, dose reduction is helpful in alleviating symptoms. In patients in whom steroid doses cannot be reduced or symptoms persist with dose reduction, directed pharmacologic therapy for the appropriate psychiatric disorder has reported to be effective in management.

7.5
Summary

Patients with large-vessel vasculitis are at risk for life and organ-threatening complications associated with both disease and the associated treatment. Maintaining awareness of these complications is a critical aspect of early diagnosis and intervention, which may be life-saving.

References

1. Hall S, Barr W, Lie JT, et al. Takayasu arteritis: a study of 32 North American patients. *Medicine (Baltimore)*. 1985;64:89-99.
2. Maksimowicz-McKinnon K, Clark T, Hoffman GS. Limitations of therapy and a guarded prognosis in an American cohort of Takayasu arteritis patients. *Arthritis Rheum*. 2007;56:1000-1009.
3. Kerr GS, Hallahan CW, Giordano J, et al. Takayasu arteritis. *Ann Intern Med*. 1994;120: 919-929.
4. Arnaud L, Haroche J, Limal N, et al. Takayasu arteritis in France: a single-center retrospective study of 82 cases comparing white, North African, and black patients. *Medicine*. 2010;89: 1-17.
5. Vanoli M, Daina E, Salvarani C, et al. Takayasu's arteritis: a study of 104 Italian patients. *Arthritis Rheum*. 2005;53:100-107.
6. Sundt TM Jr, Sharbrough FW, Piepgras DG, et al. Correlation of cerebral blood flow and electroencephalographic changes during carotid endarterectomy: with results of surgery and hemodynamics of cerebral ischemia. *Mayo Clin Proc*. 1981;56:533-543.
7. Coutts SB, Hill MD, Hu WY. Hyperperfusion syndrome: toward a stricter definition. *Neurosurgery*. 2003;53:1053-1058.
8. Ogino H, Matsuda H, Minatoya K, et al. Overview of late outcome of medical and surgical treatment for Takayasu arteritis. *Circulation*. 2008;118:2738-2747.
9. Tracci MC, Cherry KJ. Surgical treatment of great vessel occlusive disease. *Surg Clin North Am*. 2009;89:821-836.
10. Hunder GG. Giant cell (temporal) arteritis. *Rheum Dis Clin North Am*. 1990;16:399-409.
11. Nordborg E, Bengtsson BA. Epidemiology of biopsy-proven giant cell arteritis. *J Intern Med*. 1990;227(4):233-236.
12. Baldursson O, Steinsson K, Bjornsson J, et al. Giant cell arteritis in Iceland. An epidemiologic and histopathologic analysis. *Arthritis Rheum*. 1994;37:1007-1012.
13. Gran JT, Myklebust G. The incidence of polymyalgia rheumatica and temporal arteritis in the county of Aust Agder, South Norway: a prospective study 1987–94. *J Rheumatol*. 1997;24: 1739-1743.
14. Machado EB, Michet CJ, Ballard DJ, et al. Trends in incidence and clinical presentation of temporal arteritis in Olmsted County, Minnesota, 1950–1985. *Arthritis Rheum*. 1988;31: 745-749.
15. Ostberg G. Morphologic changes in large arteries in polymyalgia arteritica. *Acta Med Scand*. 1972;533(Suppl):135-164.
16. Liozon E, Herrman F, Ly K, et al. Risk factors for visual loss in giant cell (temporal) arteritis: a prospective study of 174 patients. *Am J Med*. 2001;111:211-217.
17. Birkhead NC, Wagener HP, Shick RM. Treatment of temporal arteritis with adrenal corticosteroids: results in fifty-five cases in which lesion was proved at biopsy. *JAMA*. 1957;163: 821-827.
18. Hayreh SS, Zimmerman B. Visual deterioration in giant cell arteritis patients while on high doses of corticosteroid therapy. *Ophthalmology*. 2003;110:1204-1215.
19. Salvarani C, Cimino L, Macchioni P, et al. Risk factors for visual loss in an Italian population-based cohort of patients with giant cell arteritis. *Arthritis Rheum*. 2005;53:293-297.
20. Gonzalez-Gay M, Blanco R, Rodriquez-Valverde V, et al. Permanent visual loss and cerebrovascular accidents in giant cell arteritis: predictors and response to treatment. *Arthritis Rheum*. 1998;41:1497-1504.
21. Bengtsson BA, Malmvall BE. The epidemiology of giant cell arteritis including temporal arteritis and polymyalgia rheumatica. Incidences of different clinical presentations and eye complications. *Arthritis Rheum*. 1981;24:899-904.

22. Graham E, Holland A, Avery A, et al. Prognosis in giant cell arteritis. *Br Med J.* 1981;282: 269-271.
23. Matteson EL, Gold KN, Bloch DA, et al. Long-term survival of patients with giant cell arteritis in the American College of Rheumatology giant cell arteritis classification criteria cohort. *Am J Med.* 1996;100:193-196.
24. Hoffman GS, Cid MC, Hellmann DB, et al. A multicenter, randomized, double-blind, placebo controlled trial of adjuvant methotrexate treatment for giant cell arteritis. *Arthritis Rheum.* 2002;46:1309-1318.
25. Maksimowicz-McKinnon K, Clark T, Hoffman GS. Takayasu and giant cell arteritis: a spectrum within the same disease? *Medicine.* 2009;88:221-226.
26. Salvarani C, Giannini C, Miller D, et al. Giant cell arteritis: involvement of intracranial arteries. *Arthritis Rheum.* 2006;55:985-989.
27. Gonzalez-Gay M, Vazquez-Rodriguez TR, Gomez-Acebo I, et al. Strokes at the time of disease diagnosis in a series of 287 patients with biopsy-proven giant cell arteritis. *Medicine.* 2009;88:227-235.
28. Blockmans D, de Ceuninck L, Vanderschueren S, et al. Repetitive 18 F-flurordeoxyglucose positron emission tomography in giant cell arteritis: a prospective study of 35 patients. *Arthritis Rheum.* 2006;55:131-137.
29. Nuenninghoff DM, Hunder GG, Christianson TJF, et al. Mortality of large-artery complication (aortic aneurysm, aortic dissection, and/or large-artery stenosis) in patients with giant cell arteritis. *Arthritis Rheum.* 2003;48:3532-3537.
30. Gonzalez-Gay M, Garcia-Porrua C, Pineiro A, et al. Aortic aneurysm and dissection in patients with biopsy-proven giant cell arteritis from northwestern Spain. A population-based study. *Medicine.* 2004;83:335-341.
31. Ozbek C, Yetkin U, Ergunes K, et al. Ascending aortic aneurysm in giant cell arteritis. *Int J Thorac Cardiovasc Surg.* 2009;13(2).
32. Scola CJ, Li C, Upchurch KS. Mesenteric involvement in giant cell arteritis. An underrecognized complication? Analysis of a case series with clinicoanatomic correlation. *Medicine.* 2008;87:45-51.
33. Wei L, MacDonald TM, Walker BR. Taking glucocorticoids by prescription is associated with subsequent cardiovascular disease. *Ann Intern Med.* 2004;141:764-770.
34. Piper JM, Ray WA, Daugherty JR, et al. Corticosteroid use and peptic ulcer disease: role of nonsteroidal anti-inflammatory drugs. *Ann Intern Med.* 1991;114:735-740.

Life-Threatening Presentations of ANCA-Associated Vasculitis

8

Duvuru Geetha and Philip Seo

Abstract The antineutrophil cytoplasm antibody (ANCA)-associated vasculitides are a spectrum of heterogeneous autoimmune diseases characterized by necrotizing small- and medium-vessel vasculitis and the presence of ANCA. These unique entities have a broad spectrum of organ involvement and severity, which influences the approach to diagnosis and treatment. These chronic multisystem disorders may be life-threatening if there is major organ involvement, such as acute renal failure or pulmonary hemorrhage, and require timely initiation of immunosuppression to induce and to maintain remission. Management, therefore, requires a high index of suspicion, targeted investigation, prompt treatment, and long-term follow-up, with input from multiple specialists. Long-term outcomes are influenced by chronic sequelae caused by organ damage, disease relapses, and medication-induced side effects. This chapter summarizes our current knowledge of the principal manifestations, evaluation, and evidence-based management of these disorders.

Keywords ANCA • Capillaritis • Glomerulonephritis • Vasculitis

8.1
Historical Overview

In 1954, the pathologists Gabriel Godman and Jacob Churg wrote "there are a number of disease entities with tissue changes very similar to those encountered in Wegener's granulomatosis, some of which are obviously related to it morphologically and pathogenetically. These group themselves into a compass from necrotizing and granulomatous processes without angiitis, through mixed forms, to vasculitis without granuloma."[1] Together, these disease entities are known as the ANCA-associated vasculitides, which are idiopathic autoimmune disorders that are associated with small- and medium-vessel

D. Geetha (✉)
Division of Nephrology, Johns Hopkins Bayview Medical Center,
Johns Hopkins University, 301 Mason Lord Drive, Baltimore, MD 21224, USA
e-mail: gduvura@jhmi.edu

M.A. Khamashta and M. Ramos-Casals (eds.), *Autoimmune Diseases*,
DOI: 10.1007/978-0-85729-358-9_8, © Springer-Verlag London Limited 2011

Table 8.1 Chapel Hill consensus conference definitions of the primary systemic vasculitides

Name	Definition
Polyarteritis nodosa	Necrotizing inflammation of medium-sized or small arteries without glomerulonephritis or vasculitis in arterioles, capillaries or venules
Wegener's granulomatosis	Granulomatous inflammation involving the respiratory tract, and necrotizing vasculitis affecting small to medium-sized vessels, e.g., capillaries, venules, arterioles and arteries. Necrotizing glomerulonephritis is common
Churg–Strauss syndrome	Eosinophil-rich and granulomatous inflammation involving the respiratory tract and necrotizing vasculitis affecting small to medium-sized vessels, and associated with asthma and blood eosinophilia
Microscopic polyangiitis	Necrotizing vasculitis with few or no immune deposits affecting small vessels, i.e., capillaries, venules or arterioles. Necrotizing arteritis of small and medium-sized arteries may be present. Necrotizing glomerulonephritis is very common. Pulmonary capillaritis often occurs

Source: Adapted with permission from Jennette et al.[3]

vasculitis, and linked by the presence of antineutrophil cytoplasmic antibodies (ANCA).[2] The main members of this family, as noted by Godman and Churg, include Wegener's granulomatosis, microscopic polyangiitis, and the Churg–Strauss syndrome (Table 8.1). Formally, this family could be considered to extend to renal limited vasculitis, drug-induced ANCA-associated vasculitis, and cocaine-induced midline destructive lesions (CIMDL).[4]

8.2
The ANCA-Associated Vasculitides

8.2.1
Clinical Overview

Wegener's granulomatosis is the archetype of this family, and is characterized by necrotizing granulomatous inflammation of the respiratory tract and adnexa, leading to orbital pseudotumor, chronic sinusitis, Eustachian tube dysfunction, subglottic stenosis, and cavitary pulmonary lesions, in addition to the manifestations associated more generally with the small- and medium-vessel vasculitides. Microscopic polyangiitis is associated with pulmonary capillaritis and glomerulonephritis, and is the most common cause of the pulmonary-renal syndromes, a family that includes anti-glomerular basement membrane disease (Goodpasture's syndrome), systemic lupus erythematosus, cryoglobulinemic vasculitis, and Wegener's granulomatosis (Table 8.2).[5]

Among patients with the ANCA-associated vasculitides, mortality is substantially increased among patients who are older than 65 years, or have cardiac symptoms, gastrointestinal involvement, or renal insufficiency (defined as a serum creatinine ≥ 1.7 mg/dL).[6] Long-term mortality is higher among patients with microscopic polyangiitis when compared

Table 8.2 Differential diagnosis of the pulmonary-renal syndromes

Diagnosis	Initial evaluation	Therapy
Microscopic polyangiitis	P-ANCA/MPO-ANCA	Glucocorticoids and cyclophosphamide
Wegener's granulomatosis	C-ANCA/PR3-ANCA	Glucocorticoids and cyclophosphamide
Systemic lupus erythematosus	ANA, dsDNA, C3, C4	Glucocorticoids and cyclophosphamide or mycophenolate mofetil
Goodpasture's syndrome	Anti-glomerular basement membrane antibodies	Glucocorticoids and cyclophosphamide with plasmapheresis
Cryoglobulinemic vasculitis (mixed essential cryoglobulinemia)	Serum cryoglobulins, rheumatoid factor, hepatitis C PCR	Glucocorticoids and antiviral therapies
Henoch–Schönlein purpura	IgA deposition on biopsy	Controversial; no proven role for glucocorticoids

to patients with either Wegener's granulomatosis or the Churg–Strauss syndrome,[7] although this may merely reflect the clinical manifestations commonly associated with each of these diagnoses.

8.2.2
Treatment Overview

When initially described, mortality associated with systemic Wegener's granulomatosis approached 90% in the first year after diagnosis.[8] Since that time, the introduction of immunosuppressive therapies has largely transformed the ANCA-associated vasculitides (AAV) into chronic syndromes characterized by relapse and remission. Despite substantial advances in our understanding of these complex syndromes, patients routinely suffer from both undertreatment and overtreatment. One of the great challenges that clinicians face early in the disease course is establishing the diagnosis.[9] The ANCA-associated vasculitides often mimic other disease processes, and may initially be misdiagnosed as malignancy or infection. Later in the disease course, the main challenge is differentiating disease manifestations that respond to immunosuppression from manifestations that do not.[10] This is a concern primarily because of the complications that result from overtreatment; in long-term follow-up of participants in European and American trials of primary systemic vasculitis, long-term mortality is primarily due to infection, malignancy, and cardiovascular disease, all of which can be traced back to the glucocorticoids and cytotoxic agents routinely used to treat these diseases.[11] Therefore, prompt initiation of immunosuppressive therapy is vital to the management of disease flares, but it is equally vital to recognize that not all manifestations of vasculitis will respond to immunosuppression. Learning to identify which manifestations of vasculitis are unlikely to respond to immunosuppression is the only way to avoid the toxicities inherent to overtreatment.

8.3
Management of Immunosuppression

It is important to note upfront that there are little data comparing the efficacy of different approaches to the management of acute vasculitis. Therefore, strategies that are considered to be standard in one institution may be considered optional or second-line in the next. That said, when a patient is diagnosed with a vasculitis flare that is threatening to life or the function of a vital organ, the rapid institution of high-dose glucocorticoids (often in the form of methylprednisolone 1 g IV daily for 3 days) is crucial to arrest the progression of vasculitis. Cytotoxic agents, generally in the form of oral cyclophosphamide 2 mg/kg daily, are administered for 6 months to induce remission, after which remission is maintained with an oral antimetabolite, such as methotrexate (20–25 mg/week),[12] azathioprine (2 mg/kg daily),[13] mycophenolate mofetil (1.0–1.5 g twice daily), or leflunomide (20–30 mg daily)[14]. In the elderly and in patients with a history of leukopenia or renal insufficiency, it is prudent to start with lower doses, and titrate carefully while following routine blood counts and chemistries.

One must recognize that each of these agents is accompanied by idiosyncratic toxicities which should be considered carefully prior to initiating therapy. Some common issues, however, merit specific mention. Use of cyclophosphamide is accompanied by an increased risk of *Pneumocystis jirovecii* pneumonia (PCP),[15] and chemoprophylaxis such as trimethoprim/sulfamethoxazole (one single strength tablet daily) or dapsone (100 mg daily) should be employed. Glucocorticoid-induced osteoporosis is an important cause of morbidity among patients treated with standard immunosuppression,[16] and should be treated aggressively with calcium and vitamin D supplements at first, and other therapies depending on risk of fracture.[17] Tremors, easy bruising, and diaphoresis may be seen with glucocorticoids, and may require reassurance.

For patients with active, severe systemic vasculitis who have contraindications to cyclophosphamide therapy, a handful of alternatives exist. Intravenous cyclophosphamide appears to be equivalent to oral cyclophosphamide for a variety of indications,[18] and may subject patients to a lower cumulative dose in exchange for a slight increase in long-term risk of disease flare.[19] For patients receiving intensive care who may be at high risk for infection, intravenous immunoglobulin (400 mg/kg daily for 5 days) may be an effective stopgap measure until more conventional immunosuppression may be instituted. [17]

Biologic agents may also be an effective way of avoiding the toxicities associated with cytotoxic agents. The use of tumor necrosis factor inhibitors is controversial, and although infliximab is used in many parts of the world as part of an augmentation strategy to enhance the benefit of standard steroid-sparing regimens, there appears to be no role for etanercept in these situations.[20] The greatest success of recent years belongs to rituximab (375 mg/m^2 weekly for 4 weeks), which was recently demonstrated to be as effective as cyclophosphamide for the treatment of severe Wegener's granulomatosis and microscopic polyangiitis [21] (although long-term outcomes associated with this treatment are not yet known.[22])

Exceptions to all of these general rules do exist. In particular, it should be noted that milder vasculitis flares can be treated effectively with non-cytotoxic strategies, such as methotrexate [23] or mycophenolate mofetil,[24] although these are generally inappropriate for fulminant vasculitis flares. Also, not all manifestations of vasculitis require, or will respond to, immunosuppression. These exceptions will be noted in the description of Clinical Manifestations, below.

Finally, plasma exchange (e.g., seven exchange procedures over 14 days) should be considered as an adjunctive treatment strategy, especially in patients who fail to respond sufficiently quickly to immunosuppression. Anecdotally, plasma exchange may be especially useful for the management of patients with pulmonary hemorrhage. In clinical trials, plasma exchange has also been shown to lead to a significant improvement in renal recovery among patients with severe renal insufficiency (i.e., serum creatinine ≥ 5.8 mg/dL) due to ANCA-associated glomerulonephritis.[25] Whether this benefit persists after long-term follow-up, and whether patients with other presentations might also benefit from routine use of plasma exchange, are largely unanswered questions.

8.4
Emergent Clinical Manifestations

8.4.1
Ocular

Ocular involvement is especially common among patients with Wegener's granulomatosis. Up to half of patients with Wegener's granulomatosis have ocular complaints, and an ocular manifestation is the presenting symptom in 15% of patients with this disease.[26]

8.4.1.1
Necrotizing Scleritis

The ANCA-associated vasculitides can affect any ocular structure, and have been associated with ischemic optic neuritis, retinitis, posterior scleritis, and uveitis.[27] That said, "red eye" is the most common complaint (Fig. 8.1). Although the differential is broad,[29] the primary culprits include episcleritis and scleritis, which are common manifestations of the ANCA-associated vasculitides. Episcleritis does not threaten vision, and can be treated with topical medications, such as artificial tears [30] or prednisolone acetate 1% applied every 3–4 h; patients who fail to respond to either of these may benefit from oral nonsteroidal anti-inflammatory agents. Scleritis generally will not respond to topical agents, and should be treated with systemic glucocorticoids. Because scleritis among patients with ANCA-associated vasculitis may be a harbinger of a more significant vasculitis flare, consideration should be given to simultaneously initiating an oral immunosuppressive agent, such as methotrexate, azathioprine, or mycophenolate mofetil.[31] Significant pain and scleral damage are signs of a necrotizing scleritis. This may be accompanied by peripheral corneal keratopathy ("corneal melt"). Both of these manifestations can rapidly lead to irreversible blindness, and merit therapy with cytotoxic agents.

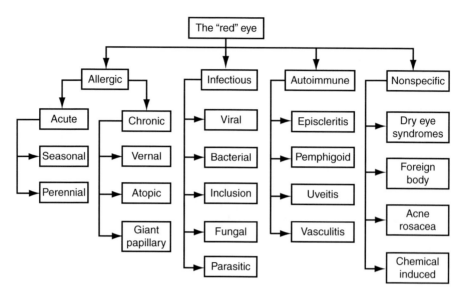

Fig. 8.1 Differential diagnosis of the red eye (From Bielory.[28] Reprinted with permission of Springer Science + Business Media)

8.4.1.2
Orbital Pseudotumor

Wegener's granulomatosis can affect any orbital or periorbital structure, but the most common manifestation is orbital pseudotumor, a retroorbital mass that consists of necro-tizing granulomatous inflammation and fibrosis (Fig. 8.2). The symptoms associated with orbital pseudotumor are due to mass effect; therefore, patients with orbital pseudo-tumor may present with ocular pain associated with proptosis or diplopia. As the mass develops, patients may develop exposure keratopathy or a compressive ocular neuropa-thy, both of which can lead to blindness if not treated. Diagnosis is generally made with imaging, using modalities such as magnetic resonance imaging. In the correct clinical setting, biopsy is generally not necessary to confirm the diagnosis. However, a number of conditions can mimic this phenomenon, including orbital cellulitis, thyroid ophthal-mopathy, sarcoidosis, lymphoid tumor, metastatic carcinoma, and IgG4-related systemic disease. In addition, an idiopathic orbital inflammatory syndrome can appear as an iso-lated condition, although this is a diagnosis of exclusion.[32] Aggressive immunosuppres-sive therapy, often with cytotoxic agents, is central to the management of orbital pseudotumor and is key to improving the discomfort associated with this diagnosis. If the eyelid cannot close completely over the eye, topical antibiotic ointments and an occlusive dressing can be used to prevent exposure keratopathy.[33] Response to immuno-suppression can be slow, and if vision is threatened, transantral or transfrontal surgical decompression may be required.[34,35]

Fig. 8.2 Magnetic resonance imaging demonstrating orbital pseudotumor of the left eye in a patient with Wegener's granulomatosis

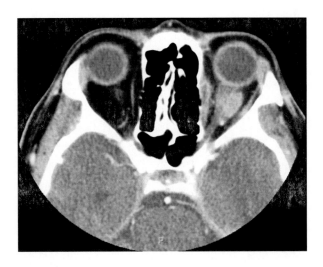

8.4.2
Otolaryngologic

More than the other ANCA-associated vasculitides, Wegener's granulomatosis is characterized by inflammation of the otolaryngologic structures, often leading to chronic sinusitis, Eustachian tube dysfunction, chondritis, and subglottic stenosis.[36]

8.4.2.1
Subglottic Stenosis

Subglottic stenosis is a narrowing of the airway at the level of the cricoid cartilage or tracheal rings that may occur as the result of trauma (e.g., intubation), but can also occur in 7–23% of patients with Wegener's granulomatosis.[37] Subglottic stenosis tends to progress independently of the other manifestations associated with Wegener's granulomatosis. This may imply that inflammation occurs with a systemic flare, but narrowing of the airway occurs as part of the healing process, as the area of inflammation turns to scar. Patients may present with dyspnea, stridor, cough, or change in voice timbre. Biopsy may not be helpful to confirm the diagnosis, as most are nonspecific. Diagnosis is generally confirmed by direct visualization, although computed tomography or pulmonary function tests (with flow-volume loops) may also be useful to follow the diagnosis longitudinally.

Regarding the management of subglottic stenosis, immunosuppression is often indicated, especially if symptoms occur in the setting of other organ involvement. Furthermore, glucocorticoids are anti-inflammatory, and may help increase airway patency. However, in cases in which the airway is critically compromised, systemic therapies may be insufficient. Direct visualization of the lesion, followed by endoscopic dilatation and steroid injection, is often the treatment of choice.[38] Laser treatment can be effective in the short term, but in the long term can lead to severe scaring and further complications.[39] In the most severe cases, open laryngotracheal reconstruction or tracheostomy, depending on urgency, should be considered.[40] In non-emergent settings, surgical intervention should be deferred until after the patient is in clinical remission.

8.4.2.2
Chondritis

Chondritis is a relatively uncommon manifestation of the ANCA-associated vasculitides; when it occurs, it is specific for Wegener's granulomatosis. Auricular chondritis presents as pain, swelling, and tenderness of the external ear that spares the ear lobe. Chondritis of the tracheal and bronchial cartilage is potentially life-threatening, leading to destruction of the tracheal rings that can cause tracheomalacia and collapse of the respiratory tract. Such involvement is common among patients with subglottic stenosis, and also requires aggressive immunosuppressive therapy, typically with a cytotoxic agent.[41]

8.4.2.3
Sensorineural Hearing Loss

Hearing loss is common in Wegener's granulomatosis and may precede the diagnosis of vasculitis by years. Sensorineural hearing loss may occur through vasculitic inflammation of the cochlear circulation, and may respond to aggressive immunosuppression, when instituted promptly[42]; a treatment trial is often warranted, along with formal hearing testing to monitor improvements objectively. Conductive hearing loss may also be seen with Wegener's granulomatosis, but is more likely to be multifactorial, owing to both age and genetics. In some cases, conductive hearing loss may be due to a serous otitis media that occurs due to Eustachian tube dysfunction, and may improve with a tympanostomy tube placement.

8.4.3
Pulmonary

Pneumocystis jirovecii pneumonia can occur in any immunosuppressed patient, and should be considered in any patient who presents with dyspnea who has not received chemoprophylaxis. Moreover, when evaluating a patient with acute dyspnea, it is helpful to consider the underlying diagnosis. Each form of the ANCA-associated vasculitides is associated with unique causes of dyspnea, and knowing which type of vasculitis the patient has may help facilitate the evaluation.

8.4.3.1
Bronchospasm

For the patient with the Churg–Strauss syndrome, the most likely cause of dyspnea is asthma. There is an old belief that as patients progress to the so-called vasculitic phase of the Churg–Strauss syndrome, the asthmatic component of this disease becomes inactive. On the contrary, many patients with the Churg–Strauss syndrome will continue to experience steroid-dependent asthma that is largely independent of the underlying vasculitis. It should be noted that patients with the Churg–Strauss syndrome may develop active bronchospasm as their glucocorticoids are tapered; therefore, it is important to initiate bronchodilator therapy prophylactically. Otherwise, the management of bronchospasm associated with the Churg–Strauss syndrome does not differ from the management of bronchospasm in other situations; it should be noted that bronchospasm in these cases will not respond to traditional immunosuppressive agents such as cyclophosphamide, which do not have a role in its management.

8.4.3.2
Pulmonary Embolism

With Wegener's granulomatosis, it is important to remember that these patients have a higher risk of venous thromboembolic events.[43] This increased risk seems to be coincident with disease flare; however, thrombus in these cases will not resolve with immunosuppression, and should be managed with conventional anticoagulation. An interesting question is whether these patients would benefit from lifelong anticoagulation, but this has not yet become standard of care.

8.4.3.3
Pulmonary Capillaritis

Although it can occur in all forms of ANCA-associated vasculitis, hemoptysis associated with pulmonary capillaritis is most characteristic of microscopic polyangiitis (Fig. 8.3).[5] This manifestation can be life-threatening, and merits urgent immunosuppressive therapy in addition to ventilator support when indicated. Patients present with hemoptysis, but progression of symptoms can be rapid. Computed tomography can be useful to evaluate the process, which is associated with an alveolar filling process, but the appearance is nonspecific. Bronchoscopy with bronchoalveolar lavage can serve a dual purpose of confirming the presence of hemosiderin-laden macrophages consistent with this diagnosis, and to evaluate for other causes of hemoptysis, including neoplasm, tuberculosis, abscess, and upper airway source.[44]

8.4.4
Cardiac

Vasculitis of the coronary arteries is an uncommon manifestation of the primary systemic vasculitides, although it has been reported. More common is accelerated coronary artery

Fig. 8.3 Computed tomography demonstrating pulmonary hemorrhage in a patient with Wegener's granulomatosis presenting with hemoptysis

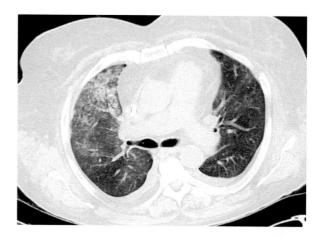

disease, likely due to prolonged use of glucocorticoids or the inflammatory state associated with the primary diagnosis.[45] Myocarditis, valvulitis, pericarditis, and arrhythmia (including complete heart block[46]) have all been reported among patients with ANCA-associated vasculitis.[47] These abnormalities, in turn, are associated with increased mortality, even among patients who are asymptomatic.[48]

8.4.4.1
Eosinophilic Myocarditis

Eosinophilic myocarditis can be found in association with several hypereosinophilic disorders, including the Churg–Strauss syndrome. It is not seen in association with the other ANCA-associated vasculitides. Eosinophilic infiltration of the myocardium leads to fibrotic injury and diminished cardiac function; one study demonstrated abnormalities in cardiac function in 62% of patients with the Churg–Strauss syndrome, although only 26% were symptomatic.[49] As with other cardiomyopathies, as cardiac function declines, the risk of arrhythmia increases. Rapid assessment and treatment of patients with active myocarditis is crucial; moreover, given the prevalence of involvement, a screening echocardiogram is warranted in all patients with a new diagnosis of the Churg–Strauss syndrome.

8.4.5
Renal

Renal involvement occurs in up to 70% of patients with Wegener's granulomatosis and microscopic polyangiitis, and may present with proteinuria, microscopic hematuria, red cell casts, or a rise in serum creatinine with rapid deterioration in renal function. However, renal insufficiency in a patient with ANCA-associated vasculitis is not always due to renal vasculitis, and other potential causes of renal dysfunction (such as acute interstitial nephritis due to trimethoprim/sulfamethoxazole or other drugs) must also be considered.[50] Renal insufficiency in patients with the Churg–Strauss syndrome, in particular, may be due to eosinophilic infiltration of the renal parenchyma, rather than a frank glomerulonephritis.

8.4.5.1
Glomerulonephritis

Glomerulonephritis is found most often in association with microscopic polyangiitis, and to a lesser extent in patients with the other ANCA-associated vasculitides (Fig. 8.4). A characteristic clinical feature is rapidly progressive deterioration in renal function resulting in end-stage renal failure. The importance of detecting glomerulonephritis early cannot be overstated, since long-term mortality correlates strongly with renal function at the time the vasculitis flare is diagnosed. Prompt diagnosis and timely initiation of induction treatment therefore is vital to management.[9]

The typical histopathology is a necrotizing and crescentic glomerulonephritis with variable amounts of extracapillary proliferation, fibrinoid necrosis, and glomerulosclerosis. Immunofluorescence is described as "pauci-immune," and biopsies are characterized by mild or absent glomerular tuft staining for one or more immunoglobulins or complement components, and few or no electron-dense deposits on electron microscopy. In general, one should consider renal biopsy to help confirm the diagnosis and determine the long-term renal prognosis. Aggressive treatment, however, should not be delayed, if evidence of active glomerulonephritis is strong.

There are case reports of patients with ANCA-associated vasculitis who also have an immune-complex mediated glomerulonephritis, such as membranous nephropathy or IgA nephropathy. ANCA-associated vasculitis can also coexist with other forms of glomerular injury, such as anti-glomerular basement membrane (anti-GBM) disease. Typically, these patients will have both circulating ANCA and circulating anti-GBM antibodies. A recent retrospective analysis of these patients suggests that they have more severe renal disease and a worse prognosis when compared to patients who have circulating ANCA alone.[51]

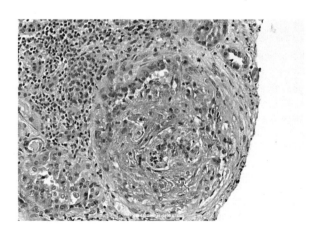

Fig. 8.4 Crescentic glomerulonephritis in a patient with microscopic polyangiitis (hematoxylin and eosin stain)

In patients who progress to end-stage renal disease, renal transplantation is an excellent option.[52] Although patients who are ANCA-negative at the time of kidney transplant may have a lower risk of vasculitis relapse, the overall relapse rate is quite low, and ANCA positivity should not be considered a contraindication to renal transplantation.[53] In some series, patients with ANCA-associated vasculitis actually fare better than patients with end-stage renal disease due to other diagnoses.[54]

8.4.6
Gastroenterological

An acute abdomen is an uncommon presentation for the ANCA-associated vasculitides, which often spare the mesenteric circulation. That said, *mesenteric ischemia* is an important consideration in this patient population. Although classically described as postprandial abdominal pain, patients may initially present with diarrhea. Early immunosuppression is key to the management of these patients; late complications, such as peritonitis and bowel perforation, are all associated with a substantial increase in mortality.[55] Both angiography and colonoscopy may be useful to confirm the diagnosis, depending on the level of symptoms experienced by the patient. Angiography further holds open the possibility of allowing angioplasty when indicated, although caution must be used, as these lesions tend to re-occlude.

8.4.7
Neurologic

Neurologic involvement is not uncommon among the ANCA-associated vasculitides, and the frequency of neurologic manifestations depends on the underlying diagnosis. One study noted that neurologic manifestations of vasculitis were present in 50.8% of patients with Wegener's granulomatosis, 36.6% of patients with microscopic polyangiitis, and 76.0% of patients with the Churg–Strauss syndrome.[56]

8.4.7.1
Mononeuritis Multiplex

Peripheral neuropathy is a common manifestation of the ANCA-associated vasculitides. Although a sensory polyneuropathy is the most common form of peripheral neuropathy observed, mononeuritis multiplex may be pathognomonic for the diagnosis of vasculitis in the correct clinical setting. Mononeuritis multiplex is particularly characteristic of the Churg–Strauss syndrome.[57] A mononeuritis multiplex affecting the peroneal nerve leads to inability to dorsiflex, a phenomenon described as a "foot drop." A mononeuritis affecting the radial nerve leads to the inability to extend the wrist, or a "wrist drop." Patients with a foot drop may comment that the affected foot slaps on the floor as they walk, or they develop a high-stepping gate to avoid this phenomenon. Both wrist drop and foot drop can be caused by other forms of nerve damage besides a mononeuritis multiplex; therefore, the diagnosis should be confirmed by nerve conduction study.[58] Prompt initiation of immuno-suppression presents the best chance of preserving motor function, although some level of residual weakness is often inevitable.

8.4.7.2
Pachymeningitis

Specific to Wegener's granulomatosis is the development of granulomatous inflammation of the meninges that leads to a chronic, granulomatous pachymeningitis. This is a relatively rare manifestation that occurs predominantly in patients with limited disease, but if allowed to progress, cranial nerve deficits can occur. Patients often present complaining of head-ache. Magnetic resonance imaging can be valuable for making this diagnosis, although it should be noted that malignancy can also present as a pachymeningitis, and biopsy should be performed if the underlying diagnosis is not clear. Because pachymeningitis may be refractory to antimetabolite treatments, cytotoxic therapies should be considered.[59]

8.4.8
Cutaneous

A broad spectrum of cutaneous manifestations are associated with the ANCA-associated vasculitides, including erythema nodosum, pyoderma gangrenosum, and Winkelman (Churg–Strauss) granuloma, although palpable purpura is the most common disease manifestation.[60]

8.4.8.1
Purpura

Approximately 5% of patients with ANCA-associated vasculitis will present with palpable purpura, caused by extravasation of red blood cells into the skin. This finding is most often described as raised and non-blanching, but can occur in a variety of forms, including ves-icles and blisters. Although not life-threatening, it may be an important harbinger of a more serious disease flare, or lead to an important opportunity to confirm the underlying diagnosis. Biopsy should be performed with immunofluorescence, which will reveal evidence of a "pauci-immune" vasculitis, which is pathognomonic for these diseases.[61]

8.4.8.2
Cutaneous Ulcers

Vasculitis that affects the medium-caliber blood vessels in the skin can lead to large cutaneous ulcerations that may mimic pyoderma gangrenosum or a number of chronic

Fig. 8.5 Cutaneous lower-extremity ulcer in a patient with ANCA-associated vasculitis

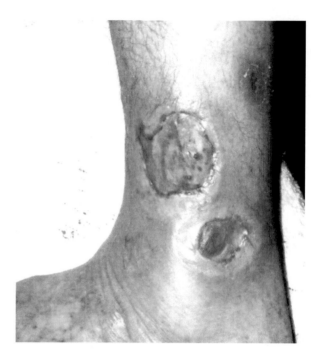

infections (Fig. 8.5).[62] Meticulous wound care, in the form of judicious debridement, colloidal dressings, and compression stockings, in addition to immunosuppression, are key to promoting appropriate wound healing. Overly aggressive debridement can paradoxically worsen these lesions. Severe peripheral arterial disease may impair wound healing, and in some cases, revascularization should be considered.[63] If allowed to fester, these lesions are at risk for superinfection; therefore, if a cutaneous ulcer fails to respond to immunosuppressive therapy, consideration should be given to re-biopsy for culture.

8.5
Conclusions

The ANCA-associated vasculitides can be challenging to diagnose and treat. An awareness of the myriad situations that may occur in association with these diagnoses, and a sensitivity toward the manifestations that do not merit treatment with systemic immunosuppression, is the clinician's best defense.

References

1. Godman G, Churg J. Wegener's granulomatosis: pathology and review of the literature. *Arch Pathol Lab Med.* 1954;58:533-553.

2. Seo P, Stone JH. The antineutrophil cytoplasmic antibody-associated vasculitides. *Am J Med.* 2004;117(1):39-50.
3. Jennette J, Falk R, Andrassy K, et al. Nomenclature of systemic vasculitides proposal of an international consensus conference. *Arthritis Rheum.* 1994;37:187-192.
4. Rachapalli SM, Kiely PD. Cocaine-induced midline destructive lesions mimicking ENT-limited Wegener's granulomatosis. *Scand J Rheumatol.* 2008;37(6):477-480.
5. Chung SA, Seo P. Microscopic polyangiitis. *Rheum Dis Clin North Am.* 2010;36(3):559-572.
6. Guillevin L, Pagnoux C, Mahr A, Le Toumelin P. The Five-Factor Score (FFS) revisited: a tool to assess the Prognoses of Polyarteritis Nodosa (PAN), Microscopic Polyangiitis (MPA), Churg-Strauss Syndrome (CSS) and Wegener's Granulomatosis (WG) based on 1108 patients from the French Vasculitis Study Group (FVSG). *Arthritis Rheum.* 2008;58(9(Suppl1)):906.
7. Lane SE, Watts RA, Shepstone L, Scott DGI. Primary systemic vasculitis: clinical features and mortality. *QJM-An Int J Med.* 2005;98(2):97-111.
8. Walton E. Giant-Cell granuloma of the respiratory tract (Wegener's granulomatosis). *Br Med J.* 1958;2:265-270.
9. Jayne D. The diagnosis of vasculitis. *Best Pract Res Clin Rheumatol.* 2009;23(3):445-453.
10. Seo P. Wegener's granulomatosis: managing more than inflammation. *Curr Opin Rheumatol.* 2008;20(1):10-16.
11. Seo P, Silva F, Hoffman GS, et al. Morbidity and mortality of Wegener's granulomatosis: data from a current multicenter longitudinal cohort. American College of Rheumatology Scientific Meeting; 2008.
12. Pagnoux C, Mahr A, Hamidou MA, et al. Azathioprine or methotrexate maintenance for ANCA-associated vasculitis. *N Engl J Med.* 2008;359(26):2790-2803.
13. Jayne D. Randomised trial of cyclophosphamide versus azathioprine during remission in ANCA-associated systemic vasculitis (CYCAZAREM). *J Am Soc Nephrol.* 1999;10:105A.
14. Metzler C, Miehle N, Manger K, et al. Elevated relapse rate under oral methotrexate versus leflunomide for maintenance of remission in Wegener's granulomatosis. *Rheumatology.* 2007;46(7):1087-1091.
15. Ognibene F, Shelhamer J, Hoffman G, et al. Pneumocystitis carinii pneumonia: a major complication of immunosuppressice therapy in patients with Wegener's granulomatosis. *Am J Respir Crit Care Med.* 1995;151:795-799.
16. Saag KG, Gehlbach SH, Curtis JR, Youket TE, Worley K, Lange JL. Trends in prevention of glucocorticoid-induced osteoporosis. *J Rheumatol.* 2006;33(8):1651-1657.
17. http://www.sheffield.ac.uk/FRAX/
18. De Groot K, Harper L, Jayne DR, et al. Pulse versus daily oral cyclophosphamide for induction of remission in antineutrophil cytoplasmic antibody-associated vasculitis: a randomized trial. *Ann Intern Med.* 2009;150(10):670-680.
19. De Groot K, Adu D, Savage CO. The value of pulse cyclophosphamide in ANCA-associated vasculitis: meta-analysis and critical review. *Nephrol Dial Transplant.* 2001;16(10):2018-2027.
20. Chung SA, Seo P. Advances in the use of biologic agents for the treatment of systemic vasculitis. *Curr Opin Rheumatol.* 2009;21(1):3-9.
21. Stone JH, Merkel PA, Seo P, et al. The RAVE-ITN Research Group. Rituximab versus cyclophosphamide for induction of remission in ANCA-associated vasculitis: a randomized controlled trial (RAVE). *Arthritis Rheum.* 2009;60(10(Suppl)):550.
22. Calabrese LH, Molloy ES. Therapy: rituximab and PML risk-informed decisions needed! *Nat Rev Rheumatol.* 2009;5(10):528-529.
23. De Groot K, Rasmussen N, Bacon PA, et al. Randomized trial of cyclophosphamide versus methotrexate for induction of remission in early systemic antineutrophil cytoplasmic antibody-associated vasculitis. *Arthritis Rheum.* 2005;52(8):2461-2469.
24. Joy MS, Hogan SL, Jennette JC, Falk RJ, Nachman PH. A pilot study using mycophenolate mofetil in relapsing or resistant ANCA small vessel vasculitis. *Nephrology, Dialysis, Transplantation: Official Publication of the European Dialysis and Transplant Association – European Renal Association*; December 2005;20(12):2725-2732.

25. Jayne DR, Gaskin G, Rasmussen N, et al. Randomized trial of plasma exchange or high-dosage methylprednisolone as adjunctive therapy for severe renal vasculitis. *J Am Soc Nephrol JASN*. 2007;18(7):2180-2188.

26. Perez VL, Chavala SH, Ahmed M, et al. Ocular manifestations and concepts of systemic vasculitides. *Surv Ophthalmol*. 2004;49(4):399-418.

27. Pakrou N, Selva D, Leibovitch I. Wegener's granulomatosis: ophthalmic manifestations and management. *Semin Arthritis Rheum*. 2006;35(5):284-292.

28. Bielory L. Allergic eye disorders. In: Liebermann PL, Blaiss MS, eds. *Atlas of Allergic Diseases, Chap. 11*. Philadelphia: Current Medicine Group; 2005.

29. Leibowitz HM. The red eye. *N Engl J Med*. 2000;343(5):345-351.

30. Williams CP, Browning AC, Sleep TJ, Webber SK, McGill JI. A randomised, double-blind trial of topical ketorolac vs artificial tears for the treatment of episcleritis. *Eye*. 2005;19(7):739-742.

31. Galor A, Thorne JE. Scleritis and peripheral ulcerative keratitis. *Rheum Dis Clin North Am*. 2007;33(4):835-854.

32. Jacobs D, Galetta S. Diagnosis and management of orbital pseudotumor. *Curr Opin Ophthalmol*. 2002;13(6):347-351.

33. Foster KW, Roberts D, Goodwin CR, Huang CC. Surgical pearl: preventing perioperative exposure keratopathy. *J Am Acad Dermatol*. 2005;53(4):707-708.

34. Garrity JA, Fatourechi V, Bergstralh EJ, et al. Results of transantral orbital decompression in 428 patients with severe Graves' ophthalmopathy. *Am J Ophthalmol*. 1993;116(5):533-547.

35. Fatourechi V, Bartley GB, Garrity JA, Bergstralh EJ, Ebersold MJ, Gorman CA. Transfrontal orbital decompression after failure of transantral decompression in optic neuropathy of Graves' disease. *Mayo Clin Proc*. 1993;68(6):552-555.

36. Illum P, Thorling K. Otological manifestations of Wegener's granulomatosis. *Laryngoscope*. 1982;92(7 Pt 1):801-804.

37. Hernandez-Rodriguez J, Hoffman GS, Koening CL. Surgical interventions and local therapy for Wegener's granulomatosis. *Curr Opin Rheumatol*. 2010;22(1):29-36.

38. Hoffman GS, Thomas-Golbanov CK, Chan J, Akst LM, Eliachar I. Treatment of subglottic stenosis, due to Wegener's granulomatosis, with intralesional corticosteroids and dilation. *J Rheumatol*. 2003;30(5):1017-1021.

39. Lebovics R, Hoffman G, Leavitt R. The management of subglottic stenosis in patients with Wegener's granulomatosis. *Laryngoscope*. 1992;102:1341-1345.

40. Gluth MB, Shinners PA, Kasperbauer JL. Subglottic stenosis associated with Wegener's granulomatosis. *Laryngoscope*. 2003;113(8):1304-1307.

41. Erickson VR, Hwang PH. Wegener's granulomatosis: current trends in diagnosis and management. *Curr Opin Otolaryngol Head Neck Surg*. 2007;15(3):170-176.

42. McCaffrey TV, McDonald TJ, Facer GW, DeRemee RA. Otologic manifestations of Wegener's granulomatosis. *Otolaryngol Head Neck Surg*. 1980;88(5):586-593.

43. Merkel PA, Lo GH, Holbrook JT, et al. Brief communication: high incidence of venous thrombotic events among patients with Wegener granulomatosis: the Wegener's Clinical Occurrence of Thrombosis (WeCLOT) Study. *Ann Intern Med*. 2005;142(8):620-626.

44. Bidwell JL, Pachner RW. Hemoptysis: diagnosis and management. *Am Fam Physician*. 2005;72(7):1253-1260.

45. Pagnoux C, Chironi G, Simon A, Guillevin L. Atherosclerosis in ANCA-associated vasculitides. *Ann NY Acad Sci*. 2007;1107:11-21.

46. Ghaussy NO, Du Clos TW, Ashley PA. Limited Wegener's granulomatosis presenting with complete heart block. *Scand J Rheumatol*. 2004;33(2):115-118.

47. Goodfield NE, Bhandari S, Plant WD, Morley-Davies A, Sutherland GR. Cardiac involvement in Wegener's granulomatosis. *Br Heart J*. 1995;73(2):110-115.

48. Oliveira GH, Seward JB, Tsang TS, Specks U. Echocardiographic findings in patients with Wegener granulomatosis. *Mayo Clin Proc*. 2005;80(11):1435-1440.

49. Dennert RM, van Paassen P, Schalla S, et al. Cardiac involvement in Churg-Strauss syndrome. *Arthritis Rheum*. 2010;62(2):627-634.
50. Choi MJ, Fernandez PC, Patnaik A, et al. Brief report: trimethoprim-induced hyperkalemia in a patient with AIDS. *N Engl J Med*. 1993;328:703-706.
51. Levy JB, Hammad T, Coulthart A, Dougan T, Pusey CD. Clinical features and outcome of patients with both ANCA and anti-GBM antibodies. *Kidney Int*. 2004;66(4):1535-1540.
52. Geetha D, Seo P. Renal transplantation in the ANCA-associated vasculitides. *Am J Transplant*. 2007;7(12):2657-2662.
53. Seo P, Stone JH. Small-vessel and medium-vessel vasculitis. *Arthritis Rheum*. 2007;57(8): 1552-1559.
54. Koening CL, Langford CA, Kirchner HL, et al. Renal graft survival and patient mortality in Wegener's granulomatosis (WG): a case/control study. *Arthritis Rheum*. 2007;56(9):2.
55. Pagnoux C, Mahr A, Cohen P, Guillevin L. Presentation and outcome of gastrointestinal involvement in systemic necrotizing vasculitides: analysis of 62 patients with polyarteritis nodosa, microscopic polyangiitis, Wegener granulomatosis, Churg-Strauss syndrome, or rheumatoid arthritis-associated vasculitis. *Medicine (Baltimore)*. 2005;84(2):115-128.
56. Travers R, Allison D, Brettie R, Hughes G. Polyarteritis nodosa: a clinical and angiographic analysis of 17 cases. *Semin Arthritis Rheum*. 1979;8:184-199.
57. Wolf J, Bergner R, Mutallib S, Buggle F, Grau AJ. Neurologic complications of Churg-Strauss syndrome – a prospective monocentric study. *Eur J Neurol*. 2009;17(4):582-588.
58. Hughes R. Peripheral nerve diseases: the bare essentials. *Pract Neurol*. 2008;8(6):396-405.
59. Fam AG, Lavine E, Lee L, Perez-Ordonez B, Goyal M. Cranial pachymeningitis: an unusual manifestation of Wegener's granulomatosis. *J Rheumatol*. 2003;30(9):2070-2074.
60. Daoud M, Hutton K, Gibson L. Cutaneous periarteritis nodosa: a clinicopathological study of 79 cases. *Br J Dermatol*. 1997;136:706-713.
61. Chen KR, Carlson JA. Clinical approach to cutaneous vasculitis. *Am J Clin Dermatol*. 2008;9(2):71-92.
62. Weenig RH, Davis MD, Dahl PR, Su WP. Skin ulcers misdiagnosed as pyoderma gangrenosum. *N Engl J Med*. 2002;347(18):1412-1418.
63. Hafner J, Schneider E, Burg G, Cassina PC. Management of leg ulcers in patients with rheumatoid arthritis or systemic sclerosis: the importance of concomitant arterial and venous disease. *J Vasc Surg*. 2000;32(2):322-329.

Severe Polyarteritis Nodosa

9

Loïc Guillevin and Gregory Pugnet

Abstract Polyarteritis nodosa (PAN) is a well-defined vasculitis that mainly affects medium-sized vessels. Over several decades, PAN and microscopic polyangiitis (MPA), which affects predominantly small-sized vessels, were considered a single entity. The Chapel Hill Consensus Conference Nomenclature clarified the matter: MPA is responsible for glomerulonephritis and lung capillaritis, while PAN is characterized by vascular nephropathy and never affects the lungs. Clinical manifestations compromising prognosis or responsible for major sequelae define severe PAN and include vascular nephropathy, malignant arterial hypertension, intestinal ischemia, liver infarction, coronary artery vasculitis, and left heart failure. The cause of death is often related to vasculitic involvement of vital internal organs, mainly gastrointestinal involvement, but also is associated with severe side effects associated with the use of immunosuppressive agents, mainly infections.

Keywords Gastrointestinal ischemia • Hypertension • Myocardial infarction • Polyarteritis nodosa

9.1
Introduction

Polyarteritis nodosa (PAN) was first described by Küssmaul and Maier.[1] For many decades, the now distinct vasculitides were considered together under the term PAN. Today, PAN is a well-defined vasculitis that mainly affects medium-sized vessels. Considering PAN etiologies, primary and secondary forms can also be discerned, as PAN can be the consequence of hepatitis B virus (HBV) infection[2,3] and sometimes of other etiological agents.[4-6] PAN is a rare disease. In a study[7] that considered only biopsy-proven forms, its annual incidence and

L. Guillevin (✉)
Department of Internal Medicine, National Referral Center for Rare
Systemic and Autoimmune Diseases: Vasculitides and Scleroderma, Hôpital Cochin, Assistance
Publique–Hôpitaux de Paris, University Paris Descartes, Inserm U1060 Paris, France
e-mail: loic.guillevin@cch.aphp.fr

M.A. Khamashta and M. Ramos-Casals (eds.), *Autoimmune Diseases*,
DOI: 10.1007/978-0-85729-358-9_9, © Springer-Verlag London Limited 2011

prevalence were, respectively, 0.7/100,000 and 6.3/100,000 inhabitants. Estimates of the annual incidence rate for PAN-type systemic vasculitides in a general population range from 4.6/1,000,000 in England,[7] 9.0/1,000,000 in Olmsted County, Minnesota, to 77/1,000,000 in a hepatitis B-hyperendemic, Alaskan Eskimo population.[8] In Seine–Saint-Denis County (a Paris suburb), PAN prevalence was estimated at 24/1,000,000 inhabitants in 2000.[9]

A close relationship has been demonstrated between PAN and HBV infection.[2] In France, contamination through infected blood transfusion has now disappeared, and intravenous drug use is also less frequent than it was 20 years ago.[10] Sexual transmission is one of the main routes for HBV transmission. Over the past few years, the frequency of HBV-related PAN (HBV–PAN) has declined to 7.3%[10] and only rare cases are now observed in developed countries. Clinical manifestations compromising prognosis or responsible for major sequelae define severe PAN. In this chapter, we review the main characteristics of severe PAN, its outcome, and treatment.

9.2
Classification

PAN predominantly affects medium-sized arteries. Over several decades, PAN and micro-scopic polyangiitis (MPA), which primarily affects small-sized vessels, especially arteri-oles, capillaries, and venules, were considered a single entity, thereby explaining why the majority of patient series published before the 1990s did not describe "pure forms" of PAN. The Chapel Hill Consensus Conference Nomenclature[11] has now clarified the matter, which was not the case for the classification criteria[12] established in 1990 by the American College of Rheumatology (ACR). MPA is responsible for glomerulonephritis and lung capillaritis; PAN is characterized by vascular nephropathy and never affects the lungs. MPA is one of the antineutrophil cytoplasm antibody (ANCA)–associated vasculitides. Because severe PAN can only be described and analysis to identify poor-prognosis factors can only be based on a phenotypically well-described disease, distinguishing between PAN and MPA is of major importance.

9.3
Clinical Manifestations

PAN can be observed in any patient, independently of age, but usually appears around 50 years, predominantly in men,[13] but can also develop in children and patients older than 65.[13-16] Early during the course of the disease, two-thirds of the patients are in poor general condition, which can be the sole manifestation. Every type of fever can be observed.

Patients usually complain of myalgias that are intense, diffuse, spontaneous, and/or induced by pressure. Arthralgias predominate in the major joints: knees, ankles, elbows, and wrists, but are rarely present in shoulders and hips. Pain can be localized to nerve territories. Muscle wasting can reflect weight loss, sometimes exceeding 20 kg, and paralysis. Patients can be bedridden due to the intensity of pain and amyotrophy. Clinical manifestations of PAN, independently of their severity, are detailed in Table 9.1.[13-15,17,18]

Table 9.1 Clinical features of PAN, expressed as percentages of the studied populations

Feature	Frohnert and Sheps[a,b14]	Leib et al.[a,b15]	Cohen et al.[a,b17]	Guillevin et al.[c13]	Pagnoux et al.[d 18]
Patients (n)	130	64	53	115	348
Mean [range] age (years)	[6–75]	47 [17–80]	54 [17–78]	51 [20–80]	51.2 [ND]
M/F ratio	1.9	1.1	1.9	1.8	1.7
General symptoms	76			96.5	93.1
• Fever		36	31	69	63.8
• Weight loss			16	87	69.5
Peripheral neuropathy	52	72	60	83.5	74.1
Myalgias	30			47	58.6
Arthralgias	58		55	55.7	48.9
Joints and muscles		73			
Cutaneous signs	58	28	58	31	49.7
Renal disease	8	63	66	29.6	50.6
Hypertension		25	14	31	34.8
Gastrointestinal tract signs	14	42	25	53	37.9
Respiratory symptoms	38	47	13	0	0
Central neuropathy	3	25		9.6	4.6
Cardiac and vascular signs	10	30	4	12.2	22.4
Eyes		3	8	1.7	8.6
Ear, nose, and throat involvement		3	0	0	0

ND not done

[a]Retrospective studies

[b]These series include PAN, MPA, and sometimes Churg–Strauss patients

[c]Only HBV–PAN

[d]PAN with and without HBV

9.3.1
Severe Manifestations

9.3.1.1
Renal Involvement

Renal manifestations of vascular nephropathy can be responsible for renal insufficiency of variable intensity, but pauci-immune crescentic glomerulonephritis is never observed. Severe or malignant arterial hypertension[18] may occur as a complication of PAN.

Acute renal insufficiency occurs early during the course of PAN or at the time of a flare. During the early phase or later, when renal failure follows chronic renal ischemic deterioration, some patients may require hemodialysis. The outcome of renal insufficiency cannot be predicted and improvement may occur. Some patients may be able to come off dialysis, but end-stage renal failure may develop years after the early manifestations of PAN.

In patients with renal involvement, angiography, when performed, shows renal infarcts, responsible for renal insufficiency, multiple stenoses, and microaneurysms of branches of digestive and renal arteries. Microaneurysms rupture rarely, spontaneously or after renal biopsy.[19-21] Renal hematoma can be extensive, and requires embolization[22,23] and even nephrectomy should it fail.[22]

9.3.1.2
Gastrointestinal Involvement

Gastrointestinal tract involvement is one of the most severe manifestations of PAN,[18] especially when associated with HBV infection.[13,24] Abdominal pain occurs in one-quarter to one-third of the patients and can be the first symptom. A majority of patients have ischemia of the small bowel, but rarely the colon or stomach. Small intestine perforation and digestive bleeding[24] are the most severe manifestations. Gastric perforations are rare[25] as are those of the esophagus.

Relapses after surgery or medical treatment are signs of poor prognosis. Digestive malabsorption and acute or chronic pancreatitis with pseudo-cysts have been described[26]; their prognoses are extremely dismal. Vasculitis of the appendix or gallbladder[27] is sometimes the first PAN symptom; its significance is not equivocal: It is sometimes a pathological curiosity without any other clinical, pathological, and/or immunological involvement of vasculitis. In other cases, cholecystitis or appendicitis is another symptom of PAN. The prognoses of these manifestations seem different, depending upon whether one or the other is the first sign of PAN or a complication of previously diagnosed and treated PAN. In the former situation, the prognosis remains good; however, when these symptoms occur during the course of PAN, they often precede other severe symptoms of gastrointestinal involvement and the prognosis is poor.

Liver involvement, such as infarction and hematomas,[28] can exist, even in the absence of HBV infection.

9.3.1.3
Cardiac Involvement

Vasculitis of the coronary arteries or their branches, or severe or malignant hypertension is responsible for cardiac manifestations. Radiological and electrocardiogram abnormalities had occurred in 40% of PAN patients, 78% of whom had histological cardiac manifestations, mainly affecting the myocardium, found subsequently during autopsy.[29]

In our experience, despite coronary artery vasculitis, angina is rare and coronary angiography is usually normal. Specific myocardial involvement is the sequential consequence of inflammation, stenosis, and/or thrombosis and, finally, coronary artery occlusion. Stenosis(es) can be seen in the main coronary arteries, as described by Küssmaul and Maier[1] (nodular coronary arteritis), and were present in 25/66 autopsies performed by Holsinger et al.[29] Although coronary aneurysms sometimes occur, ruptures are rare. Most cases have been described in infants[30] and, retrospectively, we postulate that most of them could have been Kawasaki disease misdiagnosed as PAN. Nonetheless, aneurysms cannot be excluded in adults,[31] even though we must admit never having seen one in our specialized referral center. Arterioles can also be affected, and foci of myocardial necrosis can be seen.[29]

Left heart failure is the most frequent manifestation of cardiac involvement. When cardiac insufficiency is present, it occurs early during the course of PAN. Heart enlargement was observed in a quarter of the patients in a reported series.[32] Atrioventricular block, like severe ventricular rhythm disturbances, is extremely rare. Supraventricular rhythm disturbances are more frequent than ventricular rhythm disturbances. The vasculitic process more rarely affects the pericardium, and pericarditis is usually a nonspecific satellite of myocardial involvement. Pericardial involvement is rare and asymptomatic. However, pericarditis can be the first manifestation of PAN and pericardium biopsy can make the diagnosis. Biological markers, such as brain natriuretic peptide (BNP) or its precursor protein N-terminal proBNP (NT-proBNP), could contribute to an early diagnosis of cardiac insufficiency and troponin I determination could reveal myocardial involvement.

Imaging techniques also have a major role to play, not only echocardiography, but also magnetic resonance imaging (MRI), which can detect myocardial signals of vasculitis and is able to study precisely cardiac function parameters and visualize pericardial and myocardial involvements. No literature on PAN is available, but such techniques are already being used in Churg–Strauss syndrome[33] and other vasculitides.

Arterial hypertension is present in 34–36% of PAN patients and is usually mild[13,18]; however, it should be kept in mind that it can be triggered or adversely affected by corticosteroids. Malignant hypertension was detected in 6/115 (5.2%) of our HBV–PAN patients[13] and 11/125 (4.9%) PAN patients without HBV infection.[18] Hypertension is more frequent in HBV–PAN. It responds well to angiotensin-converting-enzyme inhibitors, which improved its prognosis.[34]

9.3.2
Other Situations

9.3.2.1
Peripheral Neuropathy

Motor, sensory, or sensory–motor peripheral neuropathy, mainly distal and asymmetrical, is the most frequent neurological manifestation of PAN, observed in around 70% of the patients. Mononeuritis multiplex is common. The most frequently involved nerves are superficial peroneal, deep peroneal, radial, cubital, and/or median nerves. Paralysis occurs early, usually during the first trimester. Peripheral neuropathy can be the first manifestation of PAN.

Sensory symptoms can be predominant, mostly hypoesthesia. Deep sensory nerve transmissions are never affected. The electromyogram is characteristic of truncular axonal neuropathy. Symmetrical neuropathy is observed less frequently.

Cranial nerve palsies are extremely rare. Cerebrospinal fluid analyses are usually normal. Some clinicians consider peripheral neuropathy a severe symptom of PAN. In fact, although neuropathy can induce sequelae and severely limit function (motor and sensory), it does not aggravate prognosis. Therefore, peripheral neuropathy, when it occurs, does not require treatment intensification, which has never been proven more effective than steroids alone to obtain the regression of motor or sensory involvement.

9.3.2.2
Central Nervous System Involvement

CNS involvement is rare, but focal or generalized seizures, hemiplegia, and brain hemorrhage can be seen. The central manifestations differ according to the location and mechanisms involved: brain arteritis, aneurysm rupture, or hematoma. Computed-tomography scans are usually normal, but MRI shows T_2-weighted hypersignals in the brain, localized to the white matter. Brain angiography can show caliber irregularities more clearly, thereby orienting the diagnosis. Ischemic or hemorrhagic seizures can also be the consequence of malignant hypertension. In the first published version of the FFS, CNS involvement was one of the five severity criteria. In the revised version of the FFS,[35] CNS is no longer a criterion of poor prognosis, because CNS manifestations are rarely life-threatening, even though they can cause irreversible brain damage and loss of function.

9.3.2.3
Orchitis

This rare manifestation is one of the most characteristic of PAN,[18] and it was retained as an ACR classification criterion.[12] Noninfectious orchitis is rarely the first manifestation affecting the testicular artery. When treated immediately, orchitis may regress under steroids. Exclusive testicular involvement evokes a tumor or testicular torsion.[36]

9.3.2.4
Skin Involvement

Vascular purpura is common in PAN. Because they contain medium-sized vessels, skin nodules can be present. Cutaneous manifestations are predominantly located on the legs. Nodules are small, ranging in diameter from 0.5 to 2 cm, and found in the dermis and hypodermis. They appear and disappear within a few days. Livedo racemosa or reticularis can be observed. Post-inflammatory ischemic leg ulcers can arise and are recognized by their topography.

9.3.2.5
Peripheral Vascular Manifestations

Arterial obstruction is responsible for distal digital gangrene. Angiography can demonstrate the presence of stenoses and/or microaneurysms. Raynaud's phenomenon, when present, can remain isolated or be complicated by necrosis. In some cases, type II or III cryoglobulinemia can be present. Although cryoglobulinemia is usually detected in the setting of hepatitis C virus infection, and not PAN, it can occur in HBV–PAN, in which case, it disappears after treatment.

9.3.2.6
PAN Associated with HBV Infection

The immunological process responsible for this PAN subgroup usually manifests in less than 6 months after HBV infection.[37] Hepatitis is rarely diagnosed and remains silent before PAN onset. PAN occurrence several years after HBV contamination suggests that virus mutants could induce it. Clinical manifestations are roughly the same as those commonly seen in PAN. HBe-antigen-to-anti-HBe-antibody seroconversion usually leads to recovery. Sequelae are the consequence of vascular nephropathy.

Abdominal manifestations (53%) are common, especially surgical emergencies. Among the nine patients studied by Sergent et al.,[38] two of the three deaths were attributed to colon vasculitis. Furthermore, 31% of Eskimo patients described by McMahon et al.[8] died, and one of the four early deaths was the consequence of bowel perforation. In our study,[13] 41/115 (35.6%) patients died, 7/41 (17%) of them attributed to gastrointestinal involvement. Hepatic manifestations of PAN are moderate.

9.4
Diagnostic Approach

9.4.1
Laboratory Abnormalities

Inflammatory signs are found in more than 80% of the patients. Hypereosinophilia >1,500/mm^3 is rare. HBs antigen should be systematically sought, even though it was found in only one-third of the patients.[18]

ANCA are not detected in the sera of PAN patients and we consider that, in the context of systemic vasculitides, the presence of perinuclear-labeling P-ANCA, with anti-myeloperoxidase specificity in ELISA, should be considered exclusionary for "classic-PAN."[39]

9.4.2
Angiographic Studies

Angiography is able to visualize microaneurysms and stenoses (narrowing or tapering) in medium-sized vessels. They are not pathognomonic but are frequently present in PAN. Arterial saccular or fusiform aneurysms range in size from 1 to 5 mm and are predominantly seen in the kidneys, mesentery, and liver. These lesions may disappear with arteritis regression.[40] Angiography can be a useful diagnostic tool.

9.4.3
Histopathological Studies

Biopsies are diagnostic when they show necrotizing vasculitis. They should be oriented and preferably taken from a clinically affected organ. Skin, muscle, and nerve are the sites usually considered for biopsy. Diagnosis can also be made on surgical specimens. In patients presenting with fever, myalgias, weight loss, and other general symptoms, a muscle biopsy can be positive. Vasculitis is more frequently positive when distal muscles are biopsied.

9.5
Outcome and Prognosis

PAN is a disease that relapses more frequently in the absence of HBV infection: less than 10% of HBV–PAN patients[13] versus 28% of non-HBV–PAN patients.[18]

9.5.1
The Five-Factor Score (FFS)

The FFS comprises four clinical symptoms associated with a poor outcome (renal insufficiency [serum creatinine > 140 μmol/L], cardiomyopathy, gastrointestinal involvement, and age over 65 years) and the absence of ear, nose, and throat symptoms.[35] Those symptoms are detailed in the preceding chapter. The prognostic score was validated on 1,108 patients with systemic necrotizing vasculitides: PAN, Churg–Strauss syndrome, MPA, or Wegener's granulomatosis. Ear, nose, and throat manifestations are not relevant to evaluating PAN severity and are only pertinent for Wegener's granulomatosis and Churg–Strauss syndrome.

9.5.2
Mortality

The causes of deaths can be divided into two categories: related to vasculitis manifestations or treatment side effects. In all vasculitides, when major organs are involved, lethal complications can occur. A few patients die early from multiorgan involvement, and treatment is unable to control their disease. Death occurs during the course of PAN characterized by fever, rapid weight loss, diffuse pain, and one or several major organ involvement(s). It often occurs during the first months after disease onset and is often the consequence of gastrointestinal involvement.[18]

Adverse events are frequently responsible for deaths. Deaths occurring during the first months of the disease are often due to uncontrolled vasculitis; fatalities during the following years may be the consequence of treatment side effects. Infections are the primary cause of death and are favored by corticosteroids and/or cytotoxic agents.[18,41] Lowering drug doses and shortening treatment durations could contribute to diminishing such complications. Viral infections usually occur later. *Pneumocystis jiroveci* pneumonia has become a rare event since the systematic implementation of co-trimoxazole prophylaxis.[42]

9.6
Treatment

9.6.1
Indications of Corticosteroids Alone

Steroids alone are effective when prescribed to treat PAN without poor-prognosis factors, i.e., FFS=0,[43] and obtained survival rates similar to those of patients whose regimen combined corticosteroids and cyclophosphamide. Steroids must be combined with cytotoxic to treat severe PAN.

9.6.2
Indications of Corticosteroids and Cyclophosphamide

Steroids and immunosuppressants, especially cyclophosphamide, have transformed the prognosis of non-HBV–PAN. Corticosteroids alone were able to increase the 5-year survival rate from 10% for untreated patients to about 55% in the mid-to-late 1960s. Survival was further prolonged by adding an immunosuppressant, either azathioprine or cyclophosphamide, to the treatment regimen.

When cyclophosphamide is indicated for severe PAN, an intravenous pulse should be preferred to oral administration, as it achieves a more rapid clinical response, which is particularly important for patients with active disease. When combined with corticosteroids, intravenous cyclophosphamide should not exceed 12 pulses. At present, we recommend pulse cyclophosphamide until remission is obtained and then prescribe 12–18 months of maintenance therapy, with azathioprine or methotrexate, as has also been demonstrated for ANCA-positive systemic necrotizing vasculitides.[44,45]

9.6.3
Treatment of HBV– and Other Virus-Related–PAN

Virus-associated vasculitides require specific treatments. In the context of chronic hepatitis B, steroids and immunosuppressants can effectively treat vasculitis and the short-term outcome is comparable to strategies comprising plasma exchange (PE) and antiviral agents.[13]

However, immunosuppressants have deleterious effects: they enhance virus replication, and, over the long term, they perpetuate chronic HBV infection and facilitate progression toward cirrhosis, which may be complicated later by hepatocellular carcinoma.

Based on the efficacies of antiviral drugs against chronic hepatitis and PE for PAN, we combined the two therapies to treat HBV–PAN. The rationale of the therapeutic sequence was for initial corticosteroids to rapidly control the most severe life-threatening PAN manifestations, which are common during the first weeks of overt vasculitis, and for their abrupt withdrawal to enhance immunological clearance of HBV-infected hepatocytes and favor HBe-antigen-to-anti-HBe-antibody seroconversion, with PE to control the course of PAN.

A regimen combining an antiviral agent (vidarabine, interferon-α2b or, more recently, lamivudine) and PE to treat HBV–PAN obtained excellent overall therapeutic results within a few weeks.[13] The antiviral strategy increased the seroconversion rate from 14.7% with conventional treatment to 49.4% for patients receiving an antiviral agent and PE.[13]

9.6.4
Plasma Exchange

There is presently no argument to support the systematic prescription of plasma exchange (PE) at the time of diagnosis of non-HBV–PAN, even for patients with poor-prognosis factors. A prospective trial organized by the EUVAS Group confirmed that PE significantly improved renal function better than pulse corticosteroids in patients with ANCA-associated vasculitides with severe glomerulonephritis, but had no effect on survival.[44] Despite the lack of evidence and no prospective trial, PE is a useful tool as second-line treatment of PAN refractory to conventional therapy.

9.6.5
Biotherapies

Several biotherapies have been proposed, and some are under evaluation to treat vasculitides. All the efforts have been focused on ANCA-associated vasculitides, and the first results are encouraging. In Kawasaki disease, which shares histology with PAN, intravenous immunoglobulins have been proven effective.[46] However, intravenous immunoglobulins, antitumor necrosis factor-α (TNFα) (infliximab, etanercept and adalimumab), and anti-CD20 (rituximab) biologics have not shown any efficacy against PAN. Moreover, no rationale exists for such prescription. Therefore, it is not recommended that these treatments be prescribed outside of clinical trials.

9.6.6
Specific Treatments

Specific treatments for hypertension, pain, and motor rehabilitation are also important elements in the overall therapeutic regimen for PAN patients. Since maximal immunosuppression is given at treatment onset, prevention of opportunistic infections, like *Pneumocystis jiroveci* pneumonia, may be necessary and should be prescribed on an individual basis.[47] In the case of gastrointestinal involvement with persistent abdominal pain, despite medical treatment, exploratory surgery should be performed to look for and treat bowel perforation masked by the corticosteroid-and-immunosuppressant regimen. For these patients, it seems reasonable to administer drugs intravenously to circumvent possibly impaired drug absorption. Rapid and severe weight loss due to severe gastrointestinal involvement must be countered with parenteral nutrition. Despite the fact that weight loss has not been demonstrated to be a factor of poor prognosis, good general condition is always preferable, because it contributes to limiting the infection rate under cytotoxic agents.

References

1. Küssmaul A, Maier K. Über eine nicht bisher beschriebene eigenthümliche Arterienerkrankung (Periarteritis Nodosa), die mit Morbus Brightii und rapid fortschreitender allgemeiner Muskelähmung einhergeht. *Dtsch Arch Klin Med*. 1866;1:484-518.
2. Trépo C, Thivolet J. Hepatitis associated antigen and periarteritis nodosa (PAN). *Vox Sang*. 1970;19:410-411.
3. Prince AM, Trepo C. Role of immune complexes involving SH antigen in pathogenesis of chronic active hepatitis and polyarteritis nodosa. *Lancet*. 1971;1:1309-1312.
4. Calabrese LH. Vasculitis and infection with the human immunodeficiency virus. *Rheum Dis Clin North Am*. 1991;17:131-147.
5. Corman LC, Dolson DJ. Polyarteritis nodosa and parvovirus B19 infection. *Lancet*. 1992;339:491.
6. Mader R, Schaffer I, Schonfeld S. Recurrent poststreptococcal cutaneous polyarteritis nodosa. *Isr J Med Sci*. 1988;24:269-270.
7. Scott DG, Bacon PA, Elliott PJ, Tribe CR, Wallington TB. Systemic vasculitis in a district general hospital 1972–1980: clinical and laboratory features, classification and prognosis of 80 cases. *Q J Med*. 1982;51:292-311.
8. McMahon BJ, Heyward WL, Templin DW, Clement D, Lanier AP. Hepatitis B-associated polyarteritis nodosa in Alaskan Eskimos: clinical and epidemiologic features and long-term follow-up. *Hepatology*. 1989;9:97-101.
9. Mahr A, Guillevin L, Poissonnet M, Ayme S. Prevalences of polyarteritis nodosa, microscopic polyangiitis, Wegener's granulomatosis, and Churg-Strauss syndrome in a French urban multiethnic population in 2000: a capture-recapture estimate. *Arthritis Rheum*. 2004;51:92-99.
10. Guillevin L, Lhote F. Distinguishing polyarteritis nodosa from microscopic polyangiitis and implications for treatment. *Curr Opin Rheumatol*. 1995;7:20-24.
11. Jennette JC, Falk RJ, Andrassy K, et al. Nomenclature of systemic vasculitides. Proposal of an international consensus conference. *Arthritis Rheum*. 1994;37:187-192.
12. Lightfoot RW Jr, Michel BA, Bloch DA, et al. The American College of Rheumatology 1990 criteria for the classification of polyarteritis nodosa. *Arthritis Rheum*. 1990;33:1088-1093.
13. Guillevin L, Mahr A, Callard P, et al. Hepatitis B virus-associated polyarteritis nodosa: clinical characteristics, outcome, and impact of treatment in 115 patients. *Medicine (Baltimore)*. 2005;84:313-322.
14. Frohnert PP, Sheps SG. Long-term follow-up study of periarteritis nodosa. *Am J Med*. 1967;43:8-14.

15. Leib ES, Restivo C, Paulus HE. Immunosuppressive and corticosteroid therapy of polyarteritis nodosa. *Am J Med*. 1979;67:941-947.
16. Mouthon L, Le Toumelin P, Andre MH, Gayraud M, Casassus P, Guillevin L. Polyarteritis nodosa and Churg-Strauss angiitis: characteristics and outcome in 38 patients over 65 years. *Medicine (Baltimore)*. 2002;81:27-40.
17. Cohen RD, Conn DL, Ilstrup DM. Clinical features, prognosis, and response to treatment in polyarteritis. *Mayo Clin Proc*. 1980;55:146-155.
18. Pagnoux C, Seror R, Henegar C, et al. Clinical features and outcomes in 348 patients with polyarteritis nodosa: a systematic retrospective study of patients diagnosed between 1963 and 2005 and entered into the French Vasculitis Study Group Database. *Arthritis Rheum*. 2010;62: 616-626.
19. Akcicek F, Dilber S, Ozgen G, et al. Spontaneous perirenal hematoma due to periarteritis nodosa. *Nephron*. 1994;68:396.
20. Cornfield JZ, Johnson ML, Dolehide J, Fowler JE Jr. Massive renal hemorrhage owing to polyarteritis nodosa. *J Urol*. 1988;140:808-809.
21. Sagcan A, Tunc E, Keser G, et al. Spontaneous bilateral perirenal hematoma as a complication of polyarteritis nodosa in a patient with human immunodeficiency virus infection. *Rheumatol Int*. 2002;21:239-242.
22. Daskalopoulos G, Karyotis I, Heretis I, Anezinis P, Mavromanolakis E, Delakas D. Spontaneous perirenal hemorrhage: a 10-year experience at our institution. *Int Urol Nephrol*. 2004;36:15-19.
23. Hachulla E, Bourdon F, Taieb S, et al. Embolization of two bleeding aneurysms with platinum coils in a patient with polyarteritis nodosa. *J Rheumatol*. 1993;20:158-161.
24. Pagnoux C, Mahr A, Cohen P, Guillevin L. Presentation and outcome of gastrointestinal involvement in systemic necrotizing vasculitides: analysis of 62 patients with polyarteritis nodosa, microscopic polyangiitis, Wegener granulomatosis, Churg-Strauss syndrome, or rheumatoid arthritis-associated vasculitis. *Medicine (Baltimore)*. 2005;84:115-128.
25. Gourgoutis GD, Paguirigan AA, Berzins T. Gastric perforation in polyarteritis nodosa. Report of a patient. *Am J Dig Dis*. 1971;16:171-177.
26. Suresh E, Beadles W, Welsby P, Luqmani R. Acute pancreatitis with pseudocyst formation in a patient with polyarteritis nodosa. *J Rheumatol*. 2005;32:386-388.
27. Chen KT. Gallbladder vasculitis. *J Clin Gastroenterol*. 1989;11:537-540.
28. Nakazawa K, Itoh N, Duan HJ, Komiyama Y, Shigematsu H. Polyarteritis nodosa with atrophy of the left hepatic lobe. *Acta Pathol Jpn*. 1992;42:662-666.
29. Holsinger DR, Osmundson PJ, Edwards JE. The heart in periarteritis nodosa. *Circulation*. 1962;25:610-618.
30. Bowyer S, Mason WH, McCurdy DK, Takahashi M. Polyarteritis nodosa (PAN) with coronary aneurysms: the kawasaki-PAN controversy revisited. *J Rheumatol*. 1994;21:1585.
31. Maillard-Lefebvre H, Launay D, Mouquet F, et al. Polyarteritis nodosa-related coronary aneurysms. *J Rheumatol*. 2008;35:933-934.
32. Bletry O, Godeau P, Charpentier G, Guillevin L, Herreman G. Cardiac manifestations of periarteritis nodosa. Incidence of non-hypertensive cardiomyopathy. *Arch Mal Coeur Vaiss*. 1980;73:1027-1036.
33. Marmursztejn J, Vignaux O, Cohen P, et al. Impact of cardiac magnetic resonance imaging for assessment of Churg-Strauss syndrome: a cross-sectional study in 20 patients. *Clin Exp Rheumatol*. 2009;27(1 Suppl 52):S70-S76.
34. Cohen L, Guillevin L, Meyrier A, Bironne P, Bletry O, Godeau P. Hypertension artérielle maligne de la périartérite noueuse. Incidence, caractéristiques clinico-biologiques et pronostic d'une série de 165 patients. *Arch Mal Coeur Vaiss*. 1986;79:773-778.
35. Guillevin L, Pagnoux C, Seror R, et al. The Five-Factor Score revisited: assessment of prognoses of systemic necrotizing vasculitides based on the FVSG cohort. *Medicine (Baltimore)*. 2011;90:19-27.

36. Warfield AT, Lee SJ, Phillips SM, Pall AA. Isolated testicular vasculitis mimicking a testicular neoplasm. *J Clin Pathol.* 1994;47:1121-1123.
37. Stroup SP, Herrera SR, Crain DS. Bilateral testicular infarction and orchiectomy as a complication of polyarteritis nodosa. *Rev Urol.* 2007;9:235-238.
38. Sergent JS, Lockshin MD, Christian CL, Gocke DJ. Vasculitis with hepatitis B antigenemia: long-term observation in nine patients. *Medicine (Baltimore).* 1976;55:1-18.
39. Henegar C, Pagnoux C, Puechal X, et al. A paradigm of diagnostic criteria for polyarteritis nodosa: analysis of a series of 949 patients with vasculitides. *Arthritis Rheum.* 2008;58:1528-1538.
40. Darras-Joly C, Lortholary O, Cohen P, Brauner M, Guillevin L. Regressing microaneurysms in 5 cases of hepatitis B virus related polyarteritis nodosa. *J Rheumatol.* 1995;22:876-880.
41. Bourgarit A, Le Toumelin P, Pagnoux C, et al. Deaths occurring during the first year after treatment onset for polyarteritis nodosa, microscopic polyangiitis, and Churg-Strauss syndrome: a retrospective analysis of causes and factors predictive of mortality based on 595 patients. *Medicine (Baltimore).* 2005;84:323-330.
42. Jarrousse B, Guillevin L, Bindi P, et al. Increased risk of Pneumocystis carinii pneumonia in patients with Wegener's granulomatosis. *Clin Exp Rheumatol.* 1993;11:615-621.
43. Ribi C, Cohen P, Pagnoux C, et al. Treatment of polyarteritis nodosa and microscopic polyangiitis without poor-prognosis factors: a prospective randomized study on 124 patients. *Arthritis Rheum.* 2010;62:1186-1197.
44. Jayne D, Rasmussen N, Andrassy K, et al. A randomized trial of maintenance therapy for vasculitis associated with antineutrophil cytoplasmic autoantibodies. *N Engl J Med.* 2003;349:36-44.
45. Pagnoux C, Mahr A, Hamidou MA, et al. Azathioprine or methotrexate maintenance for ANCA-associated vasculitis. *N Engl J Med.* 2008;359:2790-2803.
46. Newburger J, Takahashi M, Beiser A, et al. A single intravenous infusion of gamma globulin as compared with four infusions in the treatment of acute Kawasaki syndrome. *N Engl J Med.* 1991;324:1633-1639.
47. Godeau B, Coutant-Perronne V, Le Thi Huong D, et al. Pneumocystis carinii pneumonia in the course of connective tissue disease: report of 34 cases. *J Rheumatol.* 1994;21:246-251.

Life-Threatening Cryoglobulinemia

10

Soledad Retamozo, Cándido Díaz-Lagares, Xavier Bosch,
Salvatore de Vita, and Manuel Ramos-Casals

Abstract Cryoglobulins are immunoglobulins that precipitate in vitro at temperatures <37°C and produce organ damage through two main etiopathogenic pathways, accumulation (hyperviscosity syndrome) and autoimmune-mediated mechanisms (vasculitis). Although cryoglobulinemia is associated with a large number of processes (mainly infections, autoimmune diseases, and cancer), the main cause is hepatitis C virus infection. Cryoglobulinemic disease is diagnosed when typical organ involvement appears in a patient with circulating cryoglobulins. Cutaneous purpura is the most indicative and frequent manifestation of cryoglobulinemic vasculitis, while the most frequently affected internal organs are the joints, kidneys, and peripheral nerves. The evolution varies widely, and the prognosis is heavily influenced not only by cryoglobulinemic damage to vital organs but also by the associated underlying diseases. Cryoglobulinemia may result in progressive (renal involvement) or acute (pulmonary hemorrhage, gastrointestinal ischemia, CNS involvement) organ damage. The mortality rate of intestinal ischemia and alveolar hemorrhage is >80% after the first episode and reaches 100% after a second episode. Unfortunately, this may be the first cryoglobulinemic involvement in almost two-thirds of cases, highlighting the complex management and very elevated mortality of these cases.

Keywords Cryoglobulinemia • Cryoglobulinemic glomerulonephritis • Intestinal ischemia • Pulmonary hemorrhage • Vasculitis

S. Retamozo (✉)
Department of Autoimmune Diseases, Laboratory of Autoimmune Diseases
Josep Font, Institut d'Investigacions Biomèdiques August Pi i Sunyer
(IDIBAPS), C/Villaroel 170, 08036 Barcelona, Spain
e-mail: soleretamozo@hotmail.com

M.A. Khamashta and M. Ramos-Casals (eds.), *Autoimmune Diseases*,
DOI: 10.1007/978-0-85729-358-9_10, © Springer-Verlag London Limited 2011

10.1
Introduction

Cryoglobulins are immunoglobulins (Ig) that precipitate when serum is incubated at lower than 37°C. Although circulating cryoglobulins are not always related to the presence of symptomatology, nearly half of the patients with cryoglobulinemia have clinical manifestations of systemic vasculitis.[1] Cryoglobulinemic vasculitis mainly affects the small- and, less frequently, medium-sized arteries and veins,[2] which are thought to be damaged by deposition of immune complexes on their walls, with the subsequent activation of the complement cascade.[3] Cryoglobulins have been observed in a wide variety of diseases, including malignancies, infections, and systemic autoimmune diseases.[4,5] A viral origin of cryoglobulinemia was long suspected, but it was not until the beginning of the 1990s that there was evidence of a close relation with the hepatitis C virus (HCV).[6-8] The distinctive etiopathogenic feature of cryoglobulinemia is an underlying B cell clonal expansion that mainly involves rheumatoid factor–secreting cells.[9,10]

In 1966, Meltzer et al.[11] described the typical clinical symptoms associated with cryoglobulinemia (purpura, arthralgia, and weakness). Subsequent studies in large series of patients[12-14] have described a broad spectrum of clinical features involving the skin, joints, kidneys, and peripheral nerves. As in other systemic vasculitides, some cryoglobulinemic patients may present with potentially life-threatening situations involving internal organs such as the kidneys, lungs, gastrointestinal tract, and central nervous system (CNS). However, there is very limited information on the prognosis and management of these patients. In this chapter, we analyze the etiology, clinical manifestations, immunological features, and outcomes of patients with life-threatening and complex situations associated with cryoglobulinemic vasculitis.

10.2
Definition of Life-Threatening Cryoglobulinemia

The following organ involvements were considered as potentially life-threatening in patients with cryoglobulinemic vasculitis:

(a) Renal failure: cryoglobulinemic glomerulonephritis presenting with raised serum creatinine >1.5 mg/dL; glomerular injury was diagnosed by renal biopsy and classified as membranoproliferative glomerulonephritis, mesangial proliferative glomerulonephritis, or focal proliferative glomerulonephritis according to previous studies[12]

(b) Gastrointestinal involvement: vasculitic involvement of the esophagus, stomach, small intestine, colon, or any intra-abdominal viscera, presenting as gastrointestinal hemorrhage, intestinal ischemia, acute pancreatitis, or acute cholecystitis

(c) Pulmonary hemorrhage leading to respiratory failure, in the absence of pulmonary edema, adult respiratory distress syndrome, infectious pneumonia, lung cancer, or granulomatous disease

(d) Central nervous system (CNS) involvement: cerebral ischemia (in the absence of hypercoagulability or cardiovascular disease), cerebral hemorrhage, spinal cord, or cranial nerve involvement

(e) Digital ischemic necrosis due to biopsy-proven vasculitic involvement
(f) Myocardial involvement: coronary vasculitic involvement leading to myocardial infarction, in the absence of cardiovascular diseases

10.3
General Characteristics

A review of literature between 1971 and April 2010 identified 311 patients with life-threatening cryoglobulinemia, 30 (10%) with more than one manifestation (Table 10.1). There were 176 (57%) women and 135 (43%) men, with a mean age at diagnosis of

Table 10.1 Epidemiologic features, associated processes, mean cryocrit, and causes of death in patients with life-threatening cryoglobulinemia, according to the clinical presentation

	Renal failure ($n=223$)	Gastrointestinal ($n=43$)	CNS involvement ($n=39$)	Pulmonary hemorrhage ($n=17$)
Sex (female) (%)	128 (58)	22 (51)	22 (56)	7 (41)
Mean age at diagnosis of cryoglobulinemic syndrome (years)	51 (25–81)	56 (28–81)	53 (30–74)	53 (36–87)
Mean age at life-threatening involvement (years)	53 (25–81)	58 (28–81)	54 (30–76)	54 (36–87)
Associated conditions (%)				
Chronic viral infection	169 (76)	35 (81)		10 (59)
HCV infection	164 (74)	34 (79)	35 (90)	9 (53)
HBV infection	5 (2)	1 (2)	2 (5)	1 (6)
Autoimmune diseases	12 (5)	4 (9)	3 (8)	2 (12)
Neoplasia	6 (3)	2 (5)	2 (5)	1 (6)
Idiopathic (essential)	36 (16)	2 (5)	4 (10)	4 (23)
Mean cryocrit (%)	9% ($n=45$)	11.8% ($n=11$)	3.2% ($n=13$)	14% ($n=10$)
Death (%)	90 (40)	13 (30)	15 (38)	12 (70)
Causes of death (%):				
Infectious processes	25 (28)	4 (12)	3 (20)	4 (33)
Cryoglobulinemia vasculitis	21 (23)	8 (61)	9 (60)	7 (58)
Chronic renal failure ($n=15$)				–
Acute renal failure ($n=3$)	–			–
Cardiovascular events	16 (18)	1 (8)	–	–
Liver-related processes	11 (12)	–	–	–
Neoplasia	5 (5)	–	3 (20)	1 (6)
Multiorganic failure	4 (4)	–	–	
Other	8 (9)			

Percentages are given in parentheses. Causes of death were classified according to the ICD-9 and ICD-10 codes *HCV* hepatitis C virus

cryoglobulinemia of 54 years (range, 25–87) and a mean age at life-threatening involvement of 55 years (range, 25–87). In 266 (86%) patients, life-threatening involvement was the first clinical manifestation of cryoglobulinemia. Severe involvement appeared after a mean time of 1.2 years (range 1–11) after the diagnosis of cryoglobulinemic vasculitis. Two hundred and forty-one (77%) patients had associated chronic viral infections, including HCV infection in 209, HBV infection in 6, HIV infection in 1, and viral coinfection in the remaining 25 patients (HCV–HIV coinfection in 21, HCV–HBV coinfection in 3, HCV–CMV coinfection in 1). Other etiologies included systemic autoimmune diseases in 19 (6%) and neoplasias in 11. In the remaining 47 (15%) cases, no etiology was identified (essential cryoglobulinemia). Treatment of the life-threatening cryoglobulinemia included corticosteroids in 210 cases, plasmapheresis in 178, immunosuppressive agents in 113, rituximab in 29, and infliximab in 2 cases. Of the 209 HCV patients, 154 received antiviral therapy (interferon (IFN-α) monotherapy in 88, combined IFN-α and ribavirin in 65, and ribavirin monotherapy in 1). Urgent surgery was performed in 15 patients. Fourteen months (range, 3–120) was a mean follow-up from the diagnosis of life-threatening cryoglobulinemia. One hundred and thirty-eight patients (44%) died due to cryoglobulinemic vasculitis in 38 (27%) (chronic renal failure in 15, ischemic colitis in 7, pulmonary hemorrhage in 6, acute renal failure in 3 patients, coronary vasculitis in 3, cerebral hemorrhages in 2, and CNS vasculitis in 2), sepsis in 34 (25%), cardiovascular disease in 17 (12%), liver processes in 12 (9%), multiorganic failure in 9 (6%), neoplasia in 8 (6%), and other complications in 20 patients (14%).

10.4
Life-Threatening Cryoglobulinemic Presentations

10.4.1
Renal Failure Due to Glomerulonephritis

Two hundred and twenty-three cases of biopsy-proven cryoglobulinemic glomerulonephritis presenting with renal failure have been reported[15-66] (Table 10.2). There were 128 (58%) women and 95 (42%) men, with a mean age at diagnosis of cryoglobulinemic vasculitis of 51 years (range, 25–87) and of 53 (range, 25–87) at diagnosis of glomerulonephritis. The mean time between diagnosis of cryoglobulinemia and life-threatening involvement was 16 months (range, 0–168). Clinical presentation consisted of nephrotic syndrome in 115 (52%) patients and nephritic syndrome (proteinuria, hypertension, general edemas) in 44 (20%), while the remaining 64 (29%) patients had an indolent presentation with asymptomatic raised creatinine levels. Renal biopsy disclosed membranoproliferative glomerulonephritis in 195 (87%) cases, mesangial proliferative glomerulonephritis in 14 (6%), focal proliferative glomerulonephritis in 9 (4%), and other histopathological lesions in 5 (2%) patients. Other cryoglobulinemic manifestations included purpura in 152 (68%) patients, articular involvement in 129 (58%), peripheral neuropathy in 83 (37%) patients, and fever in 13 (6%). Cryocrit levels were detailed in 45 patients with a mean cryocrit level of 9% (range, 0.5–80%) while cryocrit quantification was detailed in 16 (mean of 284 mg/dL, ranging from 0.19 to 2,434 mg/dL).

Table 10.2 Epidemiologic features, associated processes, mean cryocrit, and causes of death in patients with life-threatening renal cryogloblinemic involvement

	Renal failure (*n*=223) (%)
Sex (female) (%)	128 (58)
Mean age at diagnosis of cryoglobulinemia (years)	51 (25–81)
Mean age at life-threatening involvement (years)	53 (25–81)
Mean time between diagnosis of cryoglobulinemia and life-threatening involvement (months)	16 (0–168)
Associated conditions:	
HCV infection	144 (65)
HCV + HIV infection	18 (8)
HBV infection	5 (2)
HBV + HCV infection	2 (0.9)
Other associated conditions:	
Essential	36 (16)
Autoimmune diseases	12 (5)
Neoplasia	6 (3)
Mean cryocrit (%) (*n*=45)	9 (0.5–80)
Mean cryocrit (mg/dL) (*n*=16)	284 (0.19–2434)
Other cryoglobulinemic manifestations at diagnosis:	
Cutaneous purpura	152 (68)
Articular involvement	129 (58)
Peripheral neuropathy	83 (37)
Fever	13 (6)
Renal manifestations:	195 (87)
Renal failure	223 (100)
Nephrotic syndrome	115 (52)
Nephritic syndrome	44 (20)
Renal biopsy:	
Membranoproliferative glomerulonephritis	195 (87)
Mesangial proliferative glomerulonephritis	14 (6)
Focal proliferative glomerulonephritis	9 (4)
Others	5 (2)
Treatment:	
Plasma exchange	118 (53)
Corticosteroids	112 (50)
Immunosuppressive agents	61 (28)
Interferon α + ribavirin	60 (27)
Interferon α	52 (23)
Rituximab	21 (9)
Hemodialysis	21 (9)
Infliximab	2 (0.9)

(continued)

Table 10.2 (continued)

	Renal failure ($n=223$) (%)
Mean follow-up of life-threatening cryoglobulinemia (months)	18 (3–120)
Outcomes:	
Chronic renal failure	44 (20)
Relapse	14 (6)
Hemodialysis	10 (5)
Neoplasia	8 (4)
Death	90 (40)
Causes of death:	
Life-threatening cryoglobulinemia	33 (37)
Infectious processes	25 (28)
Cardiovascular events	16 (18)
Liver-related processes	11 (12)
Neoplasia	5 (5)

Specific treatment for cryoglobulinemia consisted of combined therapy including plasma exchange in 118 (53%), corticosteroids in 112 (50%) cases, immunosuppressive agents in 61 (cyclophosphamide in 50, azathioprine in 6, mycophenolate mofetil in 4, and tacrolimus in 1), antiviral agents in 98 (IFN-α monotherapy in 46, combined IFNα and ribavirin in 52), rituximab in 21 (9%), hemodialysis in 21 (9%), and infliximab in 2 (0.9%) patients. The combined therapy most frequently used was endovenous methyl-prednisolone, cyclophosphamide, and plasma exchange in 39 patients (17%), followed by methylprednisolone and cyclophosphamide in 8 (3%), and methylprednisolone and plasma exchange in 6 patients (3%). After a mean follow-up of 18 months (range, 3–120) from the diagnosis of glomerulonephritis, 23 (10%) patients developed chronic renal failure and 7 (3%) evolved to end-stage renal disease. Ninety (40%) patients died due to infectious processes in 25 (28%), cryoglobulinemic vasculitis (chronic renal failure in 15 and acute renal failure in 3) in 21 (23%), cardiovascular disease in 16 (18%), liver processes in 11 (12%), neoplasia in 5 (5%), multiorganic failure in 4 (4%), and other complications in 8 (9%) patients.

10.4.2
Gastrointestinal Vasculitis

Gastrointestinal involvement was the second life-threatening cryoglobulinemic presentation most frequently reported with 43 cases[16,18,24,35,41,48,50,53,54,65-74] (Table 10.3). There were 22 (51%) women and 21 (49%) men, with a mean age at diagnosis of cryoglobulinemic vasculitis of 56 years (range, 28–81) and a mean age at diagnosis of gastrointestinal vasculitis involvement of 58 years (range, 28–81). The mean time between diagnosis of cryoglobulinemia and life-threatening involvement was 26 months (range, 0–132).

Table 10.3 Epidemiologic features, associated processes, mean cryocrit, and causes of death in patients with life-threatening gastrointestinal cryoglobulinemia

	Gastrointestinal ($n=43$) (%)
Sex (female)	22 (51)
Mean age at diagnosis of cryoglobulinemia (years)	56 (28–81)
Mean age at life-threatening involvement (years)	58 (28–81)
Mean time between diagnosis of cryoglobulinemia to life-threatening involvement (months)	26 (0–132)
Associated conditions:	
HCV infection	25 (58)
Autoimmune diseases	4 (9)
Neoplasia	2 (5)
HCV + CMV infection	1 (2)
HBV infection	1 (2)
Mean cryocrit (%) ($n=11$)	11.8 (1–26)
Mean cryocrit (mg/dL) ($n=8$)	789 (0.18–1113)
Other cryoglobulinemic manifestations at diagnosis:	
Cutaneous purpura	29 (67)
Articular involvement	17 (39)
Peripheral neuropathy	12 (28)
Fever	8 (19)
Raynaud syndrome	5 (12)
Clinical manifestations at life-threatening diagnosis:	
Abdominal pain	43 (100)
Bloody stool	12 (28)
Intestinal perforation	3 (7)
Hematemesis	2 (5)
Hypermenorrhagia	1 (2)
Gastrointestinal manifestations:	
Intestinal ischemia	37 (86)
Cholecystitis	3 (7)
Pancreatitis	2 (5)
Adnexa and greater omentum	1 (2)
Treatment:	
Corticosteroids	34 (79)
Plasma exchange	19 (44)
Immunosuppressive agents	19 (44)
Interferon α	14 (32)
Surgery	11 (25)
Rituximab	9 (21)
Interferon α + ribavirin	4 (9)
Mean follow-up of life-threatening cryoglobulinemia (months)	11 (6–24)

(continued)

Table 10.3 (continued)

	Gastrointestinal ($n=43$) (%)
Outcomes:	
Relapse	4 (9)
Neoplasia	2 (5)
Death	13 (30)
Causes of death:	
Life-threatening cryoglobulinemia	8 (61)
Infectious processes	4 (12.5)
Others	1 (8)

10.4.2.1
Intestinal Ischemia

There were 37 (86%) patients with cryoglobulinemia intestinal ischemia (Fig. 10.1), all presenting with severe abdominal pain and general malaise with bloody stool in 12 (32%) cases, nausea and vomiting in 5 (13%), fever in 8 (23%), intestinal perforation in 3 (8%), hematemesis in 2 (5%), and hypovolemic shock in 1 patient. In 23 patients, intestinal vasculitis was confirmed histopathologically, in 6 patients, diagnosis was made by endoscopy, while in the remaining 8 cases, the diagnosis was based on the clinical and laboratory features. Other cryoglobulinemic manifestations included purpura in 25 (67%) patients, articular involvement in 14 (38%), peripheral neuropathy in 10 (27%) patients, and Raynaud phenomenon in 3 (8%). Cryocrit levels were detailed in 10 patients with a mean cryocrit level of 11.9% (range, 1–26%) while cryocrit quantification was detailed in six (mean of 1.2 mg/dL, ranging from 0.19 to 6.2 mg/dL).

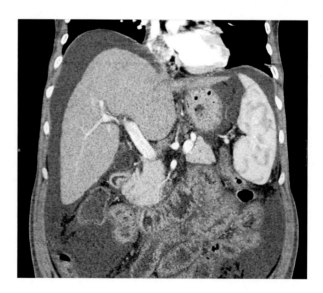

Fig. 10.1 Intestinal ischemia (diffuse edema of intestinal wall)

Treatment consisted of corticosteroids in 30 (81%) patients, plasma exchange in 17 (46%) patients, immunosuppressive agents in 14 (38%) (cyclophosphamide in 13 and azathioprine in 1), antiviral agents in 14 (38%) (IFN-α monotherapy in 10, combined IFN-α and ribavirin in 4), rituximab in 9 (24%), and surgery in 7 (19%) patients. Thirteen patients died (eight due to the cryoglobulinemic intestinal involvement, four due to an infectious process, and one due to liver involvement). Two additional patients died after a second episode of intestinal ischemia. (The first episode was successfully resolved after surgery and medical treatment).

10.4.2.2
Cryoglobulinemic Cholecystitis

Three patients presented with abdominal pain in the upper right quadrant suggestive of cholecystitis. A 47-year-old woman had history of malaise, arthralgia, palpable purpura, polyneuropathy, and Raynaud phenomenon. She had undergone cholecystectomy due to clinically suspected acute cholecystitis, and histological analysis disclosed vasculitic involvement. Hypocomplementemia, type II mixed cryoglobulinemia, HCV antibodies, and HCV RNA were detected. Remission of the cryoglobulinemia was induced with cyclophosphamide and steroids. HCV elimination with interferon did not succeed. A 64-year-old man had 1-year history of cryoglobulinemia vasculitis, which initially presented with malaise, arthralgia, fever, and polyneuropathy. He was under treatment of low-dose methyl prednisolone (4 mg/day) until his second admission with abdominal pain and fever. A cholecystectomy was performed, and histological examination of the gallbladder disclosed vasculitis of the small- and medium-sized vessels. He was treated with corticosteroids and interferon. A 66-year-old man had recurrent episodes of abdominal pain associated with blood-stained diarrhea for which he twice underwent colonoscopy without evidence of vasculitis on histological examination. He had undergone cholecystectomy due to clinically suspected acute cholecystitis, and histology of the gallbladder wall disclosed evidence of recent and old vasculitis. He had previous hepatitis B infection, being positive for anti-HBs antibody but negative for HBsAg. Hypocomplementemia and type II mixed cryoglobulinemia (cryocrit 26%) were present. His treatment consisted of corticosteroids and plasma exchange. Three patients were successfully cured of cryoglobulinemic vasculitis after surgery and medical treatment.

10.4.2.3
Cryoglobulinemic Pancreatitis

Two patients had cryoglobulinemic pancreatitis. They presented with abdominal pain, and the diagnosis was performed with abdominal CT. One patient also presented renal failure, CNS involvement, and digital ischemic necrosis, and he was treated with corticosteroids, cyclophosphamide, plasma exchange, and surgery of fingers of the left hand. The second patient was treated with corticosteroids and IFN-α monotherapy. Both patients were successfully cured of cryoglobulinemic pancreatitis with medical treatment.

10.4.2.4
Cryoglobulinemic Vasculitis of the Adnexa and Greater Omentum

A 45-year-old woman had abdominal pain and hypermenorrhagia 2 months before admission. The intraoperative abdominal situs showed multiple adhesions. The adhesions as well as both the adnexa and part of the greater omentum were resected. Histological examination of the adnexa and greater omentum specimen disclosed a necrotizing vasculitis of the small- and medium-sized vessels. She also presented malaise, fever, and mononeuritis multiplex after the surgery. Treatment consisted in corticosteroids and IFN-α monotherapy, but the outcome was not detailed.

10.4.3
CNS Involvement

Thirty-nine patients presenting with CNS involvement[16,18,22,25,31,35,41,47,50,54,65,67,75-86] (Table 10.4). There were 22 women (56%) and 17 men (44%), with a mean age at diagnosis of cryoglobulinemic vasculitis of 53 years (range, 30–74) and a mean age at diagnosis of CNS

Table 10.4 Epidemiologic features, associated processes, mean cryocrit, and causes of death in patients with cryoglobulinemic central nervous system involvement

	CNS involvement ($n=39$) (%)
Sex (female)	22 (56)
Mean age at diagnosis of cryoglobulinemia (years)	53 (30–74)
Mean age at life-threatening involvement (years)	54 (30–76)
Mean time between diagnosis of cryoglobulinemia to life-threatening involvement (months)	9 (0–60)
Associated conditions:	
HCV infection	33 (85)
Autoimmune diseases	3 (8)
HCV + HIV infection	2 (5)
Neoplasia	1 (2)
Mean cryocrit (%) ($n=13$)	3.2 (1–13)
Mean cryocrit (mg/dL) ($n=8$)	10 (0.19–13)
Other cryoglobulinemic manifestations at diagnosis:	
Cutaneous purpura	24 (61)
Peripheral neuropathy	21 (54)
Articular involvement	14 (36)
Sores in MMII	4 (10)
Neurological symptoms at presentation:	
Hemiplegic	17 (43)
Coma	11 (28)
Paraplegia	6 (15)

Table 10.4 (continued)

	CNS involvement ($n=39$) (%)
Encephalopathy	6 (15)
Seizures	4 (10)
Disturbances of the bladder	4 (10)
Generalized pyramidalism	3 (8)
Visual impairment	1 (2)
Main characteristics with life-threatening:	
Cerebral ischemia	16 (41)
CNS vasculitis	13 (33)
Cerebral hemorrhage	5 (13)
Transverse myelitis	5 (13)
Treatment:	
Corticosteroids	35 (90)
Plasma exchange	21 (54)
Immunosuppressive agents	15 (38)
Interferon α	9 (23)
Antiaggregant therapy	4 (10)
Interferon α + ribavirin	1 (2)
Infliximab (Anti TNF)	1 (2)
Mean follow-up of life-threatening cryoglobulinemia (months)	14 (6–84)
Outcomes:	
Relapse	4 (10)
Neurological damage	5 (13)
Neoplasia	4 (10)
Death	15 (38)
Causes of death:	
Life-threatening cryoglobulinemia	9 (60)
Infectious processes	3 (20)
Others	2 (13)
Neoplasia	1 (7)

cryoglobulinemic involvement of 54 years (range, 30–76). The mean time between diagnosis of cryoglobulinemia and life-threatening involvement was 9 months (range, 0–60). Twelve patients presented with another life-threatening manifestation (CNS involvement and cryoglobulinemic glomerulonephritis in 7 patients; CNS involvement, cryoglobulinemic glomerulonephritis, and pulmonary hemorrhage in two; CNS involvement, cryoglobulinemic glomerulonephritis, and digital ischemic necrosis in one; CNS involvement and digital ischemic necrosis in one; and CNS involvement, cryoglobulinemic glomerulonephritis, and intestinal ischemia in 1 patient). One patient had two coexisting CNS involvements (anterior optic neuropathy and transverse myelitis). Clinical presentation consisted of hemiplegia in 17 (43%) patients, coma in 11 (28%), paraplegia in 6 (15%), encephalopathy in 6 (15%), seizures in 4 (10%), disturbances of the bladder in 4 (10%), generalized pyramidalism in 3 patients (8%), and visual impairment in 1 (2%). CNS involvement consisted of cerebral ischemia in 16 (41%) cases, cerebral hemorrhages in 5 (13%), medullary involvement in 5 (13%), including transverse myelitis in four (three with repeated episodes) and ischemic involvement of the spinal cord and CNS vasculitis in 13 (33%) (demonstrated by magnetic resonance imaging in all patients and post-mortem study in 4). Other cryoglobulinemic manifestations included purpura in 24 (61%) patients, peripheral neuropathy in 21 (54%), articular involvement in 14 (36%), and sores in the legs in 4 patients (10%). Cryocrit levels were detailed in 13 patients with a mean cryocrit level of 3.2% (range, 1–13%) while cryocrit quantification was detailed in eight (mean of 10 mg/dL, ranging from 0.19 to 13 mg/dL).

Specific treatment for cryoglobulinemia included corticosteroids at high doses (1–1.5 mg/kg/day) in 35 (90%) patients, plasma exchange in 21 (54%), immunosuppressive agents in 15 (38%) (cyclophosphamide in 10, azathioprine in 3 and ciclosporine in 2), antiviral agents in 9 (23%) (IFN-α monotherapy in 8, combined IFN-α, and ribavirin in 1), antiaggregant therapy in 4 (10%), and infliximab in 1 patient (2%). After a mean follow-up of 14 months (range 6–84) from the diagnosis of CNS involvement, 4 patients had neurological impairment (generalized pyramidalism in three, paraplegia in two, and dysbasia, dysarthria, and spasticity in one). The patient with medullar involvement clearly improved, with a slight sensory alteration remaining at the last visit. Fifteen patients (38%) died: nine (60%) due to life-threatening cryoglobulinemia (multiorganic failure due to cryoglobulinemic vasculitis in four, cerebral hemorrhages in two cases, and CNS vasculitis in two), sepsis in three (20%), neoplasia in three (8%) (lymphoma in two and lung cancer in one).

10.4.4
Pulmonary Hemorrhage

Seventeen patients presented pulmonary hemorrhage[15,17,18,31,32,45,50,54,87-89] (Table 10.5; Fig. 10.2). There were ten (59%) men and seven (41%) women, with a mean age, at diagnosis of cryoglobulinemic vasculitis, of 53 years (range, 36–87) and of 54 (range, 36–87) at diagnosis of pulmonary hemorrhage. The mean time between diagnosis of cryoglobulinemia and life-threatening involvement was 13 months (range, 0–60). Clinical features included dyspnea and hemoptysis in eight cases, and respiratory failure in seven. All patients showed pulmonary infiltrates in the chest X-ray. Other cryoglobulinemic manifestations included purpura in seven (41%) patients, fever in four (23%), peripheral neuropathy in three (18%), and articular involvement in three (18%) patients. Cryocrit levels were detailed in 10 patients with a mean cryocrit level of 14% (range, 4–60%) while cryocrit quantification was detailed in five (mean of 1.1 mg/dL, ranging from 1 to 2.1 mg/dL).

One patient was treated conservatively with oral prednisone due to advanced age (87-year-old) and showed an insidious evolution and died 1 year later due to a second episode of pulmonary hemorrhage. The remaining 16 patients required admission to the intensive care unit (ICU) and were treated with endovenous methylprednisolone in all cases, cyclophosphamide in 8, plasma exchange in 7, and rituximab in 1. Twelve patients (70%) died, due to cryoglobulinemic vasculitis in 7 (58%) (pulmonary hemorrhage in six and multiorganic failure due to cryoglobulinemic vasculitis in one), sepsis in four (33%), and unknown in one (8%).

Table 10.5 Epidemiologic features, associated processes, mean cryocrit, and causes of death in patients with life-threatening pulmonary cryoglobulinemic involvement

	Pulmonary involvement ($n = 17$) (%)
Sex (female)	7 (41)
Mean age at diagnosis of cryoglobulinemia (years)	53 (36–87)
Mean age at life-threatening involvement (years)	54 (36–87)
Mean time between diagnosis of cryoglobulinemia to life-threatening involvement (months)	13 (0–60)
Associated conditions:	
HCV infection	8 (47)
Autoimmune diseases	2 (12)
HCV + HBV infection	1 (6)
HCV + CMV infection	1 (6)
Mean cryocrit (%) ($n = 10$)	14 (4–60)
Mean cryocrit (mg/dL) ($n = 5$)	1.1 (1–2.1)
Other cryoglobulinemic manifestations at diagnosis:	
Cutaneous purpura	7 (41)
Fever	4 (23)
Articular involvement	3 (18)
Peripheral neuropathy	3 (18)
Pulmonary manifestations at diagnosis:	
Dyspnea	8 (47)
Hemoptysis	8 (47)
Respiratory failure	7 (41)
Main characteristics with life-threatening:	
Pulmonary Hemorrhage	17 (100)
Treatment:	
Corticosteroids	16 (94)
Interferon α	1 (6)
Interferon α + ribavirin	1 (6)
Immunosuppressive agents	8 (47)
Rituximab	1 (6)
Plasma exchange	8 (47)
Mean follow-up of life-threatening cryoglobulinemia (months)	12 (8–60)
Outcomes:	
Relapse	3 (18)
Neoplasia	–
Death	12 (70)
Causes of death:	
Infectious processes	6 (50)
Life-threatening cryoglobulinemia	5 (42)
Unknown	1 (6)

Fig. 10.2 Pulmonary
hemorrhage

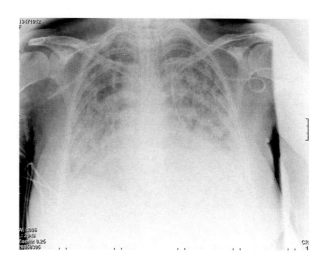

10.4.5
Digital Necrosis

There were 12 patients reported with cryoglobulinemic digital ischemic necrosis[18,24,25,35,49,67,90-92] (Table 10.6; Fig. 10.3). There were 8 (67%) men and 4 (33%) women, with a mean age at diagnosis of cryoglobulinemic vasculitis of 52 years (range, 33–70) and of 53 (range, 36–70) at diagnosis of digital ischemic necrosis. The mean time between diagnosis of cryoglobuline-mia and life-threatening involvement was 12 months (range, 0–60). Nine (75%) patients presented with feet gangrene and 3 (25%) patients with hand gangrene. All cases presented vascular ischemia diagnosed by arteriography, and in 4 patients, the diagnosis was confirmed by histological analysis. Other cryoglobulinemic manifestations included purpura in nine (75%) patients, articular involvement in 7 (58%), peripheral neuropathy in 5 (42%), and sores in MMII in 4 (33%) patients. Cryocrit levels were detailed in 2 patients with a mean cryocrit level of 2.35% (range, 4–4.5%) while cryocrit quantification was detailed in 4 (mean of 9.19 mg/dL, ranging from 0.23 to 22.8 mg/dL).

Treatment consisted of endovenous methylprednisolone (1 mg/kg/day) in ten (83%) patients, plasma exchange in seven (58%), immunosuppressive agents in seven (58%) (cyclophosphamide in four, azathioprine in one, mycophenolate mofetil in one, and cyclosporine in one), IFN-α monotherapy in six (50%), and rituximab in one (8%) patient. Urgent surgery was performed in five (42%) patients who did not respond to medical treat-ment and one patient was successfully treated with percutaneous angioplasty. After a mean follow-up of 12 months (range, 3–24) from the diagnosis of digital ischemic necrosis, five (42%) patients died: two (40%) due to life-threatening cryoglobulinemia (multiorganic failure), two (40%) due to cardiovascular disease (ischemic heart attack in one case and heart failure in one), and sepsis in one (20%).

Table 10.6 Epidemiologic features, associated processes, mean cryocrit, and causes of death in patients with digital ischemic necrosis

	Digital ischemic necrosis ($n=12$)
Sex (female)	4 (33)
Mean age at diagnosis of cryoglobulinemia (years)	52 (33–70)
Mean age at life-threatening involvement (years)	53 (36–70)
Mean time between diagnosis of cryoglobulinemia and life-threatening involvement (months)	12 (0–60)
Associated conditions:	
HCV infection	7 (58)
HCV + HBV infection	–
Autoimmune diseases	–
Mean cryocrit (%) ($n=2$)	2.35 (4.4–5)
Mean cryocrit (mg/dL) ($n=6$)	9.19 (0.23–22.8)
Main clinical cryoglobulinemia manifestations at diagnosis:	
Cutaneous purpura	9 (75)
Articular involvement	7 (58)
Peripheral neuropathy	5 (42)
Sores in MMII	4 (33)
Main characteristics with life-threatening:	
Feet gangrene	9 (75)
Distal hands gangrene	3 (25)
Treatment of life-threatening:	
Corticosteroids	10 (83)
Plasma exchange	7 (58)
Immunosuppressive agents	7 (58)
Interferon α	6 (50)
Surgery	5 (42)
Rituximab	1 (8)
Mean follow-up of life-threatening cryoglobulinemia (months)	12 (3–24)
Outcomes:	
Relapse	1 (8)
Neoplasia	1 (8)
Death	5 (42)
Causes of death:	
Life-threatening cryoglobulinemia	2 (40)
Cardiovascular disease	2 (40)
Infectious processes	1 (20)

Fig. 10.3 Digital necrosis

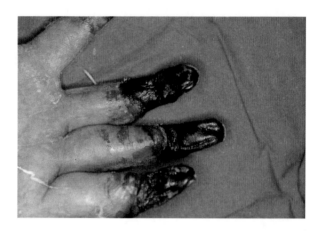

10.4.6
Myocardial Involvement

Eight cases of cryoglobulinemic myocardial involvement have been reported[16,41,49] (Table 10.7). There were four (50%) women and four (50%) men, with a mean age at diagnosis of cryoglobulinemic vasculitis of 55 years (range, 41–63) and a mean age at diagnosis of myocardial involvement of 56 years (range, 44–63). The mean time between diagnosis of cryoglobulinemia and life-threatening involvement was 12 months (range, 0–36). All patients presented ischemic heart attack demonstrated by arteriography; one patient also presented with heart failure (coronary vasculitis was demonstrated by necropsy in three). One patient presented with another life-threatening manifestations (cryoglobulinemic glomerulonephritis and digital ischemic necrosis). No patient had complicated cardiovascular risk factors. Other cryoglobulinemic manifestations included purpura in all patients, peripheral neuropathy in seven (87%), articular involvement in seven (87%), and Raynaud phenomenon in five (62%). Cryocrit levels were positive in all patients, but the values were not detailed.

Treatment consisted of corticosteroids at high doses (1–1.5 mg/kg/day) in six (75%) patients, plasma exchange in five (62%), cyclophosphamide in two (25%), and rituximab in one patient. Three (37%) patients died due to life-threatening cryoglobulinemia (coronary vasculitis).

10.4.7
Ocular Involvement

Five patients presented with ocular involvement and cryoglobulinemia[18,40,75,77,93]: Two patients (40%) had anterior optic neuropathy, retinal vasculitis in two (40%), and central retinal vein occlusion in one patient (20%). There were four (80%) men and one (20%) woman, with a mean age at diagnosis of cryoglobulinemic vasculitis of 48 years (range, 30–64) and of 49 (range, 30–64) at diagnosis of ocular involvement. The mean time between diagnosis of cryoglobulinemia and life-threatening involvement was 1 month

Table 10.7 Epidemiologic features, associated processes, mean cryocrit, and causes of death in patients with cryoglobulinemic cardiovascular involvement

	Cardiovascular disease ($n=8$)
Sex (female)	4 (50)
Mean age at diagnosis of cryoglobulinemia (years)	55 (41–63)
Mean age at life-threatening involvement (years)	56 (44–63)
Mean time between diagnosis of cryoglobulinemia and life-threatening involvement (months)	12 (0–36)
Associated conditions:	
HCV infection	3 (37)
HCV+HIV infection	–
Autoimmune diseases	–
Other cryoglobulinemic manifestations at diagnosis:	
Cutaneous purpura	8 (100)
Peripheral neuropathy	7 (87)
Articular involvement	7 (87)
Raynaud syndrome	5 (62)
Main characteristics with life-threatening:	
Myocardial infarction	5 (62)
Coronary vasculitis	3 (37)
Heart failure	1 (12)
Treatment of life-threatening:	
Corticosteroids	6 (75)
Plasma exchange	5 (62)
Immunosuppressive agents	2 (25)
Rituximab	1 (12)
Outcomes:	
Death	4 (50)
Causes of death:	
Life-threatening cryoglobulinemia	4 (100)

(range, 0–5). Four patients (80%) had associated chronic HCV infection; other etiologies included B cell lymphoma in two patients (40%) and systemic lupus erythematosus in one patient (20%). All patients were evaluated by fluorescein angiography. Clinical presentation consisted of visual loss in two patients (40%), blurry vision in two (40%), and encephalopathy in one patient. Three patients (60%) presented with another life-threatening manifestation (ocular involvement and cryoglobulinemic glomerulonephritis in two patients, and anterior optic neuropathy and transverse myelitis in one patient). Cryocrit levels were positive in all patients, but the values were not detailed.

Treatment consisted of plasma exchange in four (80%), corticosteroids at high doses (1–1.5 mg/kg/day) in three patients (60%), antiviral agents in three (60%) (IFN-α monotherapy in two and combined IFNα and ribavirin in one), cyclophosphamide in one (20%), and rituximab in one patient (20%). Four months later, one patient who had a second episode of anterior optic neuropathy was successfully treated with corticosteroids. Two patients died: one patient due to B cell lymphoma and one due to ischemic stroke.

10.5
Complex Situations

10.5.1
Coexistence with Other Systemic Vasculitis

10.5.1.1
Coexistence with Polyarteritis Nodosa (PAN)

Vasculitides are a heterogeneous group of disorders. There are diverse features, including clinical manifestations that sometimes overlap and involvement of all types of blood vessels. The prevalence of anti-HCV antibodies in patients with PAN ranges from 5% to 12%. However, since most of these PAN patients infected by HCV also had cryoglobulins in their serum, there is controversy regarding the existence of "authentic" PAN related to HCV infection. Differentiation between PAN-type and mixed cryoglobulinemia vasculitis can be difficult, since they may share the same clinical manifestations and pathologic lesions, including peripheral neuropathy, purpuric skin lesions, arthralgia, myalgia, renal involvement, and characteristics of vascular inflammatory infiltrate.[94]

Histology Evidence of Mixed Cryoglobulinemia and PAN Vasculitis

Mendez et al.[67] describe a 36-year-old man with HCV infection, positive cryoglobulins, and histological evidence of mild chronic hepatitis present with bilateral lower extremity rash associated with arthralgias. Skin biopsy disclosed leukocytoclastic vasculitis affecting small vessels. Treatment with interferon three times a week for 6 months did not show any response. He presented abdominal pain with small bowel infarction. Pathology disclosed necrotizing vasculitis affecting small vessels. An intraoperative liver biopsy noted chronic portal triaditis with the presence of fibrin thrombi in the small portal vessels. Polyarteritis nodosa was diagnosed, and plasma exchange and pulse i.v. corticosteroids resulted in incomplete response; therefore, treatment with cyclophosphamide was started. Severe ischemic colitis evolved, complicated by multiple intra-abdominal abscesses. Sepsis and acute renal and liver failure ensued, and the patient died. Canada et al.[95] describe a 53-year-old man with HCV infection undergoing cholecystectomy for presumed cholecystitis; histological examination disclosed medium-sized arteritis, consistent with PAN. The patient later developed rapidly progressive glomerulonephritis.

Kidney biopsy demonstrated cryoglobulinemia glomerulonephritis. Treatment included pulse methylprednisolone followed by oral prednisone and monthly intravenous cyclophosphamide for 6 months. The patient subsequently underwent treatment for HCV with interferon, resulting in a marked decrease in HCV RNA. The patient has had no relapse of the vasculitis, his renal function is stable, and viral load remains low after completing 36 weeks of interferon treatment. Idiopathic polyarteritis nodosa is usually treated with corticosteroids and sometimes with cyclophosphamide. Accelerated viral replication is a potential risk associated with the use of corticosteroids and cytotoxic agents when used in PAN associated with hepatitis B/C. Benefit from the combined use of plasma exchange, corticosteroids, and interferon has been reported previously in hepatitis B infections.[95] This small number does not mean that mixed cryoglobulinemia should not be listed among the causes of necrotizing vasculitis, but it makes it difficult to extract those specific features that would enable to predict which case of mixed cryoglobulinemia is associated or not with necrotizing vasculitis.[96]

Chronic HCV Infection PAN-Type Vasculitis

Cacoub et al.[94] describe ten patients who fulfilled the American College of Rheumatology criteria for PAN with multiple system clinical involvement, histological evidence of mostly medium-sized vessel necrotizing vasculitis, mixed cryoglobulinemia in all patients (type II with an IgM kappa in nine and type III in one), anti-HBc antibodies in three patients, and HCV PCR was positive in all patients except one. Disease onset was acute in all cases and patients had very severe acute clinical manifestations within a few weeks, with polyvisceral failure that was often life threatening. In the majority of these patients, the neurological involvement was a severe acute sensorimotor multifocal mononeuropathy involving all limbs. Pathological lesions involved medium- and small-sized vessels with a mixed inflammatory infiltrate of monocytes, lymphocytes, polymorphonuclear neutrophils, and a necrotizing angitis. Some distinctive features found in these patients are common in PAN but have not been reported in mixed cryoglobulinemia. They include microaneurysms (found in two patients) and renal cortical necrosis secondary to occlusion of medium-sized arteries (one patient), a known feature of PAN and unreported in cryoglobulinemia. Treatment of PAN-type vasculitis related to HCV infection consisted of corticosteroids in order to rapidly control the most severe life-threatening manifestations of systemic vasculitis. Plasma exchanges were undertaken to control the course of vasculitis by clearance of immune complexes without stimulating viral replication. Interferon-alpha was used to directly control HCV replication. Steidi et al.[97] describe a 76-year-old female patient who presented with severe peripheral neuropathy. The sural nerve biopsy revealed a severe subacute axonal neuropathy with endoneurial edema, necrotizing arteritis of medium-sized arteries with granulomatous inflammation throughout all layers of the vessel wall as well as fibrinoid media necrosis. These findings were interpreted as typically of PAN. The screening revealed chronic hepatitis C infection associated with cryoglobulinemia type II (IgG kappa IgA). After biopsy, immunosuppressive therapy with corticosteroids was started. After initial regression of paresthesias, tapering of the dose led to a relapse of symptoms. This was followed by the onset of purpura on the patient's legs. A cyclophosphamide treatment was initiated. Then, the patient started a combined treatment with interferon-alpha and ribavirin. Garcia de La Peña Lefebvre et al.[98] describe a case of a 38-year-old woman who developed systemic vasculitis after infection by HBV and HCV. The clinical and laboratory findings substantiated not only the diagnosis of polyarteritis nodosa (PAN) but also that of mixed cryoglobulinemia with a monoclonal IgM component. A deltoid muscle biopsy showed vasculitis of small- and medium-sized arteries and venules with leukocytoclasis and lymphocyte infiltrates, but no fibrinoid necrosis. An abdominal angiogram showed multiple microaneurysms of mesenteric, renal, splenic, and hepatic arteries, with multiple stenoses and visceral infarcts. HBV-related PAN was diagnosed, even though mixed cryoglobulinemia (MC) could also be considered owing to the muscle biopsy findings. The patient received a daily methylprednisolone pulse for three days, followed by oral prednisone (50 mg/day), which was rapidly tapered within 14 days. Thirteen plasma exchanges were performed within 1 month. After stopping steroids, treatment with interferon-alpha-2b (3 MU, three times a week) was prescribed for 2 months. Six weeks later, anti-HBe antibodies were detected, and cryoglobulinemia became undetectable.

These examples of highly complex situations emphasize the need to gather all relevant clinical, biological, histological, and complementary data so that the best treatment for overlapping of distinct vasculitis can be selected.[98] HCV infection may be associated with different types of systemic vasculitis (polyarteritis nodosa or mixed cryoglobulinemia). Because of the differences in clinical and pathological features and therapeutic strategy, PAN-type vasculitis should be distinguished from mixed cryoglobulinemia vasculitis in patients with HCV infection.[94]

HCV-Symptomatic Mixed Cryoglobulinemia Without Necrotizing Vasculitis

Cacoub et al.[94] described seven HCV patients with symptomatic mixed cryoglobulinemia without necrotizing vasculitis of medium- or small-sized arteries which did not fulfill criteria for PAN. The predominant extrahepatic symptom was a subacute distal polyneuropathy. No patient had life-threatening disease at entry or during the course of study. All the patients were PCR-positive for HCV. Three patients had anti-HBc antibodies, but none had HBc Ag or HBV DNA. Mixed cryoglobulinemia was found in all patients, including type II IgM kappa in six patients and type III in one patient. Neuromuscular biopsies showed an inflammatory process of medium and small vessels in all patients. The infiltrate consisted exclusively of mononuclear cell ($n=6$), and it was predominantly localized in perivascular areas. Five patients received interferon-alpha alone or associated with plasma exchanges, or with steroids and plasma exchanges. Two patients received only low-dose steroids. Three patients had slow progression of their peripheral neuropathy. Studies on medium-sized vessel vasculitis of PAN type and HCV infection association have been controversial. In this series, possible confusion between vasculitis of medium- or small-sized arteries and mixed cryoglobulinemia arises from the presence of a mixed cryoglobulin in the serum of all patients. The mechanism(s) leading to PAN or mixed-type cryoglobulinemia vasculitis in HCV patients remains unclear.[94]

10.5.1.2
Coexistence with Antineutrophil Cytoplasmic Antibody (ANCA)

The detection of ANCA has been reported in chronic hepatitis C and HCV-associated MC in few cases. Cacoub et al.[99] did not find ANCA using IFT and MPO-ANCA ELISA in 36 patients with "essential," i.e., HCV-negative, mixed cryoglobulinemia or HCV-associated mixed cryoglobulinemia. They detected P-ANCA in 2 of 15 patients with HCV infection without cryoglobulinemia and concluded that ANCA does not play a role as a marker or mediator of disease in mixed cryoglobulinemia. Bruchfield et al.[47] describe a 47-year-old female with fever, purpura, arthralgia, pleuritis, cerebral vasculitis, peripheral neuropathy, and cryoglobulinemia glomerulonephritis; C-ANCA with PR3 antibodies was detected in her. The patient received a daily methylprednisolone pulse for 3 days and combined therapy with interferon-alpha and ribavirin. Vasculitis rapidly improved, and the renal outcome was favorable. PR3-ANCA decreased to borderline levels. Didona et al.[100] describe a patient with a chronic HCV infection with mixed-type II cryoglobulinemia, cutaneous leukocytoclastic vasculitis, and P-ANCA. Asa et al.[101] describe a 49-year-old woman with a history of chronic hepatitis C virus infection with proteinuria (0.2 g/day), hematuria, renal failure (serum creatinine 1.4 mg/dL), positive antinuclear antigen, hypocomplementemia, mixed cryoglobulinemia (type III), and MPO-ANCA level was found to be high (356 EU). In renal biopsy, most glomeruli showed crescentic formation with the weak deposition of IgG, IgM, and C3 in the mesangial area and along the capillary wall. The patient was diagnosed as having systemic vasculitis associated with MPO-ANCA. Methylprednisolone pulse therapy followed by oral prednisolone (40 mg/day) effectively normalized MPO-ANCA level. Lamprecht et al.[33] describe two patients with systemic patterns vasculitis (SV). In both cases, the detection of cANCA in conjunction with glomerulonephritis and clinical signs of extrarenal vasculitis favored the diagnosis of an ANCA-associated vasculitis (AAV). However, neither patient showed characteristic clinical signs and symptoms of AAV and, especially, there was no evidence of lung involvement as typically seen in Wegener's granulomatosis (WG), microscopic polyangiitis (MPA), or Churg–Strauss syndrome (CSS). On the other hand, a nephrotic syndrome, which is a rather unusual manifestation of AAV, was observed in each of the cases. Additionally, cryoglobulinemia and hypocomplementemia (in conjunction with HCV in one of the cases) were also detected, which are characteristically not seen in AAV. The patient with crescentic glomerulonephritis suffered from urticaria vasculitis, arthritis, and pleural effusions, but HCV could not be detected. In addition, intensive interdisciplinary investigations (ophthalmology, cranial NMR, etc.) did not reveal lesions usually present in patients with AAV. The simultaneous demonstration of ANCA and cryoglobulinemia in these two vasculitic patients was at first confusing. However, complement consumption is characteristic of the groups of immune complex vasculitides (including essential cryoglobulinemic vasculitis) and exceptionally rare in ANCA-associated vasculitides (AAV), including Wegener's granulomatosis, which is most strongly associated with cANCA/PR3-ANCA. In addition, gross proteinuria is rather rare in AAV and more frequent in immune complex glomerulonephritis like essential mixed cryoglobulinemia. Thus, immunohistochemical analysis of the kidney-biopsies did in fact finally help to distinguish the different forms of vasculitis (pauci-immune *versus* immune complex). Moreover, the detection of HCV in one case guided the therapy to an immunomodulating regimen with IFN-alpha instead of traditional immunosuppressive therapy.

Clinical signs of a vasculitis and detection of cANCA or pANCA are suggestive of an ANCA-associated vasculitis (i.e.,Wegener's granulomatosis, microscopic polyangiitis, or Churg–Strauss syndrome). However, only additional investigations (complement, cryoglobulins, search for infections) and immunohistological proof of a pauci-immune or immune complex vasculitis will help to clearly establish the diagnosis of an ANCA-associated vasculitis or immune complex vasculitis, and to differentiate cases with "false-positive" ANCA. Screening for cryoglobulins and HCV infection should be performed upon first presentation in all patients with vasculitis and/or glomerulonephritis, especially when hypocomplementemia is present. Because "false-positive" cANCA can occur, histological proof of immune complex–associated lesions should be used to support the diagnosis whenever possible. If HCV-associated mixed cryoglobulinemia and (immune complex–/cryoglobulinemic-) vasculitis is demonstrated, patients can be treated with IFN-alpha if there is no life-threatening situation or risk of organ failure, whereas traditional immunosuppressive therapy and plasma exchange are still indicated in those cases of essential mixed cryoglobulinemia which are not secondary to an infection or other underlying disease.[33]

10.5.2
Hyperviscosity Syndrome

Mixed cryoglobulinemia (MC) is associated with a broad spectrum of clinical manifestations that can range from mild to life threatening in their severity. The presence of macroaggregates containing IgM rheumatoid factor and IgG could also result in a hyperviscosity state (HS) in MC, and, in fact, HS represents another clinical manifestation of MC.[102] Fifteen percent of patients with Waldenström's macroglobulinemia show HS and anemia. Although it is unusual to see HS associated with light-chain disease, it has been reported in patients with pure light-chain myeloma.[103] The increased blood viscosity in these patients is due to the aggregation of κ light chains. A patient with HS may exhibit laboratory abnormalities such as a high hematocrit, red blood cell rigidity, or a very high white blood cell count, causing resistance to blood flow. The clinical hallmarks of HS are bleeding secondary to the presence of paraproteins on the platelet surface; visual disturbances because of retinal vein distension, retinal hemorrhage or thrombosis; and signs of central nervous system involvement, such as dizziness, somnolence, or stupor. Other clinical manifestations include peripheral neuropathy, weakness, fatigue, renal failure, and congestive heart failure because of increased plasma volume. Further analysis of the data showed that the only laboratory or clinical parameter that was strongly correlated with the hemorheological factors was the cryocrit level. Ferri et al.[102] studied 19 patients before and after the removal of cryoglobulins; serum viscosity significantly decreased when the cryoglobulins were removed. The hematocrit was significantly lower in MC patients than in controls and was weakly correlated with all hemorheological parameters. On the other hand, these parameters (except for serum creatinine) were not significantly associated with clinical symptoms or organ involvement. Patent HS was present in only one case and rapidly improved after plasma exchange and cyclophosphamide therapy.

The relative rarity of HS in MC could be explained in a number of ways. It is well-known that both cellular and plasma factors play a role in blood viscosity, and there are data to indicate that the most important factors affecting blood viscosity in MC are cryoglobulin levels, temperature, and the hematocrit. However, although the amount of cryoglobulins in MC patients is much higher than in other autoimmune disorders, it only occasionally reaches the values seen in paraproteinemic states. Second, the tendency toward an increase in blood viscosity is probably compensated by a parallel decrease in the hematocrit in MC patients. Nevertheless, when hyperviscosity of the blood is present, it can contribute to the pathogenesis of some of the clinical manifestations of MC, although its role in the clinical picture remains far from clear. For this complex multisystem disease, no single treatment protocol can be established and therapy should be tailored to depending on the type of organ involved in each case. Severe cases of HS are treated with plasma exchange (PE), which is generally successful in normalizing the hemorheological parameters and in controlling the symptoms such as bleeding and headache, although to obtain sustained remission, it should be associated with conventional pharmacological therapy. Plasma exchange is also the treatment of choice for patients affected by HS secondary to either monoclonal or polyclonal cryoglobulinemia.[104]

10.5.3
Severe Peripheral Neuropathy

Although cryoglobulinemic peripheral neuropathy is often mild, we describe five patients[71,105-107] who developed severe neuropathy presentations, including falls, weakness, and painful paresthesia affecting the hands and feet, asymmetric motor neuropathy with right foot and left wrist drop, and a rapidly progressive sensory motor axonal neuropathy with clinical and electrophysiological features of mononeuritis multiplex. A sural nerve biopsy showed complete loss of myelinated nerve fibers in all patients. Four patients were infected with HCV, and one patient had essential cryoglobulinemia vasculitis. These patients received different combinations of standard therapies (corticosteroids, antiviral agents, and/or plasma exchange) with no clinical response. Further, they had a relapse of MC with peripheral neuropathy and worsening cutaneous vasculitis, accompanied by known side effects of prednisolone in one, necessitating alternative treatment with rituximab in 4 patients. Patient with essential cryoglobulinemia vasculitis experienced relief of his symptoms only with plasma exchange.

10.5.4
Cryoglobulinemic Vasculitis Exacerbated by Rituximab

Severe systemic vasculitis was exacerbated by rituximab in six patients.[60,108-110] There were three women and three men, with a mean age at diagnosis of cryoglobulinemia of 68 years (range, 58–80) and a mean age at diagnosis of systemic rituximab-related drug reactions of 69 years (range, 58–80). Four patients had associated chronic HCV infection and Waldenström's macroglobulinemia in one. Severe involvement appeared 1– 2 days after rituximab infusions in four patients, 3 weeks in one, and 16 weeks in one patient (he completed eight doses). Rituximab doses were 375 mg/m^2/week for 4 consecutive weeks in five patients and 375 mg/m^2/week was given every 2 weeks in one patient. There were two different clinical presentations: flare of *cryoglobulinemia mixta* with or without life-threatening flare of vasculitis. Renal biopsy disclosed cryoglobulinemic glomerulonephritis in four patients (67%) with renal failure, intestinal ischemia in four (67%), and heart failure in two patients (33%). One patient developed severe peripheral neuropathy and arthralgias. Other cryoglobulinemic manifestations included articular involvement in four (67%), purpura in three (50%), fever in three (50%), and peripheral neuropathy in one patient (17%). Cryocrit levels were detailed in four patients with a mean cryocrit quantification of 1.7g/l (ranging from 0.78 to 2.6 mg/dL) and cryocrit level was 63% in one patient. Treatment consisted of corticosteroids at high doses (1–1.5 mg/kg/day) in all patients, plasma exchange in three (50%), and hemodialysis in one patient. Urgent surgery was performed in one patient due to intestinal ischemia, as the patient did not respond to medical treatment; however, the patient died due to multiorgan failure. Five patients were successfully cured of flare vasculitis with medical treatment.

10.5.5
Cryoglobulinemia in Pregnancy

Presentation of cryoglobulinemia during pregnancy is exceptional. Gupta et al.[111] reported a 21-year-old primigravida at 26 weeks of pregnancy presenting with palpable macular rash in the lower extremities, without other cryoglobulinemic features. Skin biopsy disclosed leukocytoclastic vasculitis. Laboratories tests showed positive rheumatoid factor, low levels of C4, and serum monoclonal band. Immunofixation detected polyclonal immunoglobulin G and monoclonal immunoglobulin M kappa. Cryoglobulins were positive. The patient underwent plasma exchange twice within 1 week of diagnosis, followed by oral prednisolone (0.5 mg/kg) due to the reappearance of rash 2 weeks later. The patient responded well, and she delivered a healthy neonate with no evidence of any effects related to the disease or medication.

10.6
Conclusion

As in other systemic vasculitides, some cryoglobulinemic patients may present with potentially life-threatening situations involving internal organs. Cryoglobulinemia may result in progressive (renal involvement) or acute (pulmonary hemorrhage, gastrointestinal ischemia, CNS involvement) organ damage. Glomerulonephritis may result in acute renal failure in 10% of patients or may evolve progressively to chronic renal failure, a major cause of death, either directly or secondary to infection or cardiovascular disease. Ten-year survival rates of glomerulonephritis range between 33% and 49%, although the most recent series showed a rate of nearly 80% due to improved therapeutic management. The prognosis is worse in males, patients with HCV infection and those with higher cryocrit levels, low C3 levels, and raised serum creatinine at diagnosis. The mortality rate of intestinal ischemia and alveolar hemorrhage is >80% after the first episode and reaches 100% after a second episode. Unfortunately, this may be the first cryoglobulinemic involvement in almost two-thirds of cases, highlighting the complex management and very elevated mortality of these cases.

References

1. Lamprecht P, Gause A, Gross WL. Cryoglobulinemic vasculitis. *Arthritis Rheum*. 1999;42: 2507-2516.
2. Ferri C, Zignego AL, Pileri SA. Cryoglobulins. *J Clin Pathol*. 2002;55:4-13.
3. Sansonno D, Dammacco F. Hepatitis C virus, cryoglobulinaemia, and vasculitis: immune complex relations. *Lancet Infect Dis*. 2005;5:227-236.
4. Ramos-Casals M, Trejo O, García-Carrasco M, Cervera R, Font J. Mixed cryoglobulinemia: new concepts. *Lupus*. 2000;9:83-91.
5. Gorevic PD, Frangione B. Mixed cryoglobulinemia cross-reactive idiotypes: implications for the relationship of MC to rheumatic and lymphoproliferative diseases. *Semin Hematol*. 1991;28:79-94.
6. Ferri C, Greco F, Longombardo G, et al. Antibodies to hepatitis C virus in patients with mixed cryoglobulinemia. *Arthritis Rheum*. 1991;34:1606-1610.
7. Agnello V, Chung RT, Kaplan LM. A role for hepatitis C virus infection in type II cryoglobulinemia. *N Engl J Med*. 1992;327:1490-1495.
8. Ramos-Casals M, Font J. Extrahepatic manifestations in patients with chronic hepatitis C virus infection. *Curr Opin Rheumatol*. 2005;17:447-455.
9. Magalini AR, Facchetti F, Salvi L, Fontana L, Puoti M, Scarpa A. Clonality of B-cells in portal lymphoid infiltrates of HCV-infected livers. *J Pathol*. 1998;185:86-90.
10. Sansonno D, De Vita S, Iacobelli AR, Cornacchiulo V, Boiocchi M, Dammacco F. Clonal analysis of intrahepatic B cells from HCV infected patients with and without mixed cryoglobulinemia. *J Immunol*. 1998;160:3594-3601.
11. Meltzer M, Franklin EC. Cryoglobulinemia: a study of 29 patients. I. IgG and IgM cryoglobulins and factors effecting cryoprecipitability. *Am J Med*. 1966;40:828-836.
12. Trejo O, Ramos-Casals M, Garcia-Carrasco M, et al. Cryoglobulinemia: study of etiologic factors and clinical and immunologic features in 443 patients from a single center. *Medicine (Baltimore)*. 2001;80:252-262.
13. Ferri C, Sebastiani M, Giuggioli D, et al. Mixed cryoglobulinemia: demographic, clinical, and serologic features and survival in 231 patients. *Semin Arthritis Rheum*. 2004;33:355-374.
14. Sene D, Ghillani-Dalbin P, Thibault V, et al. Longterm course of mixed cryoglobulinemia in patients infected with hepatitis C virus. *J Rheumatol*. 2004;31:2199-2206.
15. Martinez J, Kohler P. Variant "Goodpasture's Syndrome": the need for immunologic criteria in rapidly progressive glomerulonephritis and hemorrhagic pneumonitis. *Ann Intern Med*. 1971;75:67-76.
16. Gorevic P, Kassab HJ, Levo Y, et al. Mixed cryoglobulinemia: clinical aspects and long-term follow-up of 40 patients. *Am J Med*. 1980;69(2):287-308.
17. Madrenas J, Vallés M, Ruiz Marcellan MC, Fort J, García Bragado F, Pelegrí A. Pulmonary hemorrhage and glomerulonephritis associated with essential mixed cryoglobulinemia. *Med Clin (Barc)*. 1989;93(7):262-264.
18. Frankel AH, Singer DR, Winearls CG, Evans DJ, Rees AJ, Pusey CD. Type II essential mixed cryoglobulinaemia: presentation, treatment and outcome in 13 patients. *Q J Med*. 1992;82(298): 101-124.

19. Johnson R, Gretch D, Yamabe H, Hart J, Bacchi C, et al. Membranoproliferative glomerulo-nephritis associated with hepatitis C virus infection. *N Engl J Med.* 1993;328:465-470.

20. Johnson R, Gretch D, Couser WG, et al. Hepatitis C virus-associated glomerulonephritis. Effect of α-interferon therapy. *Kidney Int.* 1994;46:1700-1704.

21. Tarantino A, Campise M, Banfi G, Confalonieri R, Bucci A, et al. Long-term predictors of survival in essential mixed cryoglobulinemic glomerulonephritis. *Kidney Int.* 1995;47: 618-623.

22. Petty GW, Duffy J, Houston J. Cerebral ischemia in patients with hepatitis C virus infection and mixed cryoglobulinemia. *Mayo Clin Proc.* 1996;71(7):671-678.

23. Morosetti M, Sciarra G, Meloni C, et al. Membranoproliferative glomerulonephritis and hepatitis C: effects of interferon-α therapy on clinical outcome and histological pattern. *Nephrol Dial Transplant.* 1996;11:532-534.

24. Daoud MS, el-Azhary RA, Gibson LE, Lutz ME, Daoud S, Chronic hepatitis C. cryoglobu-linemia, and cutaneous necrotizing vasculitis. Clinical, pathologic, and immunopathologic study of twelve patients. *J Am Acad Dermatol.* 1996 Feb;34:219-223.

25. Gournay J, Ferrell LD, Roberts JP, Ascher NL, Wright TL, Lake JR. Cryoglobulinemia presenting after liver transplantation. *Gastroenterology.* 1996;110:265-270.

26. Suzuki H, Hickling P, Lyons CB. A case of primary Sjögren's syndrome, complicated by cryoglobulinaemic glomerulonephritis, pericardial and pleural effusions. *Br J Rheumatol.* 1996;35(1):72-75.

27. Moses P, Krawitt E, Aziz W, Corwin H. Renal failure associated with hepatitis C virus infection: improvement in renal function after treatment with interferon-alfa. *Dig Dis Sci.* 1997;42(2):443-446.

28. Morales E, Alegre R, Herrero J, Morales J, Ortuno T, Praga M. Hepatitis-C-virus-associated cryoglobulinaemic membranoproliferative glomerulonephritis in patients infected by HIV. *Nephrol Dial Transplant.* 1997;12:1980-1984.

29. Hent R, Bergkamp F, Weening J, Dorp W. Delayed onset of membranoproliferative glomerulone-phritis in a patient with type I cryoglobulinaemia. *Nephrol Dial Transplant.* 1997;12:2155-2158.

30. D'Amico G. Renal involvement in hepatitis C infection: cryoglobulinemic glomerulonephritis. *Kidney Int.* 1998;54(2):650-671.

31. Johnson SL, Bander J. Pulmonary hemorrhage in a patient with hepatitis C induced essential mixed cryoglobulinemia. *Chest.* 1998;114:422S-425S.

32. Rodríguez-Vidigal FF, Roig Figueroa V, Pérez-Lucena E, Ledesma Jurado V, et al. Alveolar hemorrhage in mixed cryoglobulinemia associated with hepatitis C virus infection. *An Med Interna.* 1998;15(12):661-663.

33. Lamprecht P, Schmitt WH, Gross WL. Mixed cryoglobulinaemia, glomerulonephritis, and ANCA: essential cryoglobulinaemic vasculitis or ANCA-associated vasculitis? *Nephrol Dial Transplant.* 1998;13(1):213-221.

34. Cheng JT, Anderson HL Jr, Markowitz GS, Appel GB, Pogue VA, D'Agati VD. Hepatitis C virus-associated glomerular disease in patients with human immunodeficiency virus coinfection. *J Am Soc Nephrol.* 1999;10(7):1566-1574.

35. Heckmann JG, Kayser C, Heuss D, Manger B, Blum HE, Neundörfer B. Neurological mani-festations of chronic hepatitis C. *J Neurol.* 1999;246(6):486-491.

36. Misiani R, Bellavita P, Baio P, et al. Successful treatment of HCV-associated cryoglobulinaemic glomerulonephritis with a combination of interferon-alpha and ribavirin. *Nephrol Dial Transplant.* 1999;14(6):1558-1560.

37. Montagna G, Piazza V, Banfi G, et al. Hepatitis C virus-associated cryoglobulinaemic glom-erulonephritis with delayed appearance of monoclonal cryoglobulinaemia. *Nephrol Dial Transplant.* 2001;16(2):432-434.

38. Myers JP, Di Bisceglie AM, Mann ES. Cryoglobulinemia associated with Purtscher-like retinopathy. *Am J Ophthalmol.* 2001;131(6):802-804.

39. Dussol B, Moal V, Daniel L, Pain C, Berland Y. Spontaneous remission of HCV-induced cryoglobulinaemic glomerulonephritis. *Nephrol Dial Transplant.* 2001;16(1):156-159.

40. Beddhu S, Bastacky S, Johnson JP. The clinical and morphologic spectrum of renal cryoglobulinemia. *Medicine (Baltimore).* 2002;81(5):398-409.

41. Rieu V, Cohen P, André MH, et al. Characteristics and outcome of 49 patients with symptomatic cryoglobulinaemia. *Rheumatology (Oxford).* 2002;41(3):290-300.

42. Bartolucci P, Ramanoelina J, Cohen P, Mahr A, Godmer P, et al. Efficacy of the anti-TNF-alpha antibody infliximab against refractory systemic vasculitides: an open pilot study on 10 patients. *Rheumatology (Oxford).* 2002;41(10):1126-1132.

43. Zaja F, De Vita S, Russo D, et al. Rituximab for the treatment of type II mixed cryoglobulinemia. *Arthritis Rheum.* 2002;46(8):2252-2254.

44. Arzoo K, Sadeghi S, Liebman HA. Treatment of refractory antibody mediated autoimmune disorders with an anti-CD20 monoclonal antibody (rituximab). *Ann Rheum Dis.* 2002;61(10): 922-924.

45. Suzuki R, Morita H, Komukai D, et al. Mixed cryoglobulinemia due to chronic hepatitis C with severe pulmonary involvement. *Intern Med.* 2003;42(12):1210-1214.

46. Rossi P, Bertani T, Baio P, et al. Hepatitis C virus-related cryoglobulinemic glomerulonephritis: long-term remission after antiviral therapy. *Kidney Int.* 2003;63(6):2236-2241.

47. Bruchfeld A, Lindahl K, Ståhle L, Söderberg M, Schvarcz R. Interferon and ribavirin treatment in patients with hepatitis C-associated renal disease and renal insufficiency. *Nephrol Dial Transplant.* 2003;18(8):1573-1580.

48. Roccatello D, Baldovino S, Rossi D, et al. Long-term effects of anti-CD20 monoclonal antibody treatment of cryoglobulinaemic glomerulonephritis. *Nephrol Dial Transplant.* 2004; 19(12):3054-3061.

49. Ghijsels E, Lerut E, Vanrenterghem Y, Kuypers D. Anti-CD20 monoclonal antibody (rituximab) treatment for hepatitis C-negative therapy-resistant essential mixed cryoglobulinemia with renal and cardiac failure. *Am J Kidney Dis.* 2004;43(5):e34-e38.

50. Amital H, Rubinow A, Naparstek Y. Alveolar hemorrhage in cryoglobulinemia – an indicator of poor prognosis. *Clin Exp Rheumatol.* 2005;23(5):616-620.

51. Kay J, McCluskey RT. Case records of the Massachusetts General Hospital. Case 31-2005. A 60-year-old man with skin lesions and renal insufficiency. *N Engl J Med.* 2005;353(15): 1605-1613.

52. Basse G, Ribes D, Kamar N, et al. Rituximab therapy for de novo mixed cryoglobulinemia in renal transplant patients. *Transplantation.* 2005;80(11):1560-1564.

53. Koukoulaki M, Abeygunasekara SC, Smith KG, Jayne DR. Remission of refractory hepatitis C-negative cryoglobulinaemic vasculitis after rituximab and infliximab. *Nephrol Dial Transplant.* 2005;20(1):213-216.

54. Ramos-Casals M, Robles A, Brito-Zerón P, et al. Life-threatening cryoglobulinemia: clinical and immunological characterization of 29 cases. *Semin Arthritis Rheum.* 2006;36(3):189-196.

55. Quartuccio L, Soardo G, Romano G, et al. Rituximab treatment for glomerulonephritis in HCV-associated mixed cryoglobulinaemia: efficacy and safety in the absence of steroids. *Rheumatology (Oxford).* 2006;45(7):842-846.

56. Garini G, Allegri L, Carnevali ML, Iannuzzella F, Buzio C. Successful treatment of severe/active cryoglobulinaemic membranoproliferative glomerulonephritis associated with hepatitis C virus infection by means of the sequential administration of immunosuppressive and antiviral agents. *Nephrol Dial Transplant.* 2006;21(11):3333-3334.

57. Bestard O, Cruzado JM, Ercilla G, et al. Rituximab induces regression of hepatitis C virus-related membranoproliferative glomerulonephritis in a renal allograft. *Nephrol Dial Transplant.* 2006;21(8):2320-2324.

58. De Vita S, Quartuccio L, Fabris M. Rituximab in mixed cryoglobulinemia: increased experience and perspectives. *Dig Liver Dis.* 2007;39(1):S112-S115.

59. Massari M, Catania A, Magnani G. Efficacy and risk of rituximab in type II mixed cryoglobu-linemia: a significant case report. *Dig Liver Dis.* 2007;39(1):S134-S135.
60. Shaikh A, Habermann TM, Fidler ME, Kumar S, Leung N. Acute renal failure secondary to severe type I cryoglobulinemia following rituximab therapy for Waldenström's macroglobu-linemia. *Clin Exp Nephrol.* 2008;12(4):292-295.
61. Evans JT, Shepard MM, Oates JC, Sally SE, Reuben A. Rituximab-responsive cryoglobu-linemic glomerulonephritis in a patient with autoimmune hepatitis. *J Clin Gastroenterol.* 2008;42(7):862-863.
62. Okura T, Jotoku M, Miyoshi K, et al. Case of membranoproliferative glomerulonephritis due to essential cryoglobulinemia without hepatitis C virus infection. *Geriatr Gerontol Int.* 2009;9(1):92-96.
63. Meng QH, Chibbar R, Pearson D, Kappel J, Krahn J. Heat-insoluble cryoglobulin in a patient with essential type II cryoglobulinemia and cryoglobulin-occlusive membranoproliferative glomerulonephritis: case report and literature review. *Clin Chim Acta.* 2009;406(1–2):170-173.
64. Izzedine H, Sene D, Cacoub P, et al. Kidney diseases in HIV/HCV-co-infected patients. *AIDS.* 2009;23(10):1219-1226.
65. Landau DA, Scerra S, Sene D, Resche-Rigon M, Saadoun D, Cacoub P. Causes and predictive factors of mortality in a cohort of patients with hepatitis C virus-related cryoglobulinemic vasculitis treated with antiviral therapy. *J Rheumatol.* 2010;37(3):615-621.
66. Favre G, Courtellemont C, Callard P, et al. Membranoproliferative glomerulonephritis, chronic lymphocytic leukemia, and cryoglobulinemia. *Am J Kidney Dis.* 2010;55(2):391-394.
67. Méndez P, Saeian K, Rajender Reddy K, Younossi Z, et al. Hepatitis C, cryoglobulinemia, and cutaneous vasculitis associated with unusual and serious manifestations. *Am J Gastroenterol.* 2001;96:2489-2493.
68. Lamprecht P, Moubayed P, Donhuijsen K, Gause A, Gross WL. Vasculitis of adnexa, greater omentum and gallbladder as abdominal manifestations of cryoglobulinemic vasculitis. *Clin Exp Rheumatol.* 2001;19(1):112-113.
69. Lamprecht P, Lerin-Lozano C, Merz H, et al. Rituximab induces remission in refractory HCV associated cryoglobulinaemic vasculitis. *Ann Rheum Dis.* 2003;62(12):1230-1233.
70. Fine GD, Trainer TD, Krawitt EL. Gastrointestinal bleeding, cryoglobulinemia, and hepatitis C. *Am J Gastroenterol.* 2004;99(5):964-965.
71. Jun Cai FC, Ahern M, Smith M. Treatment of cryoglobulinemia associated peripheral neuropathy with rituximab. *J Rheumatol.* 2006;33:1197-1198.
72. Salamone F, Puzzo L. Intestinal HCV-related mixed cryoglobulinemia. *Gastroenterology.* 2010;138(4):e9-e10.
73. Befort P, Riviere S, Maran A, Ramos J, Lequellec A. Repeated intestinal tract perforations secondary to cryoglobulinemia and cytomegalovirus infection: a case report. *Rev Méd Interne.* 2010;31(2):167-169.
74. Quartuccio L, Petrarca A, Mansutti E, et al. Efficacy of rituximab in severe and mild abdominal vasculitis in the course of mixed cryoglobulinemia. *Clin Exp Rheumatol.* 2010;28(57):S84-S87.
75. Propst T, Propst A, Nachbauer K, et al. Papillitis and vasculitis of the arteria spinalis anterior as complications of hepatitis C reinfection after liver transplantation. *Transpl Int.* 1997;10(3):234-237.
76. Origgi L, Vanoli M, Carbone A, Grasso M, Scorza R. Central nervous system involvement in patients with HCV-related cryoglobulinemia. *Am J Med Sci.* 1998;315(3):208-210.
77. Tembl JI, Ferrer JM, Sevilla MT, Lago A, Mayordomo F, Vilchez JJ. Neurologic complica-tions associated with hepatitis C virus infection. *Neurology.* 1999;53(4):861-864.
78. Fragoso M, Carneado J, Tadurí I, Jiménez-Ortiz C. Essential mixed cryoglobulinemia as a cause of ischemic cerebrovascular accident. *Rev Neurol.* 2000;30(5):444-446.
79. Zandman-Goddard G, Levy Y, Weiss P, Shoenfeld Y, Langevitz P. Transverse myelitis associ-ated with chronic hepatitis C. *Clin Exp Rheumatol.* 2003;21(1):111-113.

80. Filippini D, Colombo F, Jann S, Cornero R, Canesi B. Central nervous system involvement in patients with HCV-related cryoglobulinemia: literature review and a case report. *Reumatismo.* 2002;54(2):150-155.

81. Chandesris MO, Gayet S, Schleinitz N, Doudier B, Harlé JR, Kaplanski G. Infliximab in the treatment of refractory vasculitis secondary to hepatitis C-associated mixed cryoglobulinaemia. *Rheumatology (Oxford).* 2004;43(4):532-533.

82. Buccoliero R, Gambelli S, Sicurelli F, et al. Leukoencephalopathy as a rare complication of hepatitis C infection. *Neurol Sci.* 2006;27(5):360-363.

83. Shibazaki K, Iguchi Y, Kimura K, Wada K, Ueno Y, Sunada Y. Paradoxical brain embolism associated with HCV-related type II mixed cryoglobulinemia. *J Clin Neurosci.* 2007;14(8):780-782.

84. Aktipi KM, Ravaglia S, Ceroni M, et al. Severe recurrent myelitis in patients with hepatitis C virus infection. *Neurology.* 2007;68(6):468-469.

85. Erro Aguirre ME, Ayuso Blanco T, Tuñón Alvarez T, Herrera Isasi M. Brain hemorrhage as a complication of chronic hepatitis C virus-related vasculitis. *J Neurol.* 2008;255(6):944-945.

86. Chen WH, Lin HS, Kao YF. Type II cryoglobulinemia and brain hemorrhage. *Clin Appl Thromb Hemost.* 2008;14(2):241-244.

87. Bombardieri S, Paoletti P, Ferri C, Di Munno O, Fornal E, Giuntini C. Lung involvement in essential mixed cryoglobulinemia. *Am J Med.* 1979;66(5):748-756.

88. Gómez-Tello V, Oñoro-Cañaveral JJ, de la Casa Monje RM, Gómez-Casero RB, et al. Diffuse recidivant alveolar hemorrhage in a patient with hepatitis C virus-related mixed cryoglobulinemia. *Intensive Care Med.* 1999;25(3):319-322.

89. Johnston SL, Dudley CR, Unsworth DJ, Lock RJ. Life-threatening acute pulmonary haemorrhage in primary Sjögren's syndrome with cryoglobulinaemia. *Scand J Rheumatol.* 2005;34(5):404-407.

90. Griffiths TA, Daniel CJ, Harris EJ Jr. Bilateral forefoot ischemia as a premonitory symptom of mixed cryoglobulinemia. *J Foot Ankle Surg.* 1996;35(3):213-217.

91. Jacq F, Emmerich J, Héron E, Lortholary O, Bruneval P, Fiessinger JN. Distal gangrene and cryoglobulinemia related to hepatitis C virus infection with presence of anticardiolipin antibodies. *Rev Méd Interne.* 1997;18(4):324-327.

92. Lo KY, Chen CY, Lee CS. Hepatitis C virus-associated type II mixed cryoglobulinemia vasculitis complicated with membranous proliferative glomerulonephritis. *Ren Fail.* 2009;31(2):149-152.

93. Chepyala P, Velchala N, Brown D, Olden K. Encephalopathy, a rare initial presentation of HCV related cryoglobulinemia. *Am J Gastroenterol.* 2009;104:S289.

94. Cacoub P, Maisonobe T, Thibault V, et al. Systemic vasculitis in patients with hepatitis C. *J Rheumatol.* 2001;28(1):109-118.

95. Canada R, Chaudry S, Gaber L, Waters B, Martinez A, Wall B. Polyarteritis nodosa and cryoglobulinemic glomerulonephritis related to chronic hepatitis C. *Am J Med Sci.* 2006;331(6):329-333.

96. Cordonnier DJ, Maurizi J, Vialtel P, et al. Mixed cryoglobulinemia with necrotizing angiitis. Apropos of 2 cases. *Rev Méd Interne.* 1989;10(3):207-215.

97. Steidl C, Baumgaertel MW, Neuen-Jacob E, Berlit P. Vasculitic multiplex mononeuritis: polyarteritis nodosa versus cryoglobulinemic vasculitis. *Rheumatol Int.* 2010 Apr 17 [Epub ahead of print].

98. Garcia de La Peña Lefebvre P, Mouthon L, Cohen P, Lhote F, Guillevin L. Polyarteritis nodosa and mixed cryoglobulinaemia related to hepatitis B and C virus coinfection. *Ann Rheum Dis.* 2001;60(11):1068-1069.

99. Cacoub P, Noel LH, Musset L, Lunel F, Opolon P, Piette JC. Anti-neutrophil cytoplasmic antibodies and mixed cryoglobulinemia. *Clin Exp Rheumatol.* 1994;12(6):693.

100. Papi M, Didona B, De Pità O, Gantcheva M, Chinni LM. Chronic hepatitis C virus infection, mixed cryoglobulinaemia, leukocytoclastic vasculitis and antineutrophil cytoplasmic antibodies. *Lupus.* 1997;6(9):737-738.

101. Asai O, Nakatani K, Yoshimoto S, et al. A case of MPO-ANCA-related microscopic polyangiitis with mixed cryoglobulinemia. *Nippon Jinzo Gakkai Shi.* 2006;48(4):377-384.

102. Ferri C, Mannini L, Bartoli V. Blood viscosity and filtration abnormalities in MC patients. *Clin Exp Rheumatol.* 1990;8:271-281.

103. Carter PW, Cohen HJ, Crawford J. Hyperviscosity syndrome in association with kappa light myeloma. *Am J Med.* 1989;86:591.

104. Della Rossa A, Tavoni A, Bombardieri S. Hyperviscosity syndrome in cryoglobulinemia: clinical aspects and therapeutic considerations. *Semin Thromb Hemost.* 2003;29(5):473-477.

105. Uppal R, Charles E, Lake-Bakaar G. Acute wrist and foot drop associated with hepatitis C virus related mixed cryoglobulinemia: rapid response to treatment with rituximab. *J Clin Virol.* 2010;47(1):69-71.

106. Wheeler RD, Sharma H, Groves M, Wren D, Sheldon J. A case study of mixed cryoglobulinaemia associated with peripheral neuropathy. *Ann Clin Biochem.* 2007;44(Pt 6):566-569.

107. Ivorra J, Muñoz S, Román-Ivorra J, Beltrán E. Treatment with rituximab in a patient with mononeuritis multiplex associated to hepatitis C infection with mixed cryoglobulinemia. *Med Clin (Barc).* 2009;132(11):444-445.

108. Pasa S, Altintas A, Cil T, Danis R, Ayyildiz O, Muftuoglu E. A case of essential mixed cryoglobulinemia and associated acquired von-Willebrand disease treated with rituximab. *J Thromb Thrombolysis.* 2009;27(2):220-222.

109. Sène D, Ghillani-Dalbin P, Amoura Z, Musset L, Cacoub P. Rituximab may form a complex with IgM kappa mixed cryoglobulin and induce severe systemic reactions in patients with hepatitis C virus-induced vasculitis. *Arthritis Rheum.* 2009;60(12):3848-3855.

110. Ruch J, McMahon B, Ramsey G, Kwaan HC. Catastrophic multiple organ ischemia due to an anti-Pr cold agglutinin developing in a patient with mixed cryoglobulinemia after treatment with rituximab. *Am J Hematol.* 2009;84(2):120-122.

111. Gupta A, Gupta G, Marouf R. Cryoglobulinemic vasculitis in pregnancy. *Int J Gynaecol Obstet.* 2008;103(2):177-178.

Behçet's Syndrome: Clinical Presentations Affecting Prognosis and Survival

11

Emire Seyahi, Koray Tascilar, and Hasan Yazici

Abstract Behçet's syndrome (BS) is a multisystem vasculitis with unknown etiology and a unique geographic distribution. It has a high prevalence in the Middle-Eastern and Mediterranean countries. Recurrent skin-mu cosa lesions and sight-threatening panuveitis are the disease hallmarks. BS may also involve joints, vessels of all types and size, the central nervous system (CNS), and the gastrointestinal system. The disease course is characterized by exacerbations and remissions. The disease runs a more severe course among young males, and the severity diminishes with age. Males are more severely affected. Ocular, vascular, and CNS involvement are the main causes of morbidity. This may result in irreversible damage such as loss of useful vision, neurological disability, and potentially fatal bleeding from pulmonary artery aneurysm or Budd–Chiari syndrome. Mortality rate is also increased in BS, especially in young males. Large vessel and parenchymal CNS disease are the main causes of death. However, an early and aggressive approach can lead to better treatment for the ocular and vascular diseases.

Keywords Arterial aneurysms • Arthritis • Behçet's syndrome • Deep vein thrombosis • Dural sinus thrombosis • Hypopyon • Neurologic disease • Oral and genital ulcers • Panuveitis • Retinal vasculitis

11.1
Introduction

As we had indicated before,[1,2] "the skeptic would challenge the inclusion of Behçet's syndrome (BS) in a textbook of systemic autoimmune disease." BS is certainly not a true to form of autoimmune disease since typical features of autoimmune diseases such as female

E. Seyahi (✉)
Cerrahpaşa Medical Faculty, Department of Internal Medicine,
Division of Rheumatology, University of Istanbul, Istanbul 36098, Turkey
e-mail: eseyahi@yahoo.com

M.A. Khamashta and M. Ramos-Casals (eds.), *Autoimmune Diseases*,
DOI: 10.1007/978-0-85729-358-9_11, © Springer-Verlag London Limited 2011

dominance, immune cytopenias, association with Raynaud or Sjögren syndrome, and premature atherosclerosis are absent.[3]

BS is a multisystemic vasculitis characterized by skin-mucosa lesions.[4] It may also involve the eyes, blood vessels of all size and types, central nervous system, and joints.[4] It is seen mainly in a distinct geography extending from Mediterranean basin and Middle East to the Far East in which Turkey has the highest prevalence rate (up to 42/ 10[4]).[4,5] The mean age of onset is usually in the third decade. Both genders are affected equally; however, the disease runs a more severe course among men.[4,6,7] The diagnosis is mainly clinical with no specific laboratory tests.[4] The clinical course is characterized by exacerbations and remissions.[4] Disease burden tends to be more pronounced in the first few years of the disease. Majority of patients goes into remission with time.[6,7] BS can cause substantial morbidity, such as blindness and debility, associated with increased mortality rate.[7]

Here, we describe various clinical manifestations that can affect prognosis and survival in BS and review the management options.

11.2
Skin-Mucosa Lesions

Skin-mucosa lesions recur in virtually every patient and are the most frequent manifestations.[2]

11.2.1
Oral Ulcers

Oral ulcers (Fig. 11.1) are present in almost all patients (~95%) and are usually the most common lesions occurring in an individual patient.[2] They commonly appear as the first disease manifestation and continue to develop after many years of disease onset although

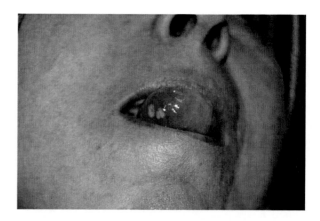

Fig. 11.1 Oral ulcers on the lower surface of the tongue

all other manifestations have faded away. Exacerbations are common when smoking is stopped[8] and among women during the menstrual cycle.[9]

They are in the form of minor oral ulcers (≤10 mm) in 85% of the cases and major ulcers (1–3 cm) in the remaining.[2] They are typically painful, usually superficial with a yellow/white base sometimes surrounded by a red halo.[2] They are usually localized at the mucous membranes of the lips, gingiva, cheeks, and tongue and less commonly at the palate, tonsils, and pharynx.

Minor ulcers heal within 1 week without scarring, whereas deeper major ulcers heal more slowly and may leave scars.[2] BS patients with chronic and destructive giant oral ulcerations could be difficult to manage.[10] Furthermore, pharyngeal stenosis ultimately leading to pneumonia and death has been reported as an unfortunate complication of retropharyngeal ulcers.[11]

11.2.2
Genital Ulcers

Genital ulcers being one of the hallmarks of BS develop in about 80–90% of the patients.[2,6,7] They usually occur during the first years of disease onset then disappear. They relapse less frequently than oral ulcers. Genital ulcers occur mostly on the scrotum (85%) and less frequently on penis, inguinal and perianal regions in men.[2] They are usually localized on major and minor labia and less frequently on the cervix and vagina in women. Similar to oral ulcers, they may be painful in a substantial portion of patients and may cause difficulty in walking and sitting. Morphologically, genital ulcers are similar to oral ulcers, but are usually deeper and larger. They usually heal in 10–30 days.[12] Caution is needed in the diagnosis and correct management because genital ulcers in BS may frequently get infected, especially among females, and healing may be delayed (Fig. 11.2). Two-thirds of genital ulcers leave scars, and larger ulcers tend to heal with more scar tissue compared to smaller ones.[12] Genital scarring is usually a strong proof for the presence of BS.[12,13] In women, these ulcers may lead to destructive lesions in the perineum and vulva. Recurrent

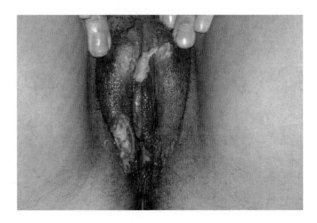

Fig. 11.2 Large ulcers with discharge on the vulva of a female patient

herpes genitalis should be remembered in the differential diagnosis as they are usually at the same site. However, their appearance and histologies are quite different than those due to BS: Herpetic lesions occur as multiple, small vesicles.

11.2.3
Papulopustular Lesions

These lesions can be found in about 85% of the patients and are usually located on the face, upper chest (Fig. 11.3), neck, shoulders, and femoral and buttock regions.[2] They usually heal within 2–3 days. Clinical and histological features of these lesions are difficult to differentiate from those seen in acne vulgaris.[14] There may be intrafollicular abscess formation. However, differing from ordinary acne, they are more commonly found in the extremities. Papulopustular lesions are more common among those patients with arthritis,[15] and recent bacteriologic studies show that these lesions may not be sterile.[16]

11.2.4
Nodular Lesions

They are observed in about 50% of patients.[2,6,7] These are painful red-purple nodules localized mostly on the shins, thighs, and rarely on the upper extremities (Fig. 11.4). Nodular lesions may be caused by two different pathologies in BS[17] (Algorithm, Fig. 11.5):

1. Erythema nodosum is more common in females and associated usually with other mucocutaneous manifestations such as oral and genital ulcers. Different than those due to other causes, erythema nodosum lesions in BS seem to be less well demarcated and are more likely to heal leaving brown pigmentation and with ulceration. Ultrasonographically, they appear as hyperechoic lesions. Histopathological examination of these lesions shows septal panniculitis associated with vasculitis in half of the cases.[18]

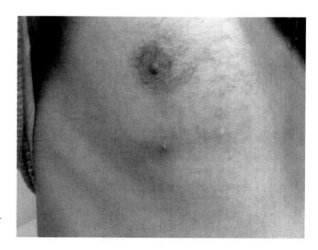

Fig. 11.3 Pustule on the upper chest of a male patient

Fig. 11.4 Red nodular lesion on the medial inferior part of tibia

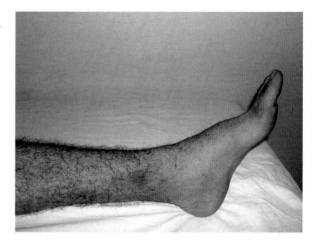

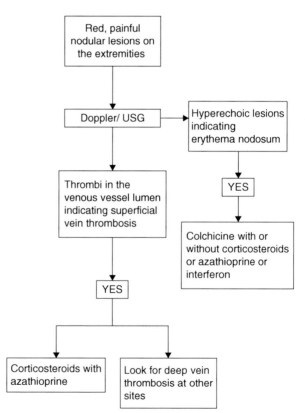

Fig. 11.5 Algorithm for diagnosis and management of erythematous nodular lesions due to Behçet's syndrome

2. Superficial thrombophlebitis is more common among male patients and have a more sinister implication since they can be associated with large vessel involvement else-where. BS patients presenting with superficial thrombophlebitis are more prone to develop dural sinus thrombi and or lower extremity deep vein thrombosis.[19,20]

On closer examination, these lesions look like beaded lesions following vein tracts. Large and small veins of the lower extremities are involved, greater saphenous being the most frequently affected. B –mode ultrasonographic pattern is hypoechoic and a Doppler study may show thrombi in the lumina of the involved vessels. Histological examination reveals organized thrombus in the lumen of the involved vein.

11.2.5
Other Mucocutaneous Manifestations

Extragenital ulcers are similar to recurrent aphthous ulcerations and develop in intertriginous regions such as infra-mammary, axillary, and interdigital regions. They almost always heal with scarring. Pyoderma gangrenosum, erythema multiforme, and Sweet lesions are other less common skin manifestations.

11.2.6
Pathergy Test

Pathergy reaction occurs in about 60% of patients.[2,6,7] A positive response is determined by a papule or pustule formation to a sterile dermal pinprick after 48 h. It is basically an exaggerated nonspecific inflammatory response to minor trauma. Male patients and those with active disease have stronger reactions.[21] It is highly specific – and almost unique for BS. However, the reproducibility is not good enough and the sensitivity is mostly around 50%. The pathergy test may be positive rarely in pyoderma gangrenosum and Sweet syndrome.

11.2.7
The Outcome in Mucocutaneous Lesions

These lesions rarely lead to serious complications, and permanent damage, however, does affect quality of life. The frequency and severity of the lesions tend to abate with time.[6,7] We had reported that the frequency of any one of the skin-mucosa manifestations decreased considerably 20 years after disease onset.[7]

11.2.8
Management of Skin-Mucosa Lesions

Local treatment by steroid preparations can be effective for oral ulcers. Colchicine has been considered to be beneficial in treating all mucocutaneous manifestations. However, a double-blind study showed that the drug was only beneficial for genital ulcers and erythema nodosum among the females.[22] Thalidomide has shown efficacy in treating all mucocutaneous lesions except the nodular lesions of BS.[23] However, caution is required because of its side effects. Our group also demonstrated that low-dose depot glucocorticoids may be effective in treating erythema nodosum in a double-blind placebo-controlled trial.[24] Azathioprine (AZA), cyclosporine A (CsA), and interferon-α (IFN-α) may all be beneficial in resistant cases.[25] Trials of topical IFN[26] and of topical CsA[27] did not demonstrate any improvement in the number, size, and healing time of oral ulcers. A prospective study reported favorable results with benzathine penicillin.[28]

Recent studies revealed that anti-TNF agents can be successfully used for various manifestations in BS. In a controlled trial among males, etanercept was effective in controlling most of the mucocutaneous manifestations of BS, whereas it did not suppress the pathergy phenomenon.[29]

Our practice in case of recalcitrant mucocutaneous disease is to switch to AZA 2.5 mg/kg from colchicine. If there is no response after 3–6 months of follow-up, interferon in a lower dose than used in uveitis (two to three million units, two to three times a week up to five million units daily) may be tried. Etanercept or infliximab may be useful in some patients. In the rare patient without nodular lesions and severe recurrent genital ulcers, a trial of thalidomide 100–300 mg/day may be appropriate. We have no experience with dapsone; however, it was shown to be effective in a double-blind trial.[30]

11.3
Joint Involvement

Joint disease in the form of mono- or oligo-arthritis or arthralgia is seen in about 30–50% of patients with BS.[31] Knees, ankles, wrists, and elbows are frequently affected. The arthritis is usually self-limited and resolves in 2–4 weeks without causing deformity or erosions on radiography. Knee synovitis causing a ruptured Baker's cyst, mimicking acute deep vein thrombophlebitis, can be observed (Algorithm, Fig. 11.6). Ultrasonographic examination is helpful in diagnosis. A pseudoseptic arthritis with extremely high leukocyte counts in the synovial fluid has also been described.[32,33]

We had reported that BS patients with arthritis were more prone to have papulopustular lesions than those without,[15] as mentioned earlier. We now believe that there is an isolated cluster in BS, which bears reactive arthritis-like features such as acne, arthritis, and enthesitis.[34] Having said that, we do not think that BS is a part of spondylarthropathies (SpA) since (a) sacroiliac joints and spine are spared, (b) there is no association with HLA B27, and (c) the clinical spectrum of eye involvement (severe panuveitis rather than anterior uveitis or conjunctivitis is seen in BS) is quite different from what is observed in the SpA.[17]

Nonsteroidal anti-inflammatory drugs and local corticosteroid injections are used frequently in management. Colchicine can be effective in both males and females as shown in controlled studies.[22] IFN-α (5 MU/3 times a week) is highly effective in treating arthritis according to one controlled study.[35] AZA and anti-TNF agents are also successful in reducing the frequency of arthritis attacks.[29,36,37] Short courses of oral prednisolone (20–30 mg/day) may be useful in more severe cases. Methotrexate and sulfasalazine may be tried in resistant cases although there are no controlled studies with these agents.

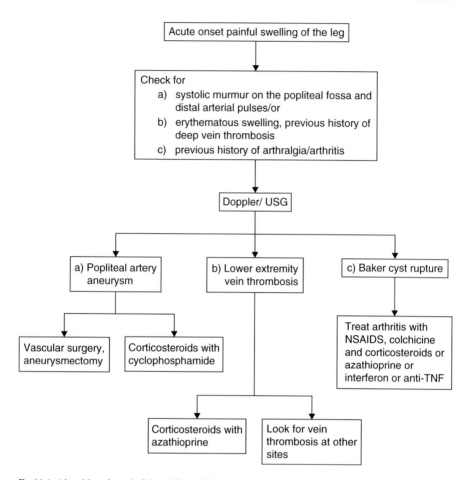

Fig. 11.6 Algorithm for painful swelling of the leg in Behçet's syndrome

11.4
Eye Disease

Eye involvement is one of the most serious manifestations and affects about 50% of the patients (males: 55%, females: 30%).[7] Young males (those with age of onset 25 years or less) are more prone to have eye disease compared to those with age of onset 25 years or more.[6] Eye disease develops within the first few years of the disease onset and runs its most severe course during these years; therefore, medical treatment should be prompt and aggressive especially during this period. The involvement is bilateral in 70–80% of patients at the beginning and becomes 90% at long term.[38] During ocular attacks, patients usually complain of ocular pain, discomfort, and visual blurring. Eye involvement in BS can be summarized as a combination of recurrent attacks of non-granulomatous uveitis and retinal vasculitis.[38] In 60% of the cases, both anterior and posterior uvea are involved.

Associated retinal vasculitis is reported to be present in ~90% of the cases. Hypopyon is observed less commonly (12%) and indicates severe outcome.[38] Fundoscopic examination may reveal choroidal and retinal exudates, hemorrhages, cytoid bodies, venous thrombosis, papilledema, and macular involvement.[38] Male gender, posterior involvement, frequent attacks, strong vitreous opacity, and exudates alongside the retinal vascular arcade are reported to be poor prognostic factors.[39,40] Recurrent inflammatory activity results in late complications such as anterior and posterior synechia, cataract, secondary glaucoma, macular degeneration, and finally phthisis bulbi.[38]

Conjunctivitis, episcleritis, and conjunctival ulcerations are rare manifestations.

The prognosis of the eye disease has been reported as poor in the past, and blindness was often considered as the eventual outcome in an average of 3 years after the onset of ocular symptoms.[41] Thirty years ago, more than half of the Japanese BS patients were reported to have lost their useful vision within 5 years of disease onset.[42] In a study from Israel, despite treatment, 75% of BS patients with uveitis had lost useful vision in 6–10 years after the onset of disease.[43] Bilateral useful vision loss was observed in 44% of males and 21% of females with eye disease at the end of 20 years in a group of patients that had registered in our clinic between 1977 and 1983.[7] Of these, 17% (25/146) of males and 10.5% (4/38) of females had bilateral useful vision loss at their initial presentation. The majority of the visual loss had already developed at the first year of disease onset (40%) and during the first 4 years following inception (42%) decreasing substantially thereafter.[7] Furthermore, about one-fourth of males and females with eye involvement were found to have unilateral loss of useful vision at the end of survey.[7] It is to be noted that the outcome of those in whom eye disease develop de-novo later during the follow-up was better, since none of the patients in this group developed bilateral loss of useful vision.[7] The outcome of 880 BS patients seen between 1980 and 1998 was similarly better: The risk of having useful vision loss at 5 and 10 years was predicted to be 21% and 30% for males whereas 10% and 17% for females, under conventional immunosuppressive treatment.[38] Accordingly, male patients who presented after 1990 were found to have a lower rate of visual loss compared to those who presented in the 1980s.[38]

Eye disease is treated with immunosuppressives, and the routine and early use of these agents has changed the visual prognosis. In this line, AZA (2.5 mg/kg/day) was found to be effective in preventing visual attacks in a double-blind controlled trial.[35,36] Moreover, there was no decrease in the mean visual acuity between the beginning and the end of the 2-year period among the AZA users.[35] When these patients were reassessed at 8 years, blindness developed significantly among less patients who initially received AZA (3/24; 13%) compared to those initially allocated to placebo (8/20; 40%) ($p=0.036$).[36] Another immunosuppressive drug that has found widespread use in the treatment of eye disease is CsA. It was superior to monthly pulses of cyclophosphamide in a single-blind study conducted in a limited number of patients.[25,44] It induces a very rapid anti-inflammatory effect in doses of 2–5 mg/kg/day, but caution is advised regarding its toxic effects such as rises in serum creatinine, hypertension, occasional episodes of neuropathy, and hearing loss. Its use is not recommended in case of concomitant CNS disease given its well-known neurotoxicity.[45,46] IFN-α offers promising results and seems to be another alternative in the management of uveitis in BS.[47] The drug was even beneficial in posterior uveitis of BS refractory to conventional medications.[48] Side effects of IFN-α include flu-like symptoms, liver enzyme elevations, cytopenias, and severe mood changes.[47,48] Anti-TNF agents (especially infliximab at 5 mg/kg) show successful results in controlling severe and resistant uveitis.[49-51] However, relapses are frequent after withdrawal.

Glucocorticoids are also used in the management of acute attacks.[25] During attacks, local steroid eye drops and mydriatics are commonly used to prevent synechiae and alleviate pain. Vitrectomy and cataract surgery are also advised in patients with complications.

11.5
Vascular Disease

Vascular disease develops in up to 25–35% of the patients and has a definite male preponderance.[6,7,52-55] Its frequency can go up to 49% among males when followed for 20 years.[7] Venous involvement is more common than arterial disease (75% vs 25%), and lower extremity deep vein thrombosis (DVT) is the most frequent manifestation.[7,53-55]

It mainly involves the venous and pulmonary circulations rather than systemic arteries. The most common manifestation is deep venous thrombosis (DVT) in a lower extremity, followed by vena cava disease, pulmonary artery disease, aortic or peripheral artery aneurysms, venous sinus thrombosis, and Budd–Chiari syndrome.[55] Bulk of the vascular involvement occurs early in the disease course (30% of events at disease onset or before fulfilling ISG criteria). However, systemic artery disease is clearly different from pulmonary artery (developing in a median of 7 years) and large vein disease with an older age at occurrence and less frequent association with deep vein thrombosis.[7,55] The 5-year probability of a new vascular event in a patient with vascular involvement is 38%.[55]

The patient with deep vein thrombosis presents with a painful and swollen calf generally on one side. It involves ultimately both sides during the follow-up. Acute venous thrombosis causes pain, erythema, and swelling, whereas chronic vein thrombosis causes varices, hyperpigmentation, skin thickening, and ulcers (Fig. 11.7). Pulmonary embolism is very rare even with thrombosis extending to inferior vena cava. Bilateral lower extremity swelling and the presence of abdominal collaterals suggest usually inferior vena cava (IVC)

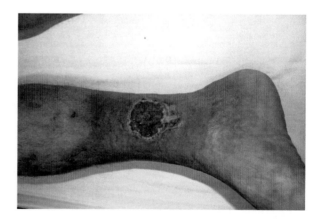

Fig. 11.7 Venous stasis ulcer on the medial lower surface of the tibia of a male Behçet patient with chronic deep vein thrombosis

disease (Fig. 11.8). IVC involvement is common in patients with Budd–Chiari syndrome. We therefore advise imaging the hepatic veins especially when there is abdominal pain and ascites in a patient with BS (Algorithm, Fig. 11.9). Superior vena cava (SVC) involvement presents with swelling in the face and upper extremities with full jugular veins without pulsation. Occasionally, patients may have dyspnea and sleep apnea disorder. Lower

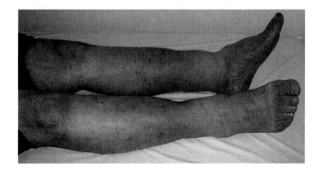

Fig. 11.8 Bilateral lower extremity swelling in male patient with inferior vena cava thrombosis

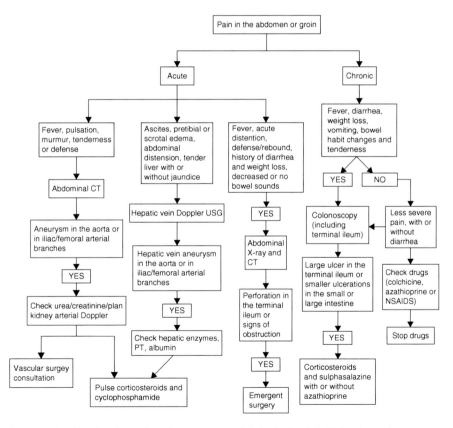

Fig. 11.9 Algorithm for diagnosis and management of abdominal pain in Behçet's syndrome

extremity deep vein thrombosis is less common than in patients with IVC disease. Despite the alarming presentation, the SVC thrombosis in BS usually has a benign course with efficient collateral circulation. It might rarely be complicated with pleural effusion and chylothorax.[56] Pulmonary artery aneurysms (PAA), the most dreaded vascular disease, presents with hemoptysis, cough, dyspnea, fever, and chest pain[57] (Algorithm, Fig. 11.10). It is always associated with high acute phase response.[57] PAA are observed as bilateral or unilateral hilar opacities on chest X-ray or thorax CT scans (Fig. 11.11). Hemoptysis may be

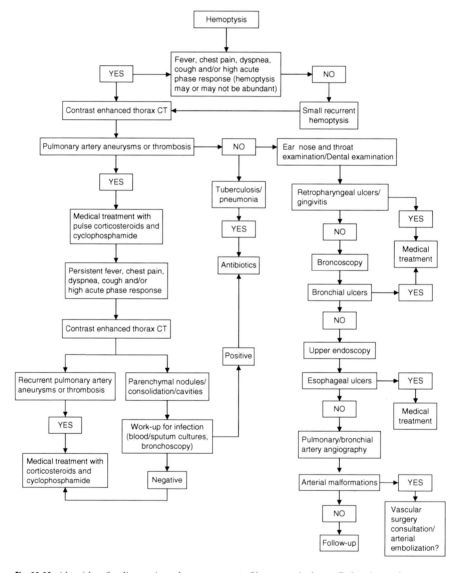

Fig. 11.10 Algorithm for diagnosis and management of hemoptysis due to Behçet's syndrome

massive leading to death; therefore, it requires emergent treatment.[58,59] Thorax CT scans of these patients may also show parenchymal nodules, consolidations, and cavities mimicking opportunistic infections (Figs. 11.11 and 11.12).[57] We recently observed that some of these patients have increased systolic pulmonary artery pressure (manuscript in preparation).

Abdominal aortic aneurysm patient with BS is a sick man in his late 30s or 40s with abdominal or back pain[55] (Algorithm, Fig. 11.9). Peripheral aneurysms present with pulsatile masses in the extremities or the neck (Algorithm, Fig. 11.6). Constitutional symptoms such as low-grade fever, loss of appetite, or an increase in the acute phase response are additional clues to the presence of arterial as well as venous disease.

Among all type of vascular involvement, Budd–Chiari syndrome has the worse outcome with a mortality rate of 60–100%.[7,60] PAA is another serious complication, leading to death by massive hemoptysis currently in about in 25–27% of patients.[57-59] Aortic and peripheral arterial aneurysms are also major causes of death because of the risk of rupture and postoperative complications.

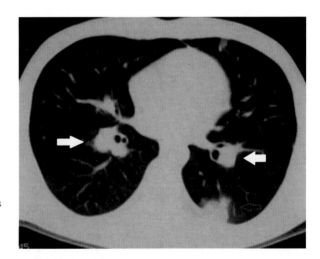

Fig. 11.11 Bilateral pulmonary artery aneurysms (*white arrows*) and peripheral nodular lesion (*red arrow*) on thorax CT

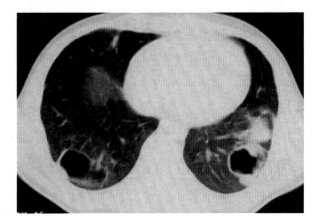

Fig. 11.12 Bilateral large cavities on thorax CT in a male patient with pulmonary artery aneurysms

Postmortem examinations revealed that the thrombi in vascular BS patients are tightly adherent to the vessel wall.[61] For this reason, we prefer not to anticoagulate BS patients with venous thrombosis. Our general approach is to treat more severe types of vascular disease such as PAA, IVC thrombosis with Budd–Chiari syndrome and abdominal, carotid, or aortic aneurysms with monthly cyclophosphamide pulses in a dose of 1,000 mg and an initial 4–8 week course of 1 mg/kg corticosteroids. Cyclophosphamide treatment is generally extended to 2 years in patients with PAA but may be of shorter duration in others. Patients with peripheral, SVC, and other type of venous thrombosis invariably receive AZA 2.5 mg/kg, which is probably of greater benefit than anticoagulation. Although there is no evidence to back it up, we generally have been prescribing low-dose aspirin but less so in recent years. Abdominal aneurysms may be managed with graft insertion, and aneurysmatic peripheral arteries may be ligated by an experienced vascular surgeon.[62] We generally administer immunosuppressive treatment both before and after the surgery as there is a considerable risk of recurrence.

11.6
Neurological Disease

There are mainly two types of neurological disease in BS: parenchymal CNS disease, which is the most common (75–80%) and dural sinus thrombosis (10–20%).[63,64] The frequency of all type of neurological involvement has been reported to be around 5% in cross-sectional studies; however, this rate doubles when a same cohort is followed for two decades.[7]

Headache is the most common neurological symptom in BS.[65] It can be due to various causes such as parenchymal CNS disease, dural sinus thrombosis, ocular inflammation, acute attacks of BS itself, and coexisting primary headaches such as migraine[65] (Algorithm, Fig. 11.13).

Parenchymal CNS disease is usually a late manifestation, developing after 5–10 years of the disease onset. Brainstem involvement is the most characteristic type of involvement.[63,64] Spinal cord and hemispheric involvement are rarely observed. Pyramidal signs, hemiparesis, behavioral–cognitive changes, and sphincter disturbances and/or impotence are the main clinical manifestations.[1,63,64] Character disorders, impairment of memory, and dementia and other psychiatric symptoms may also occur concomitantly.[66] Multiple sclerosis, sarcoidosis, and tuberculosis can be considered in the differential diagnosis in a BS patient presenting with subacute brainstem syndrome or hemiparesis.[1] However, lesions detected in the cranial MRI are often strongly suggestive of BS and usually easily help to exclude other diagnoses. The lesions in BS are generally large and extensive and located within the brainstem, extending to the diencephalon and/or basal ganglia, and less often in the periventricular and subcortical white matter.[1] In MS, however, the lesions are more discrete and smaller and are found frequently in the brainstem, supratentorially periventricular area, and corpus callosum. Moreover optic neuritis, sensory symptoms, and spinal cord involvement are infrequent in BS. Cerebrospinal fluid examinations in BS with parenchymal CNS involvement may reveal pleocytosis, modest protein increase, and low oligoclonal band positivity.[1,63]

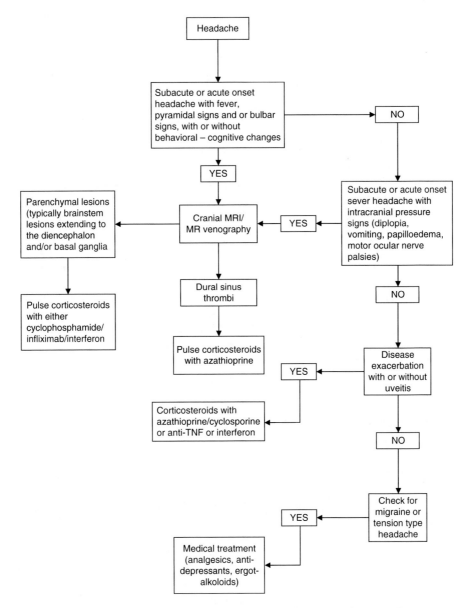

Fig. 11.13 Algorithm for diagnosis and management of headache due to Behçet's syndrome

The lesions of the nervous system may progress to produce bulbar paralysis, and this may lead often to disability and death. It is reported that the disease may follow relapsing remitting course progressing to severe disability in approximately 50% of the cases in 10 years.[64] In an outcome survey of 200 patients, almost 60% of patients with parenchymal involvement were found to be dead or dependant on another person 10 years after onset of neurological disease.[63] Poor prognostic factors were defined as abnormal cerebrospinal fluid, having parenchymal involvement, frequent attacks, and being dependant on others at admission.[63,64] Whereas, good prognostic factors were: normal CSF findings, disease course limited to single episode, non-parenchymal (dural sinus) type of involvement, and independence at admission.

Dural sinus thrombosis is usually associated with other types of venous disease[19] and has a significantly better outcome compared to parenchymal type.[1,63,64] It occurs earlier in disease course compared to parenchymal CNS type.[64] It is the predominant type of neurological involvement in juvenile BS patients.[67] Symptoms of increased intracranial pressure symptoms such as severe headache, papilledema, motor ocular nerve palsies may be seen. It can be associated rarely with fever. Eye examination will disclose bilateral swollen optic disk in most of the patients. Clinical presentations may vary according to site and rate of venous occlusions and its extent. Persistent intracranial pressure may cause optic atrophy and blindness despite treatment.[68,69]

Like almost all other manifestations, neurological involvement runs a more severe course among males. The disease is usually treated with high doses of corticosteroids and cyclophosphamide or AZA, although controlled studies with these agents in CNS disease are lacking. Interferon is reported to be effective as reported in sporadic cases[70,71] and should be considered in patients in whom a viral infection cannot be ruled out as a cause of the CNS disease.[72] In severe cases of dural sinus thrombosis with visual impairment, lumboperitoneal shunting should be considered.[69]

11.7
Other Manifestations

11.7.1
Cardiac Disease

Cardiac involvement is infrequent,[4] but may cause severe complications such as aortic regurgitation associated with aortitis, ventricular aneurysms, coronary vasculitis, and intracardiac thrombi. Intracardiac thrombi are usually associated with pulmonary vascular disease[73] and should be treated with corticosteroids and immunosuppressive agents. Atherosclerosis and associated coronary artery disease are not appreciably increased in BS.[74-76]

11.7.2
Gastrointestinal Disease

Gastrointestinal involvement is relatively rare in the Mediterranean and Middle-Eastern countries[77] compared to what is observed in the Far East.[78] It is characterized mainly by aphthous ulcerations, found especially in terminal ileum and that may cause perforation. Sulfasalazine and glucocorticoids are used in the first place. In resistant cases,

AZA can be tried with or without thalidomide.[79,80] There are case reports suggesting that anti-TNF agents could be beneficial.[81] Surgical resections are required in acute severe cases.[82]

11.7.3
Renal Disease

Glomerulonephritis and secondary amyloidosis occur rarely. Amyloidosis predominantly occurs in males and seems to be closely associated with large vessel disease and arthritis.

11.7.4
Urological Problems

Epididymitis, cystitis, and erectile dysfunction are the most common problems. Erectile dysfunction is associated mainly with parenchymal neurologic involvement.[63,64]

11.8
Mortality

In a 20-year outcome survey, we had reported a mortality rate of 10% in a cohort of 426 patients (42/426).[7] The mortality rate was significantly higher among males than females (39/286 vs 3/142, $p=0.001$).[7] Standardized mortality ratios (SMRs) were specifically increased among young males (14–24 and 25–34 years old age groups) while older males (35–50 year old age) and females had a normal life span. Furthermore, we observed that the mortality rate was highest during the first years (7 years) of disease onset and had a tendency to decrease with time. We demonstrated that patients who had died had significantly more major organ involvement (such as eye, large vessel and CNS) at disease onset compared to those who had been alive.[7] Probable causes of mortality were large vessel disease especially PAA ($n=17$), parenchymal CNS disease ($n=5$), neoplasms ($n=4$), chronic renal failure ($n=4$), ischemic heart disease ($n=3$), congestive heart failure/stroke ($n=3$), suicide ($n=2$), a traffic accident ($n=1$), and unknown ($n=3$).

Recently, French colleagues reported the outcome of 817 BS patients followed between 1974 and 2006.[83] A total of 41 (5%) died after a median follow-up of 7.7 years. The mean age at death was 34.6 ± 11.5 years and 95.1% were male. Furthermore, similar to that found in our 20-year outcome survey, the mortality rate was increased among the 15–24 years and the 25–34 years as compared to those older than 35 years. Main causes of death included arterial involvement [PAA ($n=3$), thoracic aortic aneurysm ($n=3$), myocardial infarction ($n=3$) and abdominal aortic ($n=1$) and cerebral aneurysm ($n=1$)], large venous involvement [Budd–Chiari syndrome ($n=4$), pulmonary embolism ($n=3$)], cancer ($n=6$), CNS involvement ($n=5$), and infection ($n=5$). Other causes of death included pancreatitis

($n=1$), amyloidosis ($n=1$), and thrombotic microangiopathy ($n=1$). Causes of death were unknown in four.

Mortality rates appear to be low in other series.[84-87] Kaklamani et al. observed no single death among 64 patients, during a follow-up of 30 years.[84] Benamour et al. showed a mortality rate of 3% among a cohort of 316 patients diagnosed between 1981 and 1989.[85] Yamamoto et al. reported that 22 (1%) died among 2,031 patients from Japan during the course of a single year's follow-up.[86] Similarly, seven deaths (0.3%) were observed among 2,220 patients during a follow-up of 9 years in a Korean study.[87] Causes of death were defined as intestinal involvement, large vessel disease, valvular heart disease, infection, and cerebrovascular disease.[87]

References

1. Siva A, Yazici H. Behçet's syndrome. Neurological involvement in systemic autoimmune disease. In: Erkan D, Levine SR, eds. *Handbook of Systemic Autoimmune Diseases*, vol. 3. Amsterdam: Elsevier; 2004:193.
2. Mat C, Demirkesen C, Melikoglu M, Yazici H. Behçet's syndrome. The skin in systemic autoimmune disease. In: Piercarlo Sarzi-Puttini, Doria A, Giampiero Girolomoni, Kuhn A, eds. *Handbook of Systemic Autoimmune Diseases*, vol. 5. Amsterdam: Elsevier; 2006:185.
3. Yazici H. The place of Behçet's syndrome among the autoimmune diseases. *Int Rev Immunol*. 1997;14:1-10.
4. Fresko I, Melikoglu M, Kural-Seyahi, et al. Behcet's syndrome: pathogenesis, clinical manifestations and treatment in Vasculitis by Gene. In: Ball GV, Bridges SL, eds. *Vasculitis*. 2nd ed. New York: Oxford University Press; 2008;461-480.
5. Azizlerli G, Köse AA, Sarica R, et al. Prevalence of Behçet's disease in Istanbul, Turkey. *Int J Dermatol*. 2003;42:803-806.
6. Yazici H, Tüzün Y, Pazarli H, et al. Influence of age of onset and patient's sex on the prevalence and severity of manifestations of Behçet's syndrome. *Ann Rheum Dis*. 1984;43:783-789.
7. Kural-Seyahi E, Fresko I, Seyahi N, et al. The long-term mortality and morbidity of Behcet syndrome: a 2-decade outcome survey of 387 patients followed at a dedicated center. *Medicine (Baltimore)*. 2003;82:60-76.
8. Soy M, Erken E, Konca K, Ozbek S. Smoking and Behcet's disease. *Clin Rheumatol*. 2000;19:508-509.
9. Oh SH, Han EC, Lee JH, et al. Comparison of the clinical features of recurrent aphthous stomatitis and Behçet's disease. *Clin Exp Dermatol*. 2009;34:e208-e212.
10. Mansur AT, Kocaayan N, Serdar ZA, et al. Giant oral ulcers of Behçet's disease mimicking squamous cell carcinoma. *Acta Derm Venereol*. 2005;85:532-534.
11. Hamza M. Juvenile Behçet's disease. In: Wechsler B, Godeau P, eds. *Behçet's Disease*. Amsterdam: Excerpta Medica; 1993:377-380.
12. Mat MC, Goksugur N, Engin B, et al. The frequency of scarring after genital ulcers in Behçet's syndrome: a prospective study. *Int J Dermatol*. 2006;45:554-556.
13. Hatemi I, Hatemi G, Celik AF, et al. Frequency of pathergy phenomenon and other features of Behçet's syndrome among patients with inflammatory bowel disease. *Clin Exp Rheumatol*. 2008;26(4 Suppl 50):S91-S95.
14. Ergun T, Gürbüz O, Dogusoy G, Mat C, Yazici H. Histopathologic features of the spontaneous pustular lesions of Behçet's syndrome. *Int J Dermatol*. 1998;37:194-196.

15. Diri E, Mat C, Hamuryudan V, et al. Papulopustular skin lesions are seen more frequently in patients with Behçet's syndrome who have arthritis: a controlled and masked study. *Ann Rheum Dis*. 2001;60:1074-1076.

16. Hatemi G, Bahar H, Uysal S, et al. The pustular skin lesions in Behçet's syndrome are not sterile. *Ann Rheum Dis*. 2004;63:1450-1452.

17. Yazici H. The lumps and bumps of Behçet's syndrome. *Autoimmun Rev*. 2004;3(Suppl 1): S53-S54.

18. Demirkesen C, Tüzüner N, Mat C, et al. Clinicopathologic evaluation of nodular cutaneous lesions of Behçet syndrome. *Am J Clin Pathol*. 2001;116:341-346.

19. Tunc R, Saip S, Siva A, Yazici H. Cerebral venous thrombosis is associated with major vessel disease in Behçet's syndrome. *Ann Rheum Dis*. 2004;63:1693-1694.

20. Tunc R, Keyman E, Melikoglu M, Fresko I, Yazici H. Target organ associations in Turkish patients with Behçet's disease: a cross sectional study by exploratory factor analysis. *J Rheumatol*. 2002;29:2393-2396.

21. Yazici H, Tüzün Y, Tanman AB, et al. Male patients with Behçet's syndrome have stronger pathergy reactions. *Clin Exp Rheumatol*. 1985;3:137-141.

22. Yurdakul S, Mat C, Tuzun Y, et al. A double-blind trial of colchicine in Behcet's syndrome. *Arthritis Rheum*. 2001;44:2686-2692.

23. Hamuryudan V, Mat C, Saip S, et al. Thalidomide in the treatment of the mucocutaneous lesions of the Behcet syndrome. A randomized, double-blind, placebo-controlled trial. *Ann Intern Med*. 1998;128:443-450.

24. Mat C, Yurdakul S, Uysal S, et al. A double-blind trial of depot corticosteroids in Behcet's syndrome. *Rheumatology (Oxford)*. 2006;45:348-352.

25. Yazici H, Ozyazgan Y. Medical management of Behcet's syndrome. *Dev Ophthalmol*. 1999;31:118-131.

26. Hamuryudan V, Yurdakul S, Rosenkaimer F, Yazici H. Inefficacy of topical alpha interferon in the treatment of oral ulcers of Behcet's syndrome: a randomized, double blind trial. *Br J Rheumatol*. 1991;30:395-396.

27. Ergun T, Gurbuz O, Yurdakul S, Hamuryudan V, Bekiroglu N, Yazici H. Topical cyclosporine-A for treatment of oral ulcers of Behcet's syndrome. *Int J Dermatol*. 1997;36:720.

28. Calguneri M, Kiraz S, Ertenli I, Benekli M, Karaarslan Y, Celik I. The effect of prophylactic penicillin treatment on the course of arthritis episodes in patients with Behcet's disease. A randomized clinical trial. *Arthritis Rheum*. 1996;39:2062-2065.

29. Melikoglu M, Fresko I, Mat C, et al. Short-term trial of etanercept in Behcet's disease: a double blind, placebo controlled study. *J Rheumatol*. 2005;32:98-105.

30. Sharquie KE, Najim RA, Abu-Raghif AR. Dapsone in Behçet's disease: a double-blind, placebo-controlled, cross-over study. *J Dermatol*. 2002;29:267-279.

31. Yurdakul S, Yazici H, Tuzun Y, et al. The arthritis of Behcet's disease: a prospective study. *Ann Rheum Dis*. 1983;42:505-515.

32. Volpe A, Caramaschi P, Marchetta A, Desto E, Arcar G. Pseudoseptic arthritis in a patient with Behçet's disease. *Clin Exp Rheumatol*. 2006;24:S123.

33. Humby F, Gullick N, Kelly S, Pitzalis C, Oakley SP. A synovial pathergy reaction leading to a pseudo-septic arthritis and a diagnosis of Behçet's disease. *Rheumatology (Oxford)*. 2008;47: 1255-1256.

34. Hatemi G, Fresko I, Tascilar K, et al. Increased enthesopathy among Behçet's syndrome patients with acne and arthritis: an ultrasonography study. *Arthritis Rheum*. 2008;58:1539-1545.

35. Hamuryudan V, Moral F, Yurdakul S, et al. Systemic interferon alpha 2b treatment in Behçet's syndrome. *J Rheumatol*. 1994;21:1098-1100.

36. Yazici H, Pazarli H, Barnes CG, et al. A controlled trial of azathioprine in Behcet's syndrome. *N Engl J Med*. 1990;322:281-285.

37. Hamuryudan V, Ozyazgan Y, Hizli N, et al. Azathioprine in Behcet's syndrome: effects on long-term prognosis. *Arthritis Rheum*. 1997;40:769-774.

38. Tugal-Tutkun I, Onal S, Altan-Yaycioglu R, Huseyin Altunbas H, Urgancioglu M. Uveitis in Behçet disease: an analysis of 880 patients. *Am J Ophthalmol*. 2004;138:373-380.

39. Sakamoto M, Akazawa K, Nishioka Y, Sanui H, Inomata H, Nose Y. Prognostic factors of vision in patients with Behçet disease. *Ophthalmology*. 1995;102:317-321.

40. Takeuchi M, Hokama H, Tsukahara R, et al. Risk and prognostic factors of poor visual outcome in Behcet's disease with ocular involvement. *Graefes Arch Clin Exp Ophthalmol*. 2005;243:1147-1152.

41. Mamo JG, Baghdassarian A. Behcet's disease. *Arch Ophthalmol*. 1964;71:38-48.

42. Mishima S, Masuda K, Izawa Y, Mochizuke M, Namba K. Behçet's disease in Japan: ophthalmological aspects. *Trans Am Ophthalmol Soc*. 1979;77:225-279.

43. Benezra D, Cohen E. Treatment and visual prognosis in Behçet's disease. *Br J Ophthalmol*. 1986;70:589-592.

44. Ozyazgan Y, Yurdakul S, Yazici H, et al. Low dose cyclosporin A versus pulsed cyclophosphamide in Behçet's syndrome: a single masked trial. *Br J Ophthalmol*. 1992;76:241-243.

45. Kotake S, Higashi K, Yoshikawa K, Sasamoto Y, Okamoto T, Matsuda H. Central nervous system symptoms in patients with Behcet disease receiving cyclosporine therapy. *Ophthalmology*. 1999;106:586-589.

46. Akman-Demir G, Ayranci O, Kurtuncu M, Vanli EN, Mutlu M, Tugal-Tutkun I. Cyclosporine for Behçet's uveitis: is it associated with an increased risk of neurological involvement? *Clin Exp Rheumatol*. 2008;26(4 Suppl 50):S84-S90.

47. Kotter I, Gunaydin I, Zierhut M, Stubiger N. The use of interferon alpha in Behcet disease: review of the literature. *Semin Arthritis Rheum*. 2004;33:320-335.

48. Seyahi E, Ugurlu S, Ozyazgan Y, et al. Interferon α 2b in Behçet's syndrome with severe ocular involvement. *Arthritis Rheum*. 2005;52(Suppl 9):S647.

49. Ohno S, Nakamura S, Hori S, et al. Efficacy, safety, and pharmacokinetics of multiple administration of infliximab in Behcet's disease with refractory uveoretinitis. *J Rheumatol*. 2004;31:1362-1368.

50. Sfikakis PP, Kaklamanis PH, Elezoglou A, et al. Infliximab for recurrent, sight-threatening ocular inflammation in Adamantiades-Behcet disease. *Ann Intern Med*. 2004;140:404-406.

51. Tugal-Tutkun I, Mudun A, Urgancioglu M, et al. Efficacy of infliximab in the treatment of uveitis that is resistant to treatment with the combination of azathioprine, cyclosporine, and corticosteroids in Behcet's disease: an open-label trial. *Arthritis Rheum*. 2005;52:2478-2484.

52. Hamza M. Large artery involvement in Behcet's disease. *J Rheumatol*. 1987;14:554-559.

53. Koc Y, Gullu I, Akpek G, et al. Vascular involvement in Behcet's disease. *J Rheumatol*. 1992;19:402-410.

54. Düzgün N, Ateş A, Aydintuğ OT, Demir O, Olmez U. Characteristics of vascular involvement in Behcet's disease. *Scand J Rheumatol*. 2006;35:65-68.

55. Melikoglu M, Ugurlu S, Tascilar K, et al. Large vessel involvement in Behcet's syndrome: a retrospective survey. *Ann Rheum Dis*. 2008;67(Suppl II):67.

56. Husain SJ, Sadiq F, Zubairi AB, Khan JA. Massive unilateral chylous pleural effusion: a rare initial presentation of Behcet's disease. *Singapore Med J*. 2006;47:978-980.

57. Seyahi E, Melikoglu M, Akman C, et al. Pulmonary vascular involvement in Behcet's syndrome. *Arthritis Rheum*. 2007;56(Suppl 9):S357.

58. Hamuryudan V, Yurdakul S, Moral F, et al. Pulmonary arterial aneurysms in Behçet's syndrome: a report of 24 cases. *Br J Rheumatol*. 1994;33:48-51.

59. Hamuryudan V, Er T, Seyahi E, et al. Pulmonary artery aneurysms in Behcet syndrome. *Am J Med*. 2004;117:867-870.

60. Bayraktar Y, Balkanci F, Bayraktar M, Calguneri M. Budd-Chiari syndrome: a common complication of Behçet's disease. *Am J Gastroenterol*. 1997;92:858-862.

61. Lakhanpal S, Tani K, Lie JT, Katoh K, Ishigatsubo Y, Ohokubo T. Pathologic features of Behçet's syndrome: a review of Japanese autopsy registry data. *Hum Pathol.* 1985;16:790-795.
62. Tüzün H, Beşirli K, Sayin A, Yazici H, et al. Management of aneurysms in Behçet's syndrome: an analysis of 24 patients. *Surgery.* 1997;121:150-156.
63. Akman-Demir G, Serdaroglu P, Tasci B. Clinical patterns of neurological involvement in Behcet's disease: evaluation of 200 patients. The Neuro-Behcet Study Group. *Brain.* 1999;122:2171-2182.
64. Siva A, Kantarci OH, Saip S, et al. Behcet's disease: diagnostic and prognostic aspects of neurological involvement. *J Neurol.* 2001;248:95-103.
65. Saip S, Siva A, Altintas A, et al. Headache in Behçet's syndrome. *Headache.* 2005;45:911-919.
66. Oktem-Tanör O, Baykan-Kurt B, Gürvit IH, Akman-Demir G, Serdaroğlu P. Neuropsychological follow-up of 12 patients with neuro-Behçet disease. *J Neurol.* 1999;246:113-119.
67. Seyahi E, Ozdogan H, Uğurlu S, et al. The outcome children with Behçet's syndrome. *Clin Exp Rheumatol.* 2004;22(4 Suppl 34):116.
68. Fujikado T, Imagawa K. Dural sinus thrombosis in Behçet's disease – a case report. *Jpn J Ophthalmol.* 1994;38(4):411-416.
69. Erdem H, Dinc A, Pay S, Simsek I, Uysal Y. A neuro-Behcet's case complicated with intracranial hypertension successfully treated by a lumboperitoneal shunt. *Joint Bone Spine.* 2006;73:200-201.
70. Kuemmerle-Deschner JB, Tzaribachev N, Deuter C, Zierhut M, Batra M, Koetter I. Interferon-alpha – a new therapeutic option in refractory juvenile Behçet's disease with CNS involvement. *Rheumatology (Oxford).* 2008;47:1051-1053.
71. Chroni E, Monastirli A, Polychronopoulos P, et al. Epileptic seizures as the sole manifestation of neuro-Behçet's disease: complete control under interferon-alpha treatment. *Seizure.* 2008; 17:744-747.
72. Hatemi G, Silman A, Bang D, et al. Management of Behçet disease: a systematic literature review for the European League against rheumatism evidence-based recommendations for the management of Behçet disease. *Ann Rheum Dis.* 2009;68:1528-1534.
73. Mogulkoc N, Burgess MI, Bishop PW. Intracardiac thrombus in Behçet's disease: a systematic review. *Chest.* 2000;118:479-487.
74. Ugurlu S, Seyahi E, Yazici H. Prevalence of angina, myocardial infarction and intermittent claudication assessed by Rose Questionnaire among patients with Behcet's syndrome. *Rheumatology (Oxford).* 2008;47:472-475.
75. Seyahi E, Ugurlu S, Cumali R, et al. Atherosclerosis in Behçet's syndrome. *Semin Arthritis Rheum.* 2008;38:1-12.
76. Seyahi E, Yazici H. Atherosclerosis in Behçet's syndrome. *Clin Exp Rheumatol.* 2007;25(4 Suppl 45):S1-S5.
77. Yurdakul S, Tuzuner N, Yurdakul I, Hamuryudan V, Yazici H. Gastrointestinal involvement in Behçet's syndrome: a controlled study. *Ann Rheum Dis.* 1996;55:208-210.
78. Kasahara Y, Tanaka S, Nishino M, Umemura H, Shiraha S, Kuyama T. Intestinal involvement in Behçet's disease: review of 136 surgical cases in the Japanese literature. *Dis Colon Rectum.* 1981;24:103-106.
79. Postema PT, den Haan P, van Hagen PM, van Blankenstein M. Treatment of colitis in Behçet's disease with thalidomide. *Eur J Gastroenterol Hepatol.* 1996;8:929-931.
80. Celik AF, Kural-Seyahi E, Cosgun S, Hamuryudan V, Yazici H. Thalidomide in azathioprine resistant gastrointestinal Behçet's syndrome; 3 cases. *Clin Exp Rheumatol.* 2004;22(Suppl 34):S121.
81. Travis SP, Czajkowski M, McGovern DP, Watson RG, Bell AL. Treatment of intestinal Behçet's syndrome with chimeric tumour necrosis factor alpha antibody. *Gut.* 2001;49:725-728.
82. Lee KS, Kim SJ, Lee BC, Yoon DS, Lee WJ, Chi HS. Surgical treatment of intestinal Behçet's disease. *Yonsei Med J.* 1997;38:455-460.
83. Saadoun D, Wechsler B, Desseaux K, et al. Mortality in Behçet's disease. *Arthritis Rheum.* 2010;62:2806-2812.

84. Kaklamani VG, Vaiopoulos G, Kaklamanis PG. Behcet's disease. *Semin Arthritis Rheum.* 1998;27:197-217.
85. Benamour S, Zeroual B, Bennis R, Amraoui A, Bettal S. Behçet's disease. 316 cases. *Presse Méd.* 1990;19:1485-1489.
86. Yamamoto S, Toyokawa H, Matsubara J, et al. A nation-wide survey of Behçet's disease in Japan, 1. Epidemiological survey. *Jpn J Ophthalmol.* 1974;18:282-290.
87. Park KD, Bang D, Lee ES, Lee SH, Lee S. Clinical study on death in Behçet's disease. *J Korean Med Sci.* 1993;8:241-245.

Myositis: When Weakness Can Kill

12

Patrick Gordon and Ingrid E. Lundberg

Abstract The autoimmune muscle disorders, polymyositis and dermatomyositis, mainly affect muscles, but other organs are frequently involved. The muscular involvement and even more often the extramuscular involvement may develop into severe acute and life-threatening conditions, primarily, in early disease. Life-threatening conditions may be seen due to progressive muscle weakness which in occasional individuals may affect the thoracic muscles causing respiratory failure and need assisted ventilation. The muscles of the oropharynx and upper esophageal sphincter may cause swallowing problems and aspiration. Interstitial lung disease (ILD) is the most frequent extramuscular manifestation. Most often, ILD presents as a slowly progressive disease but may in rare cases have a rapid, progressive course and develop into respiratory failure with a high mortality risk. Involvement of cardiac muscle with cardiac failure is less frequent than ILD but may also contribute to mortality. Myositis-specific autoantibodies may serve as biomarkers for extramuscular disease and as prognostic markers. Early recognition of severe forms of myositis is essential to initiation treatment with glucocorticoids in combination with other immunosuppressive agents. In severe or rapidly progressive disease, pulse doses of intravenous glucocorticoids are often advocated. However, more research is needed to identify good prognostic markers for patients with myositis.

Keywords Autoantibodies • Dermatomyositis • Interstitial lung disease • Mortality • Muscle weakness • Myositis • Polymyositis • Swallowing problems

P. Gordon (✉)
Department of Rheumatology, King's College London, 2nd Floor
Hambledon Wing East, Denmark Hill, London SE5 7RS, UK
e-mail: patrick.gordon2@nhs.net

M.A. Khamashta and M. Ramos-Casals (eds.), *Autoimmune Diseases*,
DOI: 10.1007/978-0-85729-358-9_12, © Springer-Verlag London Limited 2011

12.1
Introduction

12.1.1
Clinical and Laboratory Features in Idiopathic Inflammatory Myopathies

The idiopathic inflammatory myopathies (IIM), collectively named myositis, have a prevalence of approximately 1:20,000.[1] They are often subclassified into polymyositis, dermatomyositis, and inclusion body myositis based on their differing clinical and histopathological features. Polymyositis and dermatomyositis most often respond to immunosuppressive therapy, whereas inclusion body myositis does not. Inflammatory myopathies can present as isolated disorders but may also, in some patients, be a prominent feature of other connective tissue diseases including Sjogren's Syndrome, systemic lupus erythematosus (particularly in patients with positive anti-RNP antibodies), mixed connective tissue disease, and scleroderma. Occasionally, inclusion body myositis may occur in conjunction with connective tissue disease particularly Sjogren's Syndrome.[2]

Polymyositis and dermatomyositis are characterized clinically primarily by weakness and low muscle endurance in proximal skeletal muscles, but other organs are frequently involved, such as skin in dermatomyositis and the heart, lung, and gastrointestinal tract in both polymyositis and dermatomyositis. The onset is generally insidious over weeks to months but may be acute or semi-acute in occasional patients. The muscular involvement and even more often the extramuscular involvement may develop into the severe acute and life-threatening conditions that will be discussed in this chapter. In contrast, inclusion body myositis typically has a slower, progressive onset, over months rather than weeks, with distal as well as proximal muscle involvement and other organs are rarely affected. Therefore, acute medical problems are rarely seen in patients with inclusion body myositis and this entity will therefore not be addressed in this chapter.

Polymyositis and dermatomyositis are autoimmune disorders where the inflammatory cell infiltrates in muscle tissue are predominated by T cells, but other inflammatory cells are also present including macrophages, dendritic cells, and more rarely, B cells. There is an HLA class II association, further supporting a role of the adaptive immunity in these disorders. Moreover, autoantibodies are frequently present in polymyositis and dermatomyositis patients, and may be present in up to 80% of the patients depending on patient selection and the sensitivity of methods used for autoantibody testing. The autoantibodies that can be found in polymyositis and dermatomyositis are divided into so-called myositis-specific autoantibodies (MSA) that are mainly found in myositis patients and myositis associated autoantibodies (MAA) which can also be found in other inflammatory connective tissue diseases, for example, anti-Ro, anti-La, anti-U1RNP, anti-Ku, and anti-PM-Scl. The most frequently present MSA are the anti-tRNA-synthetases of which the anti-histidyl-tRNA-synthetase (anti-Jo-1) is the most common, being present in 20–25% of myositis patients.[3] Autoantibodies have by now been identified to seven other tRNA-synthetases (anti-PL-7 directed against threonyl-tRNA-synthetase, anti-PL12 directed against alanyl-tRNA-synthetase, anti-KS directed against asparaginyl-tRNA-synthetase, anti-OJ directed against isoleucyl-tRNA-synthetase, anti-EJ directed against glycyl-tRNA-synthetase, anti-Ha directed against tyrosyl synthetase, and the recently detected anti-Zo directed against phenylalanyl synthetase).[4] These anti-synthetase autoantibodies are associated with a clinically distinct phenotype of interstitial lung disease (ILD), nonerosive arthritis, Raynaud's phenomenon, a skin rash called mechanic's hands, and myositis.[5] The MSAs anti-Mi-2, anti-clinical amyopathic dermatomyositis (CADM) 140, and anti-p155/140 are associated with specific populations of dermatomyositis.[4] Anti-p155/140 is associated with cancer-associated dermatomyositis and juvenile dermatomyositis.[6,7] Anti-Mi-2 associated dermatomyositis has a favorable prognosis with good response to immunosuppressive treatment. Another MSA is the anti-signal recognition peptide (SRP) which is associated with a histopathological phenotype, namely, necrotizing myopathy, where inflammatory cell infiltrates are scarce. Patients with anti-SRP often have a limited response to immunosuppressive treatment.[8] Thus, the MSAs are helpful to identify clinical subsets of myositis where different organs could be involved and, in addition, have some prognostic value. As such, they are highly relevant to clinical practice. Not all of the MSAs can be tested by commercially available methods, but there is ongoing work to develop validated tests for routine clinical practice.

12.1.2
Outcome and Prognosis

Since the introduction of treatment with glucocorticoids in the 1950s, the survival in polymyositis and dermatomyositis has improved substantially. However, patients with polymyositis and dermatomyositis still have increased mortality rates, almost threefold higher compared to age- and sex-matched individuals, as reported in one of the few published population-based studies.[9] The overall standard mortality ratio (SMR) in patients with polymyositis and dermatomyositis was 2.92 (95% CI 2.48–3.44) compared to the general population in a Finnish study, which covered patients who were diagnosed between 1969 and 1985 and who had an adequate follow-up time of 10 years (in 1995).[9] In a smaller population-based study from New Zealand, the death rate was 33% after a median follow-up of 76 months.[10] The primary causes of death are cardiovascular disease, cancer, aspiration pneumonia, and respiratory failure, with varying frequencies in different cohort studies most likely depending on patient selection and variation in observation times.[11] The causes of death, with the exception of cancer, also reflect the major clinical problems in polymyositis and dermatomyositis that may lead to acute situations and that will be discussed more in depth in this chapter.

12.2
Muscle Weakness

Weakness of striated muscle is the cardinal feature of polymyositis and dermatomyositis, and the weakness may in occasional patients develop into severe weakness involving respiratory muscles and thereby become life threatening requiring assisted ventilation.

Even the diaphragm may be affected and lead to the respiratory insufficiency. Typically, these patients have restrictive lung function impairment; lung function tests demonstrate reduced lung volumes, maximal inspiratory and expiratory pressures, increased residual volume, and a normal FEV_1/VC ratio. Chest radiography or computerized tomography of the lungs may be normal. These patients may require oxygen therapy or even mechanic ventilation until the ventilation has improved.

12.3
Pulmonary Disease in Polymyositis and Dermatomyositis

Pulmonary disease is common in IIM and a major cause of death in most longitudinal series. It is a frequent cause of critical illness; in a case series of six patients admitted to ITU for inflammatory muscle disease, five were admitted for respiratory failure.[12] Respiratory failure has many potential causes in the acute setting and may be multifactorial including:

Interstitial lung disease
Acute type 1 respiratory failure due to extrinsic muscle weakness
Infection including aspiration pneumonia and atypical infection in the context of immunosuppression
Aspiration as a result of oropharyngeal disease
Other causes such as pneumothorax in the context of interstitial lung disease or bronchogenic carcinoma – a common malignancy in cancer-associated myositis

12.3.1
Interstitial Lung Disease

Interstitial lung disease (ILD) is a frequent manifestation of dermatomyositis and polymyositis detectable in up to 65% patients at presentation if carefully assessed; however, clinically significant disease is less frequent.[13-15] Mortality in IIM is higher in patients with ILD[13,16] with a survival of 85.8% at 1 year and 60.4% at 5 years reported in one series of 58 patients with ILD in a tertiary referral center.[17] In the context of interstitial lung disease, anti-Jo-1 antibodies do not have prognostic significance.[17] Reported poor prognostic factors for ILD in patients with polymyositis and dermatomyositis include an initial FVC ≤60%, a Hammond-Rich like syndrome, and a high neutrophil count on bronchoalveolar lavage.[13,15] In addition, histological diagnosis is predictive of outcome and response to therapy.[18] The main histological patterns of disease are cryptogenic organizing pneumonia (COP), nonspecific interstitial pneumonitis (NSIP), usual interstitial pneumonitis (UIP), and diffuse alveolar damage (DAD).[13] Nonspecific interstitial pneumonitis appears to be the commonest ILD histological pattern in IIM occurring in just over 80% of cases in one biopsy series (18/22).[17] However, organizing pneumonia also appears to be very frequent occurring in 38% of cases in another biopsy series.[19] Usual interstitial pneumonitis and diffuse alveolar damage are less common, respond poorly to immunosuppression, and have a poor prognosis with a survival of only 33% at 5 years in one historical case series.[18]

Cryptogenic organizing pneumonia and diffuse alveolar damage generally have an acute onset. As its name implies, organizing pneumonia has appearances not too dissimilar to infective pneumonia and in the acute phase may be mistaken for infective pneumonia causing a delay in therapy. Bronchoalveolar lavage can be helpful in excluding infection particularly in the setting of previously immunosuppressed patients. Organizing pneumonia tends to respond well to immunosuppressive therapy and is usually associated with a good prognosis[20] (Fig. 12.1). Diffuse alveolar damage in contrast has a very poor

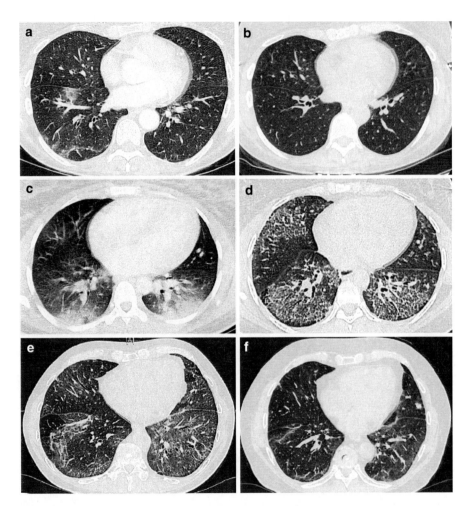

Fig. 12.1 Organizing pneumonia generally responds well to immunosuppression as in this patient with dermatomyositis at presentation (**a**) and 2 years later following immunosuppression (**b**). In contrast, a subgroup of patients with organizing pneumonia (**c**) develop a progressive fibrotic phenotype of organizing pneumonia as seen in the follow-up imaging 3 years later (**d**) despite aggressive immunosuppression including in this patient's case cyclophosphamide, rituximab, mycophenolate mofetil, and tacrolimus. Nonspecific pneumonitis shows a good response to therapy as in this patient with dermatomyositis at presentation (**e**) and 2 years later following immunosuppression (**f**)

prognosis.[20] A particularly high incidence of rapidly progressive interstitial lung disease with mortality in the order of 50% has been described in Japan in patients with anti-CADM140 antibodies and clinically amyopathic dermatomyositis.[21] However, to date, this antibody has not been described in other populations.

Nonspecific interstitial pneumonitis and usual interstitial pneumonitis generally have a more insidious presentation. Nonspecific interstitial pneumonitis in IIM generally responds well to immunosuppression with a prognosis similar to idiopathic nonspecific interstitial pneumonitis (Fig. 12.1). While idiopathic usual interstitial pneumonitis has a poor prognosis, the outcome and response to therapy of connective tissue disease associated usual interstitial pneumonitis is better than for idiopathic disease.[22]

12.3.1.1
Diagnostic Evaluation and Monitoring of Interstitial Lung Disease

IIM patients should be screened for ILD with lung function testing including CO diffusion capacity at presentation. In the vast majority of cases and all with anti-synthetase antibodies, a HRCT scan should be performed in addition to a plain chest X-ray as the latter is a poor screen for ILD. If this is not done, quite significant interstitial lung disease can be easily missed in this group of patients who frequently have very poor mobility due to muscle weakness and therefore may not complain of breathlessness until quite an advanced stage of lung disease. Patients with anti-Jo-1 or other anti-synthetase antibodies have a particularly high incidence of interstitial lung disease. In this group, interstitial lung disease may precede the muscle symptoms or be the major clinical symptom with little muscle weakness. Findings on high-resolution computerized tomography generally correlate well with histological findings on biopsy.[20,23] Therefore, due to the significant potential morbidity associated with open lung biopsy, lung biopsy is only indicated in a minority of patients in the context of known underlying IIM.

Serial lung function tests including CO transfer should be performed in all patients with ILD to monitor the progress of the disease and thus guide therapy. Bronchoalveolar lavage is a useful tool to assess alveolar inflammation and exclude infection. Krebs von den Lungen-6 (KL-6), a glycoprotein expressed on type II alveolar pneumocytes and alveolar macrophages, has been identified as a potential biomarker for interstitial lung disease. Levels are raised in patients with ILD including connective tissue disease–related ILD, hypersensitivity pneumonitis, and idiopathic interstitial pneumonia.[24,25] Several studies have also demonstrated significantly higher levels in patients with active disease.[24,25] A small study in patients with IIM showed particularly high levels in patients with diffuse alveolar damage.[24]

12.3.2
Respiratory Muscle Weakness

Respiratory muscle weakness is a frequent manifestation of dermatomyositis and polymyositis but is easily missed in the context of severe disease particularly if patients also have coexistent interstitial lung disease. In addition to breathlessness on exertion, patients may complain of breathlessness on lying flat or daytime somnolence due to overnight hypoventilation.

The vital capacity is the standard method to assess and monitor muscle weakness at the bedside. Sniff nasal inspiratory pressure (SNIP) is another reliable, noninvasive, and reproducible method for the assessment and monitoring of respiratory muscle strength. In amyotrophic lateral sclerosis, SNIP has been shown to be a better predictor of ventilatory failure than vital capacity assessments.[26] In IIM, respiratory muscle weakness has little effect on $PaCO_2$ until it drops below 50% of the predicted strength at which stage there is a linear relationship.[27] Hypercapnic respiratory failure in IIM due to muscle weakness alone does not generally occur until respiratory muscle strength is <40% predicted and is not generally severe until it is <30% predicted.[27] However, it may occur earlier in patients with coexistant lung disease such as ILD.[27] In contrast, severe hypercapnia may occur in patients with a vital capacity of >55% of predicted.[27] As such, where available, SNIP measurements should be used in addition to vital capacity to better predict the need for ventilatory support.

Even in patients with good daytime $PaCO_2$, nocturnal hypoventilation may occur. Therefore, in patients with low measures of vital capacity and/or SNIP, it is advisable to perform overnight pulsoximetry to screen for nocturnal hypoventilation. In patients with nocturnal hypoventilation or mild hypercapnic respiratory failure, noninvasive positive pressure ventilation may be preferable to invasive ventilation.

12.4
Gastrointestinal Tract Involvement

12.4.1
Dysphagia and Aspiration

The oropharynx and upper esophageal sphincter comprise of skeletal muscle and may therefore also be affected in IIM. Dysphagia is a frequent problem in IIM which is not always clinically obvious and should proactively be screened for. Undetected disease can lead to recurrent aspiration and aspiration pneumonia. Patients may lose a significant amount of weight prior to presentation due to poor food intake. Thus not surprisingly, dysphagia has been shown to be a poor prognostic factor in polymyositis.[16] Patients often do not attribute their symptoms to muscle weakness and silent aspiration is frequent, particularly in children.[28] Notably a recent study failed to show an association between swallow score and limb weakness by manual muscle testing or general disease activity as assessed by physician visual analogue scale in juvenile dermatomyositis.[28] As such, screening for dysphagia should be part of the assessment in all patients with IIM, even if limb weakness is mild. The commonest symptoms described in a retrospective study of 62 patients with IIM-associated dysphagia were "difficulty eating solid and dry foods" (96%), "food sticking in the throat" (85%), and "coughing while eating" (75%).[29] Other symptoms include quiet nasal speech, recent weight loss, recurrent chest infections, and the need to make several attempts to swallow a bolus of food.

12.4.2
Diagnostic Evaluation of Dysphagia

Where there is concern, a speech therapist's input is mandatory to confirm the diagnosis and assess the safety of a patient's swallow. Basic screening includes confirming the upward and forward movement of the larynx on swallowing water and the presence or absence of coughing after the swallow. Video fluoroscopic assessment of swallow is considered the gold standard, but even this cannot reliably detect all cases of aspiration as the texture and consistency of food also plays a part. Frequent findings on video fluoroscopy are pharyngeal pooling, impaired tongue retraction, impaired laryngeal elevation, and abnormal cricopharyngeal function.[29] Fiber-optic nasopharyngeal endoscopy may also provide useful additional information. In severe disease, a nasogastric tube is required for feeding and patients need to expectorate their own saliva. Generally, oropharyngeal muscle weakness responds well to immunosuppressive therapy although it frequently lags behind peripheral muscle recovery. Thus, although nasogastric tubes are uncomfortable, it is advisable to defer more permanent invasive solutions for feeding such as gastrostomy tubes for several months. In this way, the risks associated with gastrostomy placement can be avoided in the majority of patients.

12.5
Heart Involvement

Cardiovascular manifestations constitute a major cause of death in myositis with a cumulative survival rate after 8 years of 44.2% in patients with cardiac involvement, compared to 87% for those without clinical heart disease.[30] The most common cardiac manifestations that may cause death are heart failure, arrhythmia, cardiac arrest, and myocardial infarction. Patients with myositis do not only have an increased risk of myocardial infarction but also of another type of arterial event namely cerebrovascular accidents, according to a recent Canadian study.[31]

Cardiac involvement, in particular subclinical electrocardiogram (ECG) changes, is frequently seen in polymyositis and dermatomyositis, although clinically manifest heart problems are uncommon.[32] The overall occurrence of heart involvement varies between 6% and 75% depending on patient selection and methods used to detect cardiac involvement. Controlled studies are lacking as to whether overall cardiac involvement is more common than in age-matched healthy individuals. The most frequently reported clinically manifest cardiac problem is congestive heart failure, observed in between 3% and 45% of myositis patients. Cardiac involvement may be present at the time of myositis diagnosis when it can be the predominating symptom although cardiac manifestations may also occur in later phases of disease.[33]

Some heart manifestations are more likely to be associated with myositis. The heart is a muscle, and this muscle may be affected by inflammation and myocarditis, leading to cardiomyopathy. The histopathology of the myocarditis in polymyositis and dermatomyositis resembles the inflammation in the skeletal muscle with mononuclear inflammatory cell infiltrates localized to the endomysium and to the perivascular areas and degeneration of cardiac myocytes.

Rhythm disturbances and coronary artery disease as well as involvement of the small vessels of the myocardium are more common clinical manifestations of heart involvement in myositis than myocarditis. Other severe cardiac manifestations that may lead to acute situations are conduction abnormalities that may lead to complete heart block.

12.5.1
Diagnostic Evaluation of Cardiac Involvement

As arrhythmias and conduction abnormalities are common manifestations in polymyositis and dermatomyositis patients, an electrocardiogram (ECG) is recommended at the time of myositis diagnosis. *Echocardiography* is also recommended when clinically indicated. The frequency of echocardiographic abnormalities, left ventricular diastolic dysfunction (LVDD), hyperdynamic heart and mitral valve prolapse varies between 14% and 62% in patients with polymyositis and dermatomyositis.[34,35] More recently, new imaging techniques have been used to detect cardiac involvement including *Technetium 99 m-pyrophosphate scintigraphy* which permits detection of left ventricular wall abnormalities and *Gadolinium diethylenetriaminepentaacetic acid–enhanced magnetic resonance imaging* which detects myocardial inflammation. There are case reports suggesting the usefulness of these methods, but the sensitivity and specificity of these techniques to detect cardiac involvement in myositis are still unknown.

12.5.1.1
Blood Tests to Be Used to Detect Heart Involvement

Elevated creatine kinase (CK)-MB is not specific for heart involvement as there is an upregulation of this enzyme in regenerating skeletal muscle fibers. Of the cardiac troponin isoforms, the cardiac troponin-I (cTnI) has the highest specificity to detect myocardial involvement, whereas the other cardiac troponin isoforms, troponin C (cTnC) and troponin T (cTnT), are less specific.[36] They are also expressed in differentiated adult skeletal muscles, and high levels in sera have been reported in various myopathies.

In some studies, the presence of anti-SRP antibodies was associated with an increased risk of developing cardiac involvement,[37] but this was not confirmed in a more recent study.[8] Recently, a case of myocarditis with heart failure was reported in the early phase of myositis in a young man with anti-Jo-1 and anti-SSA antibodies.[38] The cardiac failure responded promptly to treatment with glucocorticoids. Cardiac involvement has rarely been reported in patients with anti-Jo-1 antibodies, whereas anti-SSA antibodies in patients with connective tissue disease seem to confer an increased risk of developing arrhythmias compared to anti-SSA negative patients.[39] These reports suggest that some MSAs may confer a greater risk of patients developing cardiac manifestations in polymyositis and dermatomyositis, but these observations need to be confirmed in larger cohorts. In addition, longitudinal clinical data are needed to evaluate whether there are biomarkers that can be used as prognostic markers for cardiac involvement in myositis.

12.6
Peripheral Vascular Involvement

Peripheral vascular involvement with a manifestation such as Raynaud's phenomenon is common in polymyositis and dermatomyositis, particularly in patients with the so-called anti-synthetase syndrome. Severe vascular involvement is rare in adult dermatomyositis or polymyositis, even though the inflammatory infiltrates in muscle tissue in dermatomyositis typically have a perivascular distribution. True vasculitis is rarely seen in adults with dermatomyositis but may be present in children with juvenile dermatomyositis. Vasculitis may give rise to cutaneous ulcers or in rare cases vasculitis of the gut.

12.7
Pharmacological Treatment of Polymyositis and Dermatomyositis

The correct diagnosis is clearly essential for appropriate therapy. However, a major cause for treatment resistance, particularly in polymyositis, is an incorrect diagnosis. Inclusion body myositis does not respond to immunosuppressive therapy and may be very difficult to distinguish from polymyositis at onset, even on muscle biopsy. Many noninflammatory myopathies can mimic polymyositis in the early phase (e.g., acid maltase deficiency and fascioscapulohumeral dystrophy). As such, a careful clinical assessment of the patient is essential in conjunction with a muscle biopsy. In particular, the distribution of weakness assessing the facial muscles (including whistling) and distal flexors is imperative for diagnosis, and subsequent reassessment at a later date is required in patients resistant to treatment. Malignancy is increased particularly in dermatomyositis and in addition to requiring therapy in its own right may impact therapeutic decisions for the myositis.

In patients with severe disease in whom a concomitant infection is reasonably excluded, intravenous pulsed methylprednisolone 500–1,000 mg daily for 3 days should be considered. While this is a common strategy for many autoimmune inflammatory diseases including SLE and vasculitis, there is no randomized control study showing its efficacy in IIM. In a small non-randomized partially retrospective study, 11 of 25 patients were treated with pulsed methylprednisolone 500 mg daily for 3 days repeated weekly 3–9 times in addition to standard therapy.[40] A greater proportion of these patients remained in remission at 6 months and long term (the latter in the subset with disease longer than 24 months). They also had a shorter time to normalization of their creatine kinase.[40] While this suggests efficacy of pulsed methylprednisolone, we do not advocate the high number and frequency of methylprednisolone pulses used routinely in this study due to the cumulative risks including infection and avascular necrosis associated with high-dose steroids.

Oral prednisolone is generally commenced at a dose of 0.5–1 mg/kg daily in severe disease, although in patients with mild disease, lower doses may be used. Again, there are no placebo-controlled studies demonstrating the efficacy of prednisolone, but historical data are convincing enough to make a controlled study unjustifiable. The dose is subsequently reduced monthly by approximately 20% of the preceding month's dose and according to response. Side effects are common, and most experts recommend combination therapy with another immunosuppressive agent, most often azathioprine or methotrexate; although randomized controlled trials are lacking, there is some evidence for these agents in support of their steroid-saving potency.

Methotrexate is commonly used as a first-line immunosuppressant in dermatomyositis and polymyositis, although due to concerns relating to lung toxicity, it is generally avoided in patients with significant interstitial lung disease. It had equal efficacy to cyclosporine A in a randomized trial, and there are many case series suggesting its efficacy.[41-43] In an open partially retrospective study of 53 patients with juvenile dermatomyositis, children treated with methotrexate had a median time to discontinuation of prednisolone of 10 months compared to 27 months in the control group and a significantly lower cumulative prednisolone dose as a result.[44]

Azathioprine is also a common first-line immunosuppressant used in IMM. Open-label follow-up of a small randomized placebo control trial of azathioprine therapy in polymyositis and dermatomyositis showed a better long-term outcome in the patients treated with azathioprine after 3 years.[45,46] In idiopathic interstitial pulmonary fibrosis, there is evidence for triple therapy with low-dose prednisolone, azathioprine, and the antioxidant, n-acetylcysteine.[47] Azathioprine has also been used in interstitial lung disease associated with IIM, and based on the data in idiopathic interstitial pulmonary fibrosis, additional therapy with the antioxidant n-acetylcysteine should be considered in view of its low toxicity and potential benefit.[47]

Tacrolimus has been reported as efficacious in case reports and case series in refractory IIM, particularly anti-synthetase syndrome with lung disease.[48-50] Similarly, cyclosporine A has been suggested in case series to be efficacious particularly in patients with interstitial lung disease.[51,52] Increasingly mycophenolate mofetil is being used in inflammatory myositis although data are very much restricted to case series and reports.[53,54]

In patients with severe disease, induction therapy with cyclophosphamide should be considered. While there is good evidence for its use in related conditions such as systemic lupus erythematosus, evidence is limited to case series in dermatomyositis and polymyositis. In terms of ILD, there are randomized control data for the efficacy of oral cyclophosphamide in scleroderma-associated interstitial lung disease and also a case series suggesting efficacy in IIM-associated interstitial lung disease.[55,56] Cyclophosphamide therapy is usually effective at the Eurolupus dose of 500 mg by intravenous infusion fortnightly for six doses in IMM.[57] While the risk of hemorrhagic cystitis and subsequent bladder carcinoma is low at this dose, in the order of 1%, these are serious complications and it is therefore our practice to give Mesna therapy which is generally well tolerated.[57]

Intravenous immunoglobulin (IVIG) is the only therapy that has been shown to be beneficial in a randomized control study in dermatomyositis. This small study showed a benefit from IVIG therapy in dermatomyositis patients at 3 months.[58] It is thought to be particularly beneficial in patients with dysphagia although the evidence is limited to case series.[59] However, these beneficial effects on performance and muscle inflammation could not be confirmed in a more recent study.[60] IVIG in these studies were given at a dose of 2 g/kg patient weight; split over 5 days, although it may be given over a shorter number of days. Prior to IVIG therapy, the patient's immunoglobulin A (IgA) levels need to be checked to avoid IgA deficiency–related anaphylactic reactions in previously unknown IgA-deficient patients. In acutely ill patients, IVIG has the advantage that it can be given in combination with steroids and other immunosuppressants. It is also relatively safe in patients in whom concomitant infection is suspected and other therapies are contraindicated.

In refractory cases, rituximab is also being increasingly used. It is presently undergoing assessment in a large randomized placebo control study of patients with polymyositis, dermatomyositis, and juvenile dermatomyositis. However, to date, the evidence for its efficacy is limited to case series.[61]

12.8
Summary

Polymyositis and dermatomyositis may display life-threatening features both due to severe muscle weakness, mainly when affecting respiratory and pharyngeal muscles, and due to involvement of internal organs. The most common extramuscular features that may become life-threatening are interstitial lung disease and cardiac involvement. Some myositis-specific autoantibodies have a high predictive value for interstitial lung disease, but there are no biomarkers to date that have a prognostic value or can predict who will develop life-threatening disease. Therefore, patients with polymyositis or dermatomyositis need to be monitored carefully for lung and heart involvements. Notably, these extramuscular manifestations can precede muscle involvement and may occasionally be the predominating clinical feature of the so-called amyopathic or hypomyopathic dermatomyositis and thereby cause a diagnostic challenge not limited to rheumatologists. Mild symptoms of dermatomyositis may easily be overlooked but can raise awareness of potentially life-threatening lung involvement.

References

1. Bernatsky S, Joseph L, Pineau CA, et al. Estimating the prevalence of polymyositis and dermatomyositis from administrative data: age, sex and regional differences. *Ann Rheum Dis.* 2009;68(7):1192-1196.
2. Kanellopoulos P, Baltoyiannis C, Tzioufas AG. Primary Sjogren's syndrome associated with inclusion body myositis. *Rheumatology (Oxford).* 2002;41(4):440-444.
3. Brouwer R, Hengstman GJ, Vree Egberts W, et al. Autoantibody profiles in the sera of European patients with myositis. *Ann Rheum Dis.* 2001;60(2):116-123.
4. Gunawardena H, Betteridge ZE, McHugh NJ. Myositis-specific autoantibodies: their clinical and pathogenic significance in disease expression. *Rheumatology (Oxford).* 2009;48(6):607-612.
5. Love LA, Leff RL, Fraser DD, et al. A new approach to the classification of idiopathic inflammatory myopathy: myositis-specific autoantibodies define useful homogeneous patient groups. *Medicine (Baltimore).* 1991;70:360-374.
6. Chinoy H, Fertig N, Oddis CV, et al. The diagnostic utility of myositis autoantibody testing for predicting the risk of cancer-associated myositis. *Ann Rheum Dis.* 2007;66:1345.
7. Targoff IN, Mamyrova G, Trieu EP, et al. A novel autoantibody to a 155-kd protein is associated with dermatomyositis. *Arthritis Rheum.* 2006;54(11):3682-3689.

8. Hengstman GJ, ter Laak HJ, Vree Egberts WT, et al. Anti-signal recognition particle autoantibodies: marker of a necrotising myopathy. *Ann Rheum Dis.* 2006 Dec;65(12):1635-8. Epub 2006 May 5.

9. Airio A, Kautiainen H, Hakala M. Prognosis and mortality of polymyositis and dermatomyositis patients. *Clin Rheumatol.* 2006;25:234-239.

10. Lynn SJ, Sawyers SM, Moller PW, O'Donnell JL, Chapman PT. Adult-onset inflammatory myopathy: North Canterbury experience 1989–2001. *Intern Med J.* 2005;35:170-173.

11. Lundberg IE, Forbess CJ. Mortality in idiopathic inflammatory myopathies. *Clin Exp Rheumatol.* 2008;26(5 Suppl 5):S109-S114.

12. Sherer Y, Shepshelovich D, Shalev T, et al. Outcome of patients having dermatomyositis admitted to the intensive care unit. *Clin Rheumatol.* 2007;26(11):1851-1855.

13. Kang EH, Lee EB, Shin KC, et al. Interstitial lung disease in patients with polymyositis, dermatomyositis and amyopathic dermatomyositis. *Rheumatology (Oxford).* 2005;44(10):1282-1286.

14. Fathi M, Dastmalchi M, Rasmussen E, Lundberg IE, Tornling G. Interstitial lung disease, a common manifestation of newly diagnosed polymyositis and dermatomyositis. *Ann Rheum Dis.* 2004;63(3):297-301.

15. Marie I, Hachulla E, Cherin P, et al. Interstitial lung disease in polymyositis and dermatomyositis. *Arthritis Rheum.* 2002;47(6):614-622.

16. Danko K, Ponyi A, Constantin T, Borgulya G, Szegedi G. Long-term survival of patients with idiopathic inflammatory myopathies according to clinical features: a longitudinal study of 162 cases. *Medicine (Baltimore).* 2004;83(1):35-42.

17. Douglas WW, Tazelaar HD, Hartman TE, et al. Polymyositis-dermatomyositis-associated interstitial lung disease. *Am J Respir Crit Care Med.* 2001;164(7):1182-1185.

18. Takizawa H, Hidaka N, Akiyama K, et al. Clinicopathological studies on interstitial lung disease in polymyositis-dermatomyositis. *Nihon Kyobu Shikkan Gakkai Zasshi.* 1985;23(5):528-536.

19. Tansey D, Wells AU, Colby TV, et al. Variations in histological patterns of interstitial pneumonia between connective tissue disorders and their relationship to prognosis. *Histopathology.* 2004;44(6):585-596.

20. Tazelaar HD, Viggiano RW, Pickersgill J, Colby TV. Interstitial lung disease in polymyositis and dermatomyositis. Clinical features and prognosis as correlated with histologic findings. *Am Rev Respir Dis.* 1990;141(3):727-733.

21. Sato S, Hirakata M, Kuwana M, et al. Autoantibodies to a 140-kd polypeptide, CADM-140, in Japanese patients with clinically amyopathic dermatomyositis. *Arthritis Rheum.* 2005;52(5):1571-1576.

22. Park JH, Kim DS, Park IN, et al. Prognosis of fibrotic interstitial pneumonia: idiopathic versus collagen vascular disease-related subtypes. *Am J Respir Crit Care Med.* 2007;175(7):705-711.

23. Arakawa H, Yamada H, Kurihara Y, et al. Nonspecific interstitial pneumonia associated with polymyositis and dermatomyositis: serial high-resolution CT findings and functional correlation. *Chest.* 2003;123(4):1096-1103.

24. Bandoh S, Fujita J, Ohtsuki Y, et al. Sequential changes of KL-6 in sera of patients with interstitial pneumonia associated with polymyositis/dermatomyositis. *Ann Rheum Dis.* 2000;59: 257-262.

25. Kobayashi J, Kitamura S. KL-6: a serum marker for interstitial pneumonia. *Chest.* 1995;108: 311-315.

26. Lyall RA, Donaldson N, Polkey MI, Leigh PN, Moxham J. Respiratory muscle strength and ventilatory failure in amyotrophic lateral sclerosis. *Brain.* 2001;124(Pt 10):2000-2013.

27. Braun NM, Arora NS, Rochester DF. Respiratory muscle and pulmonary function in polymyositis and other proximal myopathies. *Thorax.* 1983;38(8):616-623.

28. McCann LJ, Garay SM, Ryan MM, Harris R, Riley P, Pilkington CA. Oropharyngeal dysphagia in juvenile dermatomyositis (JDM): an evaluation of videofluoroscopy swallow study (VFSS) changes in relation to clinical symptoms and objective muscle scores. *Rheumatology.* 2007;46(8):1363-1366.

29. Oh TH, Brumfield KA, Hoskin TL, Stolp KA, Murray JA, Basford JR. Dysphagia in inflammatory myopathy: clinical characteristics, treatment strategies, and outcome in 62 patients. *Mayo Clin Proc.* 2007;82(4):441-447.
30. Gonzalez-Lopez L, Gamez-Nava JI, Sanchez L, et al. Cardiac manifestations in dermatopolymyositis. *Clin Exp Rheumatol.* 1996;14(4):373-379.
31. Tisseverasinghe A, Bernatsky S, Pineau CA. Arterial events in persons with dermatomyositis and polymyositis. *J Rheumatol.* 2009;36(9):1943-1946.
32. Lundberg IE. The heart in dermatomyositis and polymyositis. *Rheumatology (Oxford).* 2006;45(4):iv18-iv21.
33. Odabasi Z, Yapundich R, Oh SJ. Polymyositis presenting with cardiac manifestations: report of two cases and review of the literature. *Clin Neurol Neurosurg.* 2010;112(2):160-163.
34. Gonzales-Lopez L, Gamez-Nava JI, Sanchez L, et al. Cardiac manifestations in dermatopolymyositis. *Clin Exp Rheumatol.* 1996;14:373-379.
35. Gottdiener JS, Sherber HS, Hawley RJ, Engel WK. Cardiac manifestations in polymyositis. *Am J Cardiol.* 1978;41(7):1141-1149.
36. Aggarwal R, Lebiedz-Odrobina D, Sinha A, Manadan A, Case JP. Serum cardiac troponin T, but not troponin I, is elevated in idiopathic inflammatory myopathies. *J Rheumatol.* 2009;36(12):2711-2714.
37. Love LA, Leff RL, Fraser DD, et al. A new approach to the classification of idiopathic inflammatory myopathy: myositis-specific autoantibodies define useful homogeneous patient groups. *Medicine (Baltimore).* 1991;70(6):360-374.
38. Tahiri L, Guignard S, Pinto P, Duclos M, Dougados M. Antisynthetases syndrome associated with right heart failure. *Joint Bone Spine.* 2009;76(6):715-717.
39. Lazzerini PE, Capecchi PL, Guideri F, et al. Comparison of frequency of complex ventricular arrhythmias in patients with positive versus negative anti-Ro/SSA and connective tissue disease. *Am J Cardiol.* 2007;100(6):1029-1034.
40. Matsubara S, Sawa Y, Takamori M, Yokoyama H, Kida H. Pulsed intravenous methylprednisolone combined with oral steroids as the initial treatment of inflammatory myopathies. *J Neurol Neurosurg Psychiatry.* 1994;57(8):1008.
41. Vencovsky J, Jarosova K, Machacek S, et al. Cyclosporine A versus methotrexate in the treatment of polymyositis and dermatomyositis. *Scand J Rheumatol.* 2000;29(2):95-102.
42. Zieglschmid-Adams ME, Pandya AG, Cohen SB, Sontheimer RD. Treatment of dermatomyositis with methotrexate. *J Am Acad Dermatol.* 1995;32(5 Pt 1):754-757.
43. Metzger AL, Bohan A, Goldberg LS, Bluestone R, Pearson CM. Polymyositis and dermatomyositis: combined methotrexate and corticosteroid therapy. *Ann Intern Med.* 1974;81(2):182-189.
44. Ramanan AV, Campbell-Webster N, Ota S, et al. The effectiveness of treating juvenile dermatomyositis with methotrexate and aggressively tapered corticosteroids. *Arthritis Rheum.* 2005;52(11):3570-3578.
45. Bunch TW. Prednisone and azathioprine for polymyositis: long-term followup. *Arthritis Rheum.* 1981;24(1):45-48.
46. Bunch TW, Worthington JW, Combs JJ, Ilstrup DM, Engel AG. Azathioprine with prednisone for polymyositis. A controlled, clinical trial. *Ann Intern Med.* 1980;92(3):365-369.
47. Demedts M, Behr J, Buhl R, et al. High-dose acetylcysteine in idiopathic pulmonary fibrosis. *N Engl J Med.* 2005;353(21):2229-2242.
48. Ochi S, Nanki T, Takada K, et al. Favorable outcomes with tacrolimus in two patients with refractory interstitial lung disease associated with polymyositis/dermatomyositis. *Clin Exp Rheumatol.* 2005;23(5):707-710.
49. Wilkes MR, Sereika SM, Fertig N, Lucas MR, Oddis CV. Treatment of antisynthetase-associated interstitial lung disease with tacrolimus. *Arthritis Rheum.* 2005;52(8):2439-2446.
50. Guglielmi S, Merz TM, Gugger M, Suter C, Nicod LP. Acute respiratory distress syndrome secondary to antisynthetase syndrome is reversible with tacrolimus. *Eur Respir J.* 2008;31(1):213-217.

51. Maeda K, Kimura R, Komuta K, Igarashi T. Cyclosporine treatment for polymyositis/ dermatomyositis: is it possible to rescue the deteriorating cases with interstitial pneumonitis? *Scand J Rheumatol.* 1997;26(1):24-29.
52. Nawata Y, Kurasawa K, Takabayashi K, et al. Corticosteroid resistant interstitial pneumonitis in dermatomyositis/polymyositis: prediction and treatment with cyclosporine. *J Rheumatol.* 1999;26(7):1527-1533.
53. Majithia V, Harisdangkul V. Mycophenolate mofetil (CellCept): an alternative therapy for autoimmune inflammatory myopathy. *Rheumatology (Oxford).* 2005;44(3):386-389.
54. Pisoni CN, Cuadrado MJ, Khamashta MA, Hughes GR, D'Cruz DP. Mycophenolate mofetil treatment in resistant myositis. *Rheumatology (Oxford).* 2007;46(3):516-518.
55. Yamasaki Y, Yamada H, Yamasaki M, et al. Intravenous cyclophosphamide therapy for progressive interstitial pneumonia in patients with polymyositis/dermatomyositis. *Rheumatology (Oxford).* 2007;46(1):124-130.
56. Tashkin DP, Elashoff R, Clements PJ, et al. Cyclophosphamide versus placebo in scleroderma lung disease. *N Engl J Med.* 2006;354(25):2655-2666.
57. Martin-Suarez I, D'Cruz D, Mansoor M, Fernandes AP, Khamashta MA, Hughes GR. Immunosuppressive treatment in severe connective tissue diseases: effects of low dose intravenous cyclophosphamide. *Ann Rheum Dis.* 1997;56(8):481-487.
58. Dalakas MC, Illa I, Dambrosia JM, et al. A controlled trial of high-dose intravenous immune globulin infusions as treatment for dermatomyositis. *N Engl J Med.* 1993;329(27): 1993-2000.
59. Marie I, Hachulla E, Levesque H, et al. Intravenous immunoglobulins as treatment of life threatening esophageal involvement in polymyositis and dermatomyositis. *J Rheumatol.* 1999;26(12):2706-2709.
60. Helmers SB, Dastmalchi M, Alexanderson H, et al. Limited effects of high-dose intravenous immunoglobulin (IVIG) treatment on molecular expression in muscle tissue of patients with inflammatory myopathies. *Ann Rheum Dis.* 2007;66(10):1276-1283.
61. Rios FR, Callejas Rubio JL, Sanchez Cano D, Saez Moreno JA, Ortego Centeno N. Rituximab in the treatment of dermatomyositis and other inflammatory myopathies. A report of 4 cases and review of the literature. *Clin Exp Rheumatol.* 2009;27(6):1009-1016.

Complicated Sarcoidosis: Challenges in Dealing with Severe Manifestations

13

Robert P. Baughman and Hilario Nunes

Abstract Sarcoidosis can affect any part of the body. Dyspnea and cough are the most common symptoms, and advanced lung disease can lead to significant morbidity and some mortality. The causes of dyspnea in sarcoidosis include not only direct lung parenchymal involvement, but also airway disease, cardiac disease, and pulmonary hypertension. The treating physician needs to identify the cause of dyspnea, since therapy differs depending on the cause. Over the past few years, multiple treatment regimens have been developed for pulmonary sarcoidosis. Neurologic disease is a less common but significant cause of morbidity in sarcoidosis. Patients with neurosarcoidosis may present with solely neurologic disease. Identifying that sarcoidosis is the cause of the neurologic impairment is important, as therapy exists for treatment of neurosarcoidosis.

Keywords Infliximab • Methotrexate • Neurosarcoidosis • Prednisone • Pulmonary hypertension • SURT

13.1
Introduction

Sarcoidosis is a granulomatous disease of unknown etiology which can affect any organ. Pulmonary involvement is the most common manifestation of the disease.[1] However, other organs can be affected, including the skin, eyes, brain, and heart. The multisystem nature of sarcoidosis can lead to complex diagnostic and therapeutic decisions. In this chapter, we review management of lung and nervous system manifestations. We also discuss the differential diagnosis as well as therapeutic approach.

R.P. Baughman (✉)
Department of Medicine, University of Cincinnati Medical Center,
1001 Holmes, Eden Avenue, Cincinnati, OH 45267, USA
e-mail: bob.baughman@uc.edu

M.A. Khamashta and M. Ramos-Casals (eds.), *Autoimmune Diseases*,
DOI: 10.1007/978-0-85729-358-9_13, © Springer-Verlag London Limited 2011

13.2
Respiratory Failure

While pulmonary disease is the most common manifestation of sarcoidosis, respiratory failure is relatively unusual. However, pulmonary disease is the most common cause of death from sarcoidosis.[2] Table 13.1 lists the possible reasons for increasing respiratory distress in a sarcoidosis patient. The multiple causes of dyspnea highlight the multiorgan nature of sarcoidosis.

13.2.1
Parenchymal Lung Disease

In the assessment of parenchymal lung disease as the cause of respiratory disease, the clinician has two major tools: chest imaging and pulmonary function testing. While both provide information in identifying advanced lung disease, neither is the "gold standard" in defining severe respiratory disease.

Thoracic involvement is usually classified using the Scadding staging system based on chest roentgenogram.[3] Patients with fibrosis of the lung are classified as stage 4. This pattern is usually associated with worsening lung function and more severe symptoms.[4] While not all patients with stage four chest roentgenograms have severe respiratory disease, most patients who die from pulmonary sarcoidosis have a stage 4 pattern on their chest roentgenogram.[2]

One of the difficulties of using the Scadding system is the only modest agreement between readers in staging the chest roentgenogram.[5] Another difficulty is that a patient may have only limited areas of fibrosis and no symptoms. There is also the problem with mixed disease. This is often more apparent on CT scan. Patients who have areas of honeycombing and traction bronchiectasis representing fibrosis may have other areas of nodular infiltrates which may still be reversible with treatment (Fig. 13.1).[6]

Pulmonary function testing includes spirometry and lung diffusion of carbon monoxide (DLCO). Spirometry provides both the forced expiratory volume in one second (FEV-1) and the forced vital capacity (FVC). The FVC is a reasonable measure of lung volume, and

Table 13.1 Causes of respiratory distress in a sarcoidosis patient

- Directly from sarcoidosis organ involvement
  - Parenchymal airway disease
  - Pulmonary hypertension
  - Upper airway
  - Compression of airway/vasculature by lymph nodes
  - Cardiac
  - Skeletal/diaphragmatic muscle weakness
- Consequence of treatment
  - Infections
- Other causes
  - Pulmonary embolism

Fig. 13.1 Example of CT with fibrosis and reversible infiltrates

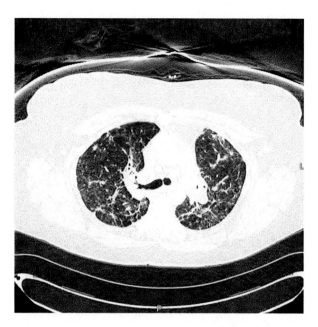

a reduced FVC implies restrictive disease. The FEV-1/FVC ratio detects airway obstruction. While sarcoidosis is often considered a restrictive disease, a significant proportion of patients have airway obstruction with a reduced FEV-1/FVC.[4,7]

There are several causes of restrictive disease and reduced FVC. Pulmonary fibrosis is associated with a reduced FVC. One can also see reduced FVC due to phrenic nerve disease[8] and/or skeletal muscle weakness.[9] In one study, muscle weakness was a better predictor of the level of dyspnea than other physiologic measures of lung function.[9] Obesity will also lead to reduced FVC. The DLCO should be reduced to a greater degree than the FVC in patients with pulmonary fibrosis, while the ratio is normal to increased in patients with obesity or muscle weakness. Marked reduction of the DLCO compared to the FVC suggests pulmonary hypertension.[10,11] This reduction of DLCO out of proportion to FVC has also been used to detect pulmonary hypertension in scleroderma patients.[12]

In one prospective study, patients with a FVC of less than 1.5 l (about 30% of predicted value) had increased mortality over those with higher FVC values.[2] However, once patients are identified with advanced lung disease and referred for lung transplant, the FVC was not predictive of mortality.[13]

All patients with significant respiratory symptoms and evidence of parenchymal lung disease should be considered for systemic therapy.[14] A stepwise approach to systemic therapy has been proposed.[15] Figure 13.2 shows this approach as applied to a patient with significant respiratory disease. Table 13.2 summarizes the initial and maintenance doses of several of the drugs used to manage complex sarcoidosis. The standard treatment is corticosteroids. In the United States, this is usually prednisone. Various starting doses of prednisone have been used. In one study, it was found that prednisone at 20 mg daily was sufficient to treat pulmonary disease and higher doses were not associated with any greater response.[16]

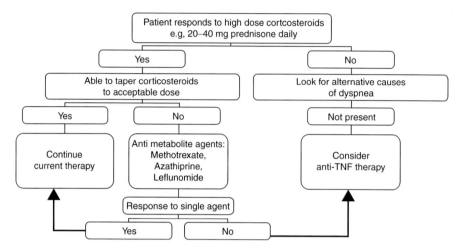

Fig. 13.2 A stepwise approach to treatment of advanced pulmonary sarcoidosis. Patients are initially treated with corticosteroids such as prednisone. Further decisions regarding treatment depend on the response to prednisone, as well as side effects from the drug

Corticosteroids are associated with significant toxicity. Many of these are dose related, and the toxicity is often cumulative. Steroid-sparing alternatives have been used for many years in the management of sarcoidosis.[15] These include methotrexate,[17] azathioprine,[18] and lefulnomide.[19] Methotrexate has been the most widely studied drug,[20] including a double-blind placebo-controlled trial.[21] In a recent Delphi survey, methotrexate was the most commonly employed steroid-sparing agent by pulmonary physicians who specialized in sarcoidosis.[22] While widely used, only about two thirds of patients will respond to methotrexate.[17] This is similar to the rate encountered with other antimetabolites.[19,23]

As noted in Table 13.2, patients being treated with methotrexate should undergo routine monitoring with complete blood counts and liver function studies. These are usually done every 2–3 months.[24] One should also monitor renal function. Methotrexate is mostly cleared by the kidneys, and impaired function can lead to unexpected high levels. The drug is also associated with liver toxicity.[25] While liver function test monitoring alone has been useful in rheumatoid arthritis patients treated with methotrexate,[26] its role in sarcoidosis is still unclear.[25] While some clinicians consider performing a liver biopsy for every gram of cumulative dose,[24] others tend to only perform biopsy when faced with unexplained worsening liver function.[27] The gastrointestinal toxicity from methotrexate may be minimized by concomitant use of folic acid.[28] The usual dose is 1 mg a day, but higher doses may be employed.

Azathioprine has been a widely used drug for various interstitial lung diseases. For sarcoidosis, the literature has been fairly limited.[18,23] However, because of its limited liver toxicity, it has been a useful alternative to methotrexate. Patient monitoring includes complete blood count. Patients with thiopurine S-methyltransferase (TPMT) deficiency can develop severe neutropenia when treated with azathioprine.[29] Genotyping of TPMT is available and has proved useful in some situations to predict which patients will develop leucopenia from the drug. A recent analysis suggested that TMPT genotyping may be

Table 13.2 Commonly used doses and monitoring of drugs for complex sarcoidosis

Drug	Initial dosage	Maintenance dose	Common toxicity	Suggested monitoring	Comments
Prednisone[a]	20–40 mg daily	<10 mg daily	Weight gain Hypertension Osteoporosis Diabetes mellitus Infections	Bone density vital signs	Cumulative toxicity
Methotrexate	10–15 mg once a week	10–15 mg once a week	Neutropenia Nausea Hepatotoxicity Pulmonary toxicity Infection	Monitor every 2–3 months: complete blood count, liver and renal function	Do not give with impaired renal function
Azathiprine	50–250 mg daily	50–250 mg daily	Neutropenia Nausea Infection	Monitor every 2–3 months: complete blood count	Thiopurine S-methyl-transferase genotyping may be useful
Leflunomide	10–20 mg daily	10–20 mg daily	Neutropenia Nausea Hepatotoxicity Neuropathy Infection	Monitor every 2–3 months: complete blood count, liver function	If develops significant toxicity, consider chlestyramine to remove drug[35]
Infliximab[b]	Two doses of 3–5 mg/kg 2 weeks apart	3–5 mg/kg every 4–6 weeks	Allergic reaction, Infection, Congestive heart failure, possible increased risk for malignancy	Tuberculin skin testing[c] prior to initiating therapy, close monitoring during infusion	Do not give to patients with NYHC 3 or 4 heart failure, adalimumab may be given to patients who develop reactions to infliximab

[a]Other corticosteroids may also be used at equivalent doses
[b]Other anti-TNF drugs (adalimumab or golibmumab) may also be used
[c]A *M. tuberculosis*–specific interferon gamma assay may be used as an alternative[44]

useful depending on the dosage of azathioprine employed and the incidence of TMPT deficiency in the population being treated.[30]

Leflunomide has also been found a useful alternative to methotrexate in some sarcoidosis patients.[19] The drug appears to cause less pulmonary toxicity than methotrexate,[31] but a drug-induced interstitial lung disease can still be encountered.[32] Hepatic toxicity can be seen with the drug. The rate appears similar to that encountered with methotrexate. Peripheral neuropathy has been reported in patients taking leflunomide.[33, 34] Besides withdrawal of the drug, it is recommended that cholestyramine be given to help remove the drug more rapidly.[35]

Biologic agents have been developed which block tumor necrosis factor (TNF). Among these have been the monoclonal antibodies directed against TNF: infliximab, adalimumab, and golibmumab. Of these three anti-TNF drugs, infliximab has been the most widely studied and used. After the original report of successful use of infliximab for sarcoidosis,[36] there have been a large number of reports of the utility of this drug for various forms of difficult to treat sarcoidosis.[37] There have been two double-blind, randomized trials of infliximab for pulmonary sarcoidosis.[38,39] Both of these studies demonstrated benefit of the drug over placebo. Also, the more impaired the patient, the larger the response to anti-TNF therapy. In addition to advanced pulmonary disease, infliximab has been shown to be useful for refractory neurosarcoidosis.[40] In a large study examining sarcoidosis patients with *lupus pernio*, infliximab was superior to all other agents.[41] Patients with forced vital capacity of less than 70% of predicted, moderate-to-severe dyspnea, *lupus pernio*, and neurologic disease would be expected to particularly benefit from anti-TNF therapy.[37] Recently, it was reported that patients with an elevated C-reactive protein were more likely to respond to therapy.

Infliximab is associated with significant toxicity. This includes an increased risk for reactivation of tuberculosis.[42] This risk can be minimized by screening for latent tuberculosis. In rheumatoid arthritis, a tuberculin skin test is usually adequate for identifying patients at risk for reactivation of tuberculosis.[43] For patients already on immunosuppressant therapy, *M. tuberculosis*–specific interferon gamma assay may be more effective in detecting latent tuberculosis.[44] For all anti-TNF agents, one should avoid treating patients with advanced congestive heart failure. In addition, there appears to be an increased risk for malignancy with these agents. All the anti-TNF agents should be considered teratogenic based on animal studies. Given all their toxicity, the drugs are usually reserved for more advanced sarcoidosis.

The anti-TNF treatments are not curative for sarcoidosis. While less than half of patients had objective evidence of relapse within 6 months of discontinuing 24 weeks of infliximab for pulmonary sarcoidosis,[38] most clinicians feel these drugs should be given for a more prolonged period.[37] One center reported that more than 90% of their sarcoidosis patients had a clinically significant relapse when infliximab was withdrawn.[45]

13.2.2
Pulmonary Hypertension

Respiratory distress in advanced sarcoidosis patients may also be due to pulmonary hypertension. In studies of all sarcoidosis patients, pulmonary hypertension was identified in 5–15% of patients.[46,47] However, in studies of dyspneic patients, the incidence of pulmonary hypertension was over 50%.[10,11] There are several reasons for pulmonary hypertension in sarcoidosis patients. These include left ventricular dysfunction, pulmonary fibrosis, and compression of pulmonary vasculature by mediastinal and hilar adenopathy. Granulomatous involvement of arterial and venous pulmonary systems has also been found.[48]

Table 13.3 lists some of the features associated with pulmonary hypertension in sarcoidosis patients. For a dyspneic patient, evaluation for pulmonary hypertension should be considered if one or more of the features in Table 13.3 are present. Patients with unexplained dyspnea may have none of these features and still have pulmonary hypertension.

Echocardiography is commonly employed to detect pulmonary hypertension. The tricuspid regurgitant jet can be used to estimate the pulmonary artery (PA) systolic pressure. In about a third of patients, the tricuspid valve cannot be adequately visualized, and therefore, an estimate of PA systolic pressure cannot be made.[49] In addition, echocardiography has been found to be an inaccurate estimate of pulmonary artery pressure in various interstitial lung diseases.[50,51] In sarcoidosis, the echocardiogram poorly correlates with estimated PA systolic pressure.[10,49] Shown in Fig. 13.3 is a direct comparison of PA systolic pressure as estimated by echocardiography compared to the directly measured pressure. There were cases in which the echocardiogram estimated a normal pressure, while an elevated pressure

Table 13.3 Features predicting sarcoidosis-associated pulmonary hypertension

- Advanced lung disease by chest X-ray[11,46,52]
- Reduced DLCO[10,11,46]
- Hypoxemia
    - Reported in one study[87]
    - Not found in another study[11]
- Desaturation with 6 MW
    - Reported in one study[47]
    - Not found in another study[88]
- Reduced 6 MWD[47,88]

DLCO diffusion in lung of carbon monoxide, *6 MW* six minute walk distance; *6MWD* six minute walk distance

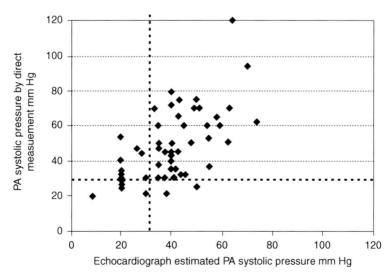

Fig. 13.3 Comparison of pulmonary artery (*PA*) estimated systolic pressure by echocardiography to directly measured PA systolic pressure at right heart catheterization for patients studied at the University of Cincinnati. The dotted lines indicted a PA pressure of 30 mmHg

was found. Indirect evidence of pulmonary hypertension such as right ventricular dilation was found to be also unreliable in identifying all patients with sarcoidosis-associated pulmonary hypertension.[52]

In the sarcoidosis patient who appears to have pulmonary hypertension, a cardiac catheterization helps determine whether the cause is left ventricular dysfunction or arterial disease. Those patients who have pulmonary hypertension due to left ventricular disease have a significantly better prognosis than those with pulmonary arterial hypertension.[49] This is in part because there are better treatments for left ventricular disease.

There are several treatments available for treatment of pulmonary arterial hypertension. There are several reports on these drugs being used to treat sarcoidosis-associated pulmonary hypertension. Of the prostanoids, systemic epoprostenol[53] and inhaled iloprost[54] have both been reported as effective. Sildenafil has been reported as improving pulmonary hemodynamics in a small group of patients with advanced lung disease.[55] The endothelin receptor antagonist bosentan has been reported effective in some cases.[10,56] The largest series reported to date has shown that a stepwise approach to treatment in these patients often leads to improved hemodynamics and 6 min walk distance.[57]

13.2.3
Upper Airway Disease

Sarcoidosis of the upper respiratory tract (SURT) can lead to airway narrowing.[58,59] This can include upper airway (Fig. 13.4), trachea, and large bronchi. Patients may have endobronchial stenosis of the proximal bronchi (ESPB) which leads to respiratory impairment.[58] These patients may be confused with asthma, especially if wheezing from the fixed airway obstruction is heard.

In evaluating the dyspneic sarcoidosis patient, one should look for evidence of upper airway disease. Proximal airway involvement is often seen in conjunction with sinus involvement.[59] Sarcoidosis patients with *lupus pernio*, cutaneous lesions involving the

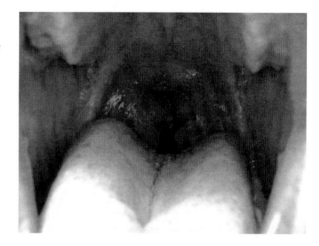

Fig. 13.4 Increase in tonsillar size by granulomatous involvement in 21-year-old Caucasian female. Patient complained of being unable to sleep lying down. Biopsy revealed noncaseating granuloma. Cultures were negative for bacteria, mycobacteria, or fungus. Tonsils regressed to normal size within a month of systemic corticosteroid therapy

Fig. 13.5 Facial lesions of patient with *lupus pernio* with maculopapular lesions on nose and cheeks (**a**). Patient also has subglottic stenosis (**b**)

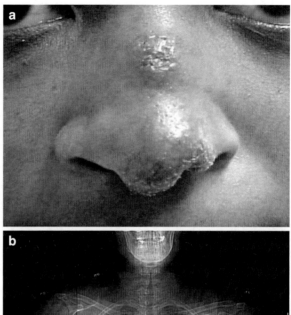

nose, cheeks, and around the eyes, often have SURT.[60,61] Figure 13.5 is an example of a patient with *lupus pernio* (Fig. 13.5a)who developed subglottic stenosis (Fig. 13.5b). Auscultation of the neck may reveal stridor, a high pitched sound similar to wheezing. Stridor is predominantly an inspiratory sound, whereas wheezing is predominantly an expiratory sound. Also, stridor is more prominent over the neck than chest.[62] The presence of stridor suggests upper airway narrowing, as seen in this case.

Pulmonary function tests are usually abnormal in patients with ESPB. In one series, pure obstructive pattern was seen in two thirds of patients, while restrictive or mixed were seen in the rest.[58] Radiologic imaging can be useful in identifying upper airway[63] or proximal bronchial airway obstruction.[59] Routine chest roentgenogram may provide information about large airway disease (Fig. 13.5b). CT scan of the chest has proved a useful tool on evaluating advance pulmonary sarcoidosis.[64] In patients with ESPB, abnormalities of the airways are usually detected by careful evaluation of the CT scan.[58,65] In some settings, the use of a sagittal view may provide better visualization of the airway narrowing (Fig. 13.6).

Endoscopy is the definitive method for diagnosing endobronchial obstruction. The usual appearance on bronchoscopy is a diffuse airway narrowing. The airway may have a cobblestone appearance suggesting carcinoma, but in sarcoidosis, there are usually multiple stenotic areas.[58] Stenosis can be smooth, especially as fibrosis has occurred. Patients

Fig. 13.6 Reconstructed
sagittal view of patient
with sarcoidosis and
endobronchial stenosis
of the proximal bronchi.
Narrowing of the right upper
lobe can be seen in this view
(Courtesy of Dr. Robert
Dales)

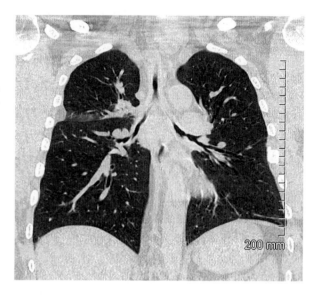

with endobronchial sarcoidosis often have cough. Endobronchial biopsy of the abnormal airway usually reveals granumolatous involvement.[66] Extrinsic compression of the airway by enlarged lymph nodes can lead to airway narrowing. In that case, the bronchial mucosa will appear normal. The differential diagnosis of a stenotic airway includes Wegener's granulomatosis, tuberculosis, deep fungal infections such as histoplasmosis, and cancer.[59]

Local therapy for patient with one or two critical stenotic areas may be helpful. This includes intralesional injection of corticosteroids. This has been reported as successful in patients with laryngeal sarcoidosis.[67] Dilation and stenting may also be useful.[68] However, most patients can be controlled by systemic therapy.[59] This may include steroid-sparing agents such as methotrexate.[69] One study compared the onset of systemic treatment to clinical outcome. In the patients with delayed treatment, moderate-to-severe symptoms persisted in 60% of patients, while in those treated within 3 months of diagnosis of ESPB, only 15% had symptoms and all were classified as mild.[58]

13.2.4
Other Causes of Dyspnea

Infection is a major complication of sarcoidosis. This is usually a consequence of immuno-suppressive therapy for the sarcoidosis. In a retrospective study of 753 sarcoidosis patients seen at one clinic over an 18-month period, seven patients (0.9%) developed fungal infections: two each with *Histoplasma capsulatum* and *Blastomyces dermatitidis* and three others with *Cryptococcus neoformans*. There were no documented cases of *M. tuberculosis* or invasive *Aspergillus*.[70] All cases occurred in patients on corticosteroids and four of seven were on methotrexate, the most commonly used cytotoxic agent in that clinic. In this series, none of the 24 patients treated with infliximab developed deep fungal infections, but the use of anti-TNF agents is a risk for serious infection with fungi and *M. tuberculosis*.

The traction bronchiectasis seen in stage 4 sarcoidosis can lead to *Aspergillus* and other fungi forming mycetomas in these cavities (Fig. 13.7). In one series, aspergillomas were diagnosed in about 1% of patients over an 18-month period.[70] Mycetomas can cause bleeding that may be massive and even fatal. Treatment for aspergillomas includes resection when possible. However, most patients have extensive fibrotic disease, which makes them poor candidates for surgery. Alternatives include systemic antifungal agents such as

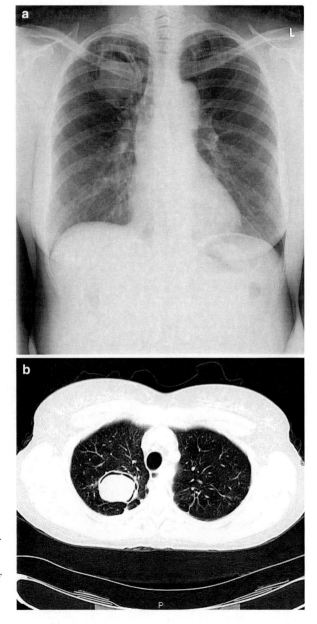

Fig. 13.7 Patient with stage 4 sarcoidosis and upper lobe cavity. Mycetoma in cavity with subsequent cultures identifying *Aspergillus nigrans*. (**a**) Posterior-anterior chest roentgenogram. (**b**) Representative CT image demonstrating the characteristic crescent sign of air between the mycetoma and the cavity wall

itraconazole and vorconazole.[71,72] Also, local instillation of amphotericin has been used in selective cases.[73] For patients with massive bleeding, bronchial embolization may also be useful.

13.3
Neurologic Disease

Neurologic disease occurs in 5–15% of sarcoidosis patients.[1,74] It is associated with significant morbidity. The manifestations of neurosarcoidosis vary considerably, but the most common areas affected are the cranial nerves, leptomeninges, base of the brain, and spinal cord. Table 13.4 summarizes the most common findings in four large series of neurosarcoidosis.

There are two presentations for possible neurosarcoidosis patient. The first is the patient who presents with neurologic disease for which the differential includes sarcoidosis. The second is for the patient with known sarcoidosis who presents with neurologic symptoms which could be due to sarcoidosis. In both cases, the evidence for neurosarcoidosis is the same. The evaluation of a patient with possible neurosarcoidosis therefore includes a focused history and physical examination, MRI imaging, and in some cases, an examination of the cerebral spinal fluid. The two major strategies proposed for the diagnosis of neurosarcoidosis are shown in Table 13.5. The specific criteria have been modified to clarify and expand some of the testing available today. For example, Zajicek et al. state that criteria for systemic sarcoidosis could include positive Gallium scan and chest imaging.[75] In an update by one of the coauthors of that report, they propose adding an elevated CD4/CD8 ratio of lymphocytes retrieved by bronchoalveolar lavage.[76] Likewise, chest imaging compatible with sarcoidosis would include not only bilateral hilar adenopathy,[14] but also the peribronchial thickening and peripheral nodularity seen on CT scan of the chest.[77] Positive emission transmission (PET) scanning has been shown to be helpful in the diagnosis of sarcoidosis.[78]

Table 13.4 Most common areas of involvement in neurosarcoidosis

	Lower et al.[80]	Zajicek et al.[75]	Pawate et al.[81]	Joseph and Scolding[76]
Number of cases	71	68	54	30
Select cranial nerves				
Optic neuritis	7 (10%)	35%	24 (35%)	27%
Facial paralysis	39 (55%)	18%	6 (11%)	18%
Hearing loss	2 (3%)	7%	5 (9%)	8%
Other common manifestations				
Pan hypo pit/diabetes insipidus	6 (8%)	5%	1 (2%)	17%
Meningeal	2 (3%)	11%	NR	22%
Spinal cord	NR	27%	NR	18%
Peripheral neuropathy	3 (4%)	NR	1 (2%)	NR

Patients may have more than one area involved

Table 13.5 Criteria for the diagnosis of neurosarcoidosis

	Zajicek et al.[75]	Judson et al.[79]
Definite	Granulomas found in a biopsy of the neurosystem Plus Clinical presentation suggestive of neurosarcoidosis	Any one of the following: 1. Positive MRI imaging with uptake in brainstem or meninges 2. Cerebral spinal fluid with increased lymphocytes or protein 3. Seventh nerve paralysis 4. Diabetes insipidus Plus Exclusion of other possible diagnosis
Probable	Clinical presentation suggestive of neurosarcoidosis And any of the following: 1. Elevated CSF protein or cells with presence of oligoclonal bands 2. MRI imaging compatible with neurosarcoidosis Plus Evidence of systemic sarcoidosis by one of following: 1. Positive histology 2. Positive Kviem 3. At least two indirect indicators of sarcoidosis (a) Positive gallium or PET scan (b) Chest imaging (e.g., bilateral hilar adenopathy) Elevated serum ACE	Any one of the following: 1. Other abnormalities on MRI imaging 2. Unexplained neuropathy 3. Positive electromyelogram Plus Exclusion of other possible diagnosis
Possible	Clinical presentation suggestive of neurosarcoidosis where above criteria are not met	Either 1. Unexplained headaches 2. Peripheral nerve radiculopathy
For all cases	Exclusion of other possible diagnosis	Exclusion of other possible diagnosis Plus Histologic confirmation of sarcoidosis in one or more organ (does not have to be nervous system)

Source: Adapted and modified from Lower and Weiss [74], Zajicek et al. [75], Joseph and Scolding [76], Judson et al. [79]

Both groups divided the diagnostic criteria into definite, probable, or possible. For definite neurosarcoidosis, Zajicek required a histologic confirmation of granulomas from the nervous system.[75] The criteria of Judson et al.[79] required histologic confirmation for all three categories. However, it does classify known cases of sarcoidosis who have a compatible clinical presentation of neurosarcoidosis as definite neurosarcoidosis. For example, a patient with mediastinal adenopathy and a positive lymph node biopsy for granulomas that

Fig. 13.8 MRI with enhancement of dura by gadolinium due to neurosarcoidosis

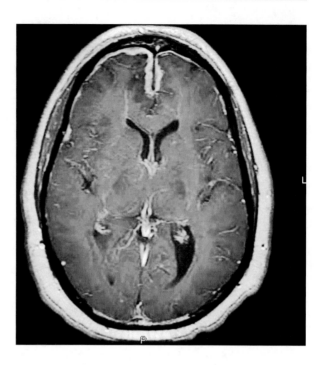

also has lymphocytic meningitis would be considered definite neurosarcoidosis (Fig. 13.8). In most series, authors combine definite and probable together.

The group of possible neurosarcoidosis will include patients without neurosarcoidosis. In some cases, the clinician may choose to still treat such a patient as a neurosarcoidosis case. Zajicek et al. included patients who could have isolated neurosarcoidosis symptoms with no confirmation of sarcoidosis.[75] On the other hand, Judson et al.[79] required that the patient have biopsy confirmed sarcoidosis, but considered a patient as possible neurosarcoidosis if, for example, they had headache not related to other causes.

The MRI and CT scan are the two most common imagings in neurosarcoidosis. In several reports, the MRI has been found to be superior to CT scan in detecting lesions.[75,76,80,81] However, it should be noted that between 11% and 33% of cases will have a normal MRI at time of evaluation.[75,76,80,81] Among the reasons for a normal MRI after initial treatment is that treatment can normalize the MRI.[82] Also, some of the series used older MRI techniques. With the new scanning algorithms, more lesions may be detected.[74] With this increased sensitivity, however, there is reduced specificity.

The most common findings on MRI are white matter lesions, parenchymal lesions (sometimes a single lesion), meningeal enhancement, optic nerve lesion, hydrocephalus, and spinal cord lesions.[74,75] Figure 13.8 demonstrates dural enhancement by gadolinium of a patient with dural involvement from neurosarcoidosis. Spinal disease is recognized to occur in up to a quarter of patients with neurosarcoidosis.[75] The lesions are often multiple and may occur with other central lesions.[83] Imaging of the entire spine increases the number of cases detected.[74]

Treatment for sarcoidosis always depends on symptoms. In neurosarcoidosis, the presentation may help direct therapy. For a patient with seventh cranial nerve paralysis, the outcome is quite good.[80] Many of these patients will resolve their paralysis with a short course of corticosteroids. Unfortunately, for most patients with neurosarcoidosis, there is a high rate of relapse unless long-term therapy is maintained. The use of a steroid-sparing agent such as methotrexate or azathioprine has been reported as effective in over half of the cases in which they were used.[75,80,84] Cyclophosphamide has been useful in the treatment of cases of refractory neurosarcoidosis.[80,85] In other cases, combinations of cytotoxic agents have proved useful in controlling disease.[83] Infliximab has been used increasingly in cases of refractory neurosarcoidosis.[40,86] Given the rapid onset of action and its effectiveness in refractory cases, clinicians are increasingly employing infliximab in patients who fail to be controlled by prednisone alone for their neurosarcoidosis.

Long-standing inflammation from neurosarcoidosis may lead persistent neurologic deficits after successful treatment. In one series of spinal sarcoidosis, only half of patients who have paraplegia at time of presentation recover muscle function.[83] The clinician must monitor response to treatment to determine whether therapy has resolved inflammation. In most cases, adequate therapy will resolve inflammatory changes seen on MRI.[82] Serial neurologic examinations also help determine if the deficit is further improving during treatment.

Hydrocephalus can occur as the result of meningeal disease. Ventriculoperitoneal shunting is the treatment for this (Fig. 13.9). There may be a granulomatous reaction to the shunt, so most patients with shunts will require long-term therapy for their sarcoidosis.

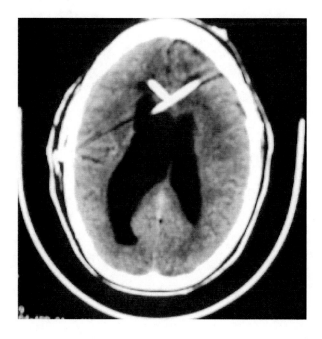

Fig. 13.9 MRI of brain of patient with neurosarcoidosis. Hydrocephalus seen with ventricular-peritoneal shunt in place

13.4
Conclusion

Sarcoidosis is a complex, multiorgan disease. Patients may present with various complaints. In addition, the cause of a particular symptom, such as dyspnea, can be due to multiple factors. In evaluating the sarcoidosis patient, the clinician has to consider more than just their area of expertise, but the entire patient.

References

1. Baughman RP, Teirstein AS, Judson MA, et al. Clinical characteristics of patients in a case control study of sarcoidosis. *Am J Respir Crit Care Med*. 2001;164:1885-1889.
2. Baughman RP, Winget DB, Bowen EH, et al. Predicting respiratory failure in sarcoidosis patients. *Sarcoidosis*. 1997;14:154-158.
3. Scadding JG. Prognosis of intrathoracic sarcoidosis in England. *Br Med J*. 1961;4:1165-1172.
4. Yeager H, Rossman MD, Baughman RP, et al. Pulmonary and psychosocial findings at enrollment in the ACCESS study. *Sarcoidosis Vasc Diffuse Lung Dis*. 2005;22(2):147-153.
5. Baughman RP, Shipley R, Desai S, et al. Changes in chest roentgenogram of sarcoidosis patients during a clinical trial of infliximab therapy: comparison of different methods of evaluation. *Chest*. 2009;136:526-535.
6. Abehsera M, Valeyre D, Grenier P, et al. Sarcoidosis with pulmonary fibrosis: CT patterns and correlation with pulmonary function. *AJR Am J Roentgenol*. 2000;174(6):1751-1757.
7. Sharma OP, Johnson R. Airway obstruction in sarcoidosis. A study of 123 nonsmoking black American patients with sarcoidosis. *Chest*. 1988;94(2):343-346.
8. Robinson LR, Brownsberger R, Raghu G. Respiratory failure and hypoventilation secondary to neurosarcoidosis. *Am J Respir Crit Care Med*. 1998;157(4 Pt 1):1316-1318.
9. Baydur A, Alsalek M, Louie SG, et al. Respiratory muscle strength, lung function, and dyspnea in patients with sarcoidosis. *Chest*. 2001;120(1):102-108.
10. Baughman RP, Engel PJ, Meyer CA, et al. Pulmonary hypertension in sarcoidosis. *Sarcoidosis Vasc Diffuse Lung Dis*. 2006;23:108-116.
11. Sulica R, Teirstein AS, Kakarla S, et al. Distinctive clinical, radiographic, and functional characteristics of patients with sarcoidosis-related pulmonary hypertension. *Chest*. 2005;128(3):1483-1489.
12. Steen V, Medsger TA Jr. Predictors of isolated pulmonary hypertension in patients with systemic sclerosis and limited cutaneous involvement. *Arthritis Rheum*. 2003;48(2):516-522.
13. Shorr AF, Davies DB, Nathan SD. Predicting mortality in patients with sarcoidosis awaiting lung transplantation. *Chest*. 2003;124(3):922-928.
14. Hunninghake GW, Costabel U, Ando M, et al. ATS/ERS/WASOG statement on sarcoidosis. American Thoracic Society/European Respiratory Society/World Association of Sarcoidosis and other Granulomatous Disorders. *Sarcoidosis Vasc Diffuse Lung Dis*. 1999;16:149-173.
15. Baughman RP, Costabel U, du Bois RM. Treatment of sarcoidosis. *Clin Chest Med*. 2008;29(3):533-548.
16. McKinzie BP, Bullington WM, Mazur JE, et al. Efficacy of short-course, low-dose corticosteroid therapy for acute pulmonary sarcoidosis exacerbations. *Am J Med Sci*. 2010;339(1):1-4.
17. Lower EE, Baughman RP. Prolonged use of methotrexate for sarcoidosis. *Arch Intern Med*. 1995;155:846-851.
18. Muller-Quernheim J, Kienast K, Held M, et al. Treatment of chronic sarcoidosis with an azathioprine/prednisolone regimen. *Eur Respir J*. 1999;14(5):1117-1122.

19. Baughman RP, Lower EE. Leflunomide for chronic sarcoidosis. *Sarcoidosis Vasc Diffuse Lung Dis.* 2004;21:43-48.
20. Paramothayan S, Lasserson T, Walters EH. Immunosuppressive and cytotoxic therapy for pulmonary sarcoidosis. *Cochrane Database Syst Rev.* 2003;(3):CD003536.
21. Baughman RP, Winget DB, Lower EE. Methotrexate is steroid sparing in acute sarcoidosis: results of a double blind, randomized trial. *Sarcoidosis Vasc Diffuse Lung Dis.* 2000;17:60-66.
22. Schutt AC, Bullington WM, Judson MA. Pharmacotherapy for pulmonary sarcoidosis: a Delphi consensus study. *Respir Med.* 2010;104(5):717-723.
23. Baughman RP, Lower EE. Alternatives to corticosteroids in the treatment of sarcoidosis. *Sarcoidosis.* 1997;14:121-130.
24. Baughman RP, Lower EE. A clinical approach to the use of methotrexate for sarcoidosis. *Thorax.* 1999;54:742-746.
25. Baughman RP, Koehler A, Bejarano PA, et al. Role of liver function tests in detecting methotrexate-induced liver damage in sarcoidosis. *Arch Intern Med.* 2003;163(5):615-620.
26. Kremer JM, Alarcon GS, Lightfoot RW Jr, et al. Methotrexate for rheumatoid arthritis. Suggested guidelines monitoring liver toxicity. American College of Rheumatology. *Arthritis Rheum.* 1994;37(3):316-328.
27. Vucinic VM. What is the future of methotrexate in sarcoidosis? A study and review. *Curr Opin Pulm Med.* 2002;8(5):470-476.
28. Morgan SL, Baggott JE, Vaughn WH, et al. Supplementation with folic acid during methotrexate therapy for rheumatoid arthritis. *Ann Intern Med.* 1994;121:833-841.
29. Lennard L, Van Loon JA, Weinshilboum RM. Pharmacogenetics of acute azathioprine toxicity: relationship to thiopurine methyltransferase genetic polymorphism. *Clin Pharmacol Ther.* 1989;46(2):149-154.
30. Hagaman JT, Kinder BW, Eckman MH. Thiopurine *S*-methyltranferase testing in idiopathic pulmonary fibrosis: a pharmacogenetic cost-effectiveness analysis. *Lung.* 2010;188(2):125-132.
31. Emery P, Breedveld FC, Lemmel EM, et al. A comparison of the efficacy and safety of leflunomide and methotrexate for the treatment of rheumatoid arthritis. *Rheumatology (Oxford).* 2000;39(6):655-665.
32. Savage RL, Highton J, Boyd IW, et al. Pneumonitis associated with leflunomide: a profile of New Zealand and Australian reports. *Intern Med J.* 2006;36(3):162-169.
33. Kho LK, Kermode AG. Leflunomide-induced peripheral neuropathy. *J Clin Neurosci.* 2007;14(2):179-181.
34. Martin K, Bentaberry F, Dumoulin C, et al. Neuropathy associated with leflunomide: a case series. *Ann Rheum Dis.* 2005;64(4):649-650.
35. Rozman B. Clinical pharmacokinetics of leflunomide. *Clin Pharmacokinet.* 2002;41(6):421-430.
36. Baughman RP, Lower EE. Infliximab for refractory sarcoidosis. *Sarcoidosis Vasc Diffuse Lung Dis.* 2001;18:70-74.
37. Baughman RP, Lower EE, Drent M. Inhibitors of tumor necrosis factor (TNF) in sarcoidosis: who, what, and how to use them. *Sarcoidosis Vasc Diffuse Lung Dis.* 2008;25:76-89.
38. Baughman RP, Drent M, Kavuru M, et al. Infliximab therapy in patients with chronic sarcoidosis and pulmonary involvement. *Am J Respir Crit Care Med.* 2006;174(7):795-802.
39. Rossman MD, Newman LS, Baughman RP, et al. A double-blind, randomized, placebo-controlled trial of infliximab in patients with active pulmonary sarcoidosis. *Sarcoidosis Vasc Diffuse Lung Dis.* 2006;23:201-208.
40. Moravan M, Segal BM. Treatment of CNS sarcoidosis with infliximab and mycophenolate mofetil. *Neurology.* 2009;72(4):337-340.
41. Stagaki E, Mountford WK, Lackland DT, et al. The treatment of lupus pernio: results of 116 treatment courses in 54 patients. *Chest.* 2009;135(2):468-476.
42. Keane J, Gershon S, Wise RP, et al. Tuberculosis associated with infliximab, a tumor necrosis factor-alpha neutralizing agent. *N Engl J Med.* 2001;345:1098-1104.

43. Gomez-Reino JJ, Carmona L, Angel DM. Risk of tuberculosis in patients treated with tumor necrosis factor antagonists due to incomplete prevention of reactivation of latent infection. *Arthritis Rheum*. 2007;57(5):756-761.

44. Matulis G, Juni P, Villiger PM, et al. Detection of latent tuberculosis in immunosuppressed patients with autoimmune diseases performance of a mycobacterium tuberculosis antigen specific IFN-gamma assay. *Ann Rheum Dis*. 2007;67(1):84-90.

45. Panselinas E, Rodgers JK, Judson MA. Clinical outcomes in sarcoidosis after cessation of infliximab treatment. *Respirology*. 2009;14(4):522-528.

46. Handa T, Nagai S, Miki S, et al. Incidence of pulmonary hypertension and its clinical relevance in patients with sarcoidosis. *Chest*. 2006;129(5):1246-1252.

47. Bourbonnais JM, Samavati L. Clinical predictors of pulmonary hypertension in sarcoidosis. *Eur Respir J*. 2008;32(2):296-302.

48. Nunes H, Humbert M, Capron F, et al. Pulmonary hypertension associated with sarcoidosis: mechanisms, haemodynamics and prognosis. *Thorax*. 2006;61(1):68-74.

49. Baughman RP, Engel PJ, Taylor L, et al. Survival in sarcoidosis associated pulmonary hypertension: the importance of hemodynamic evaluation. *Chest*. 2010;138(5):1078-1085.

50. Arcasoy SM, Christie JD, Ferrari VA, et al. Echocardiographic assessment of pulmonary hypertension in patients with advanced lung disease. *Am J Respir Crit Care Med*. 2003;167(5):735-740.

51. Nathan SD, Shlobin OA, Barnett SD, et al. Right ventricular systolic pressure by echocardiography as a predictor of pulmonary hypertension in idiopathic pulmonary fibrosis. *Respir Med*. 2008;102(9):1305-1310.

52. Rizzato G, Pezzano A, Sala G, et al. Right heart impairment in sarcoidosis: haemodynamic and echocardiographic study. *Eur J Respir Dis*. 1983;64(2):121-128.

53. Fisher KA, Serlin DM, Wilson KC, et al. Sarcoidosis-associated pulmonary hypertension: outcome with long-term epoprostenol treatment. *Chest*. 2006;130(5):1481-1488.

54. Baughman RP, Judson MA, Lower EE, et al. Inhaled iloprost for sarcoidosis associated pulmonary hypertension. *Sarcoidosis Vasc Diffuse Lung Dis*. 2009;26:110-120.

55. Milman N, Burton CM, Iversen M, et al. Pulmonary hypertension in end-stage pulmonary sarcoidosis: therapeutic effect of sildenafil? *J Heart Lung Transplant*. 2008;27(3):329-334.

56. Foley RJ, Metersky ML. Successful treatment of sarcoidosis-associated pulmonary hypertension with bosentan. *Respiration*. 2008;75(2):211-214.

57. Barnett CF, Bonura EJ, Nathan SD. Treatment of sarcoidosis-associated pulmonary hypertension: a two-center experience. *Chest*. 2009;135:1455-1461.

58. Chambellan A, Turbie P, Nunes H, et al. Endoluminal stenosis of proximal bronchi in sarcoidosis: bronchoscopy, function, and evolution. *Chest*. 2005;127(2):472-481.

59. Baughman RP, Lower EE, Tami T. Upper airway. 4: Sarcoidosis of the upper respiratory tract (SURT). *Thorax*. 2010;65(2):181-186.

60. Spiteri MA, Matthey F, Gordon T, et al. Lupus pernio: a clinico-radiological study of thirty-five cases. *Br J Dermatol*. 1985;112(3):315-322.

61. Baughman RP, Judson MA, Teirstein A, et al. Chronic facial sarcoidosis including lupus pernio: clinical description and proposed scoring systems. *Am J Clin Dermatol*. 2008;9(3):155-161.

62. Baughman RP, Loudon RG. Stridor: differentiation from asthma or upper airway noise. *Am Rev Respir Dis*. 1989;139(6):1407-1409.

63. Braun JJ, Imperiale A, Riehm S, et al. Imaging in sinonasal sarcoidosis: CT, MRI, (67)Gallium scintigraphy and (18)F-FDG PET/CT features. *J Neuroradiol*. 2010;37(3):172-181.

64. Hennebicque AS, Nunes H, Brillet PY, et al. CT findings in severe thoracic sarcoidosis. *Eur Radiol*. 2005;15(1):23-30.

65. Naccache JM, Lavole A, Nunes H, et al. High-resolution computed tomographic imaging of airways in sarcoidosis patients with airflow obstruction. *J Comput Assist Tomogr*. 2008;32(6):905-912.

66. Shorr AF, Torrington KG, Hnatiuk OW. Endobronchial biopsy for sarcoidosis: a prospective study. *Chest*. 2001;120(1):109-114.

67. Krespi YP, Mitrani M, Husain S, et al. Treatment of laryngeal sarcoidosis with intralesional steroid injection. *Ann Otol Rhinol Laryngol*. 1987;96(6):713-715.
68. Fouty BW, Pomeranz M, Thigpen TP, et al. Dilatation of bronchial stenoses due to sarcoidosis using a flexible fiberoptic bronchoscope. *Chest*. 1994;106(3):677-680.
69. Zeitlin JF, Tami TA, Baughman R, et al. Nasal and sinus manifestations of sarcoidosis. *Am J Rhinol*. 2000;14(3):157-161.
70. Baughman RP, Lower EE. Fungal infections as a complication of therapy for sarcoidosis. *QJM*. 2005;98:451-456.
71. Dannaoui E, Garcia-Hermoso D, Naccache JM, et al. Use of voriconazole in a patient with aspergilloma caused by an itraconazole-resistant strain of Aspergillus fumigatus. *J Med Microbiol*. 2006;55(Pt 10):1457-1459.
72. De Beule K, De Doncker P, Cauwenbergh G, et al. The treatment of aspergillosis and aspergilloma with itraconazole, clinical results of an open international study (1982–1987). *Mycoses*. 1988;31(9):476-485.
73. Judson MA, Stevens DA. The treatment of pulmonary aspergilloma. *Curr Opin Investig Drugs*. 2001;2(10):1375-1377.
74. Lower EE, Weiss KL. Neurosarcoidosis. *Clin Chest Med*. 2008;29(3):475-492.
75. Zajicek JP, Scolding NJ, Foster O, et al. Central nervous system sarcoidosis – diagnosis and management. *QJM*. 1999;92(2):103-117.
76. Joseph FG, Scolding NJ. Neurosarcoidosis: a study of 30 new cases. *J Neurol Neurosurg Psychiatry*. 2009;80(3):297-304.
77. Akbar JJ, Meyer CA, Shipley RT, et al. Cardiopulmonary imaging in sarcoidosis. *Clin Chest Med*. 2008;29(3):429-443.
78. Teirstein AS, Machac J, Almeida O, et al. Results of 188 whole-body fluorodeoxyglucose positron emission tomography scans in 137 patients with sarcoidosis. *Chest*. 2007;132(6):1949-1953.
79. Judson MA, Baughman RP, Teirstein AS, et al. Defining organ involvement in sarcoidosis: the ACCESS proposed instrument. *Sarcoidosis Vasc Diffuse Lung Dis*. 1999;16:75-86.
80. Lower EE, Broderick JP, Brott TG, et al. Diagnosis and management of neurologic sarcoidosis. *Arch Intern Med*. 1997;157:1864-1868.
81. Pawate S, Moses H, Sriram S. Presentations and outcomes of neurosarcoidosis: a study of 54 cases. *QJM*. 2009;102:449-460.
82. Dumas JL, Valeyre D, Chapelon-Abric C, et al. Central nervous system sarcoidosis: follow-up at MR imaging during steroid therapy. *Radiology*. 2000;214(2):411-420.
83. Bradley DA, Lower EE, Baughman RP. Diagnosis and management of spinal cord sarcoidosis. *Sarcoidosis Vasc Diffuse Lung Dis*. 2006;23(1):58-65.
84. Agbogu BN, Stern BJ, Sewell C, et al. Therapeutic considerations in patients with refractory neurosarcoidosis. *Arch Neurol*. 1995;52:875-879.
85. Doty JD, Mazur JE, Judson MA. Treatment of corticosteroid-resistant neurosarcoidosis with a short-course cyclophosphamide regimen. *Chest*. 2003;124(5):2023-2026.
86. Sodhi M, Pearson K, White ES, et al. Infliximab therapy rescues cyclophosphamide failure in severe central nervous system sarcoidosis. *Respir Med*. 2009;103(2):268-273.
87. Shorr AF, Helman DL, Davies DB, et al. Pulmonary hypertension in advanced sarcoidosis: epidemiology and clinical characteristics. *Eur Respir J*. 2005;25(5):783-788.
88. Baughman RP, Sparkman BK, Lower EE. Six-minute walk test and health status assessment in sarcoidosis. *Chest*. 2007;132(1):207-213.

Complex Situations in Patients with Adult-Onset Still's Disease

14

Petros V. Efthimiou, Manil Kukar, and Olga Petryna

Abstract Adult-onset Still's disease (AOSD) is a rare systemic inflammatory disorder of unknown etiology, characterized by quotidian or double quotidian fever, a peri-febrile cutaneous eruption, polyarthritis, and multiorgan involvement. AOSD is a challenging disease with protean disease manifestations and rare, albeit potentially life-threatening, complications. In such cases, prompt diagnosis and treatment may prove life-saving.

The purpose of this chapter is to review the diagnosis and management of challenging clinical situations in AOSD patients that are associated with significant morbidity and mortality and to provide the readers with information that could aid their decision-making process.

Keywords Adult-Onset Still's Disease (AOSD) • Complications • Interleukin (IL)-1 • Reactive hemophagocytic syndrome (RHS) • Still's arthritis • Still's rash

14.1
Introduction

Adult-onset Still's disease (AOSD) is a rare systemic inflammatory disorder of unknown etiology with a protean clinical presentation. Symptoms include a quotidian or double quotidian fever, a peri-febrile cutaneous eruption, polyarthritis and, in severe cases, multiorgan involvement. Pro-inflammatory cytokines such as interleukin (IL)-1, IL-6, and IL-18, interferon (IFN)-γ, tumor necrosis factor (TNF), and macrophage colony–stimulating factor are elevated in patients with AOSD and are thought to have a major role in the pathogenesis of the disease.[1] High index of clinical suspicion and careful investigation are required to make an early diagnosis so that aggressive treatment can be initiated. There is no single diagnostic test for AOSD; rather, the diagnosis is based on sets of clinical and laboratory criteria. Several

P.V. Efthimiou (✉)
Rheumatology Division, Lincoln Medical and Mental Health Center,
234 E. 149th Street, New York, NY 10451, USA
e-mail: pe53@cornell.edu

M.A. Khamashta and M. Ramos-Casals (eds.), *Autoimmune Diseases*,
DOI: 10.1007/978-0-85729-358-9_14, © Springer-Verlag London Limited 2011

sets of classification criteria have been published for AOSD. They have all been developed from retrospective data and classify criteria as major or minor. Table 14.1 compares the most recent Fautrel criteria[3] with the widely used original Yamaguchi's criteria.[2]

Diagnosis of AOSD usually necessitates the exclusion of infectious, neoplastic, and other autoimmune diseases. The diseases to exclude have been described in Table 14.2.

AOSD management greatly depends on the severity and chronicity of symptoms and the predominant disease pattern, systemic, or arthritic. Initial attacks may be effectively treated with short courses of systemic corticosteroids and may never recur. Persistent

Table 14.1 AOSD diagnostic criteria

Yamaguchi et al.[2]	Fautrel et al.[3]
Major	
Arthralgia >2 weeks	Spiking fever >39°
Fever >39°, intermittent ≥1 week	
Typical rash	Arthralgia Transient erythema
WBC ≥10,000 (≥80,000 granulocytes)	Pharyngitis
	PMNs ≥80%
	Glycosylated ferritin ≤20%
Minor	
Sore throat	Maculopapular rash
Lymphadenopathy and/or splenomegaly	Leucocytes >10 × 10⁹ /L
Abnormal Liver function tests	
(−)ve RF and ANA	
Diagnostic combination	
Exclusion criteria	
– Infections	
– Malignancies	
– Other rheumatic diseases	
Diagnosis: 5 criteria (at least 2 major)	4 major or 3 major+2 minor

Table 14.2 Diagnostic guidelines for hemophagocytic lymphohistiocytosis (HLH) aka hemophago-cytic syndrome

Clinical criteria	Fever
	Splenomegaly
Laboratory criteria	Cytopenia (affecting >2 of 3 lineages in the peripheral blood)
	Hemoglobin <90 g/l
	Platelets <100 × 109/l
	Neutrophils <1.0 × 109/l
	Hypertriglyceridemia and/or hypofibrinogenemia (fasting triglycerides ≥2.0 mmol/l or ≥3 SD of the normal value for age, fibrinogen ≤1.5 g/l or ≤3 SD)
Histopathologic criteria	Hemophagocytosis in bone marrow or spleen or lymph nodes. No evidence of malignancy

disease with frequent recurrent attacks with systemic symptoms (fever, rash) or differentiation into the chronic articular pattern is associated with significant morbidity and requires chronic suppressive treatment with systemic corticosteroids, often in combination with traditional Disease-Modifying anti-Rheumatic Drugs (DMARDS) or the newer biologic agents that offer a more targeted approach.

The purpose of this chapter is to review the management of challenging clinical situations in AOSD patients that may be associated with significant morbidity and mortality and to provide the readers with information that may aid their decision-making process.

14.2
Reactive Hemophagocytic Syndrome (RHS)

RHS, otherwise known as macrophage activation syndrome (MAS), is a rare but potentially fatal condition, which is characterized by acute fever; hepatosplenomegaly; lymphadenopathy; pancytopenia; and raised levels of serum ferritin, triglycerides, and liver enzymes (Table 14.3). The prevalence of RHS in AOSD may be as high as 12%, as suggested by

Table 14.3 Complications of AOSD

Pulmonary
- Pleural effusion
- Transient pulmonary infiltrates
- Interstitial lung disease
- Acute respiratory distress syndrome
- Diffuse alveolar hemorrhage

Cardiovascular
- Pericarditis
- Myocarditis
- Pulmonary artery hypertension

Reticuloendothelial system (RES)
- Macrophage activation syndrome
- Autoimmune hepatitis
- Acute liver failure

Vasculopathy
- Cutaneous Polyarteritis nodosa
- Thrombotic microangiopathy

Coagulopathy
- Portal vein thrombosis
- Thrombotic thrombocytopenic purpura
- Disseminated intravascular coagulation

Neurological
- Miller Fisher syndrome
- Peripheral neuropathy

Arlet et al.[4] The possible triggering factors for RHS include drugs, viruses [Epstein Barr Virus (EBV), cytomegalovirus (CMV), parvovirus], autoimmune disorders [rheumatoid arthritis (RA), systemic lupus erythematosus], lymphomas, and leukemias.[5] The hallmark of this syndrome is excessive activation and proliferation of T lymphocytes and macrophages with massive hypercytokinemia with high levels of interleukin-1β, interleukin-6, interferon-γ, and TNF-α. This activation cascade produces an overwhelming inflammatory reaction. RHS can occur at any time during the course of AOSD. Moreover, a simultaneous diagnosis of AOSD and RHS is not uncommon. Flares of AOSD and RHS may be clinically indistinguishable, with the exception of a higher frequency of pleuritis and ARDS in RHS. Biological findings are certainly more sensitive in evoking the diagnosis of RHS during flares of AOSD. Leucopenia or thrombocytopenia is uncommon in AOSD and hence can serve as an alert. Raised serum triglyceride level is considered to be a good marker of the hemophagocytic syndrome,[6] but it has not been specifically analyzed in flares of AOSD.

The treatment of secondary RHS has included a variety of chemotherapeutic and immunosuppressive agents including corticosteroids, cyclosporine, and intravenous gamma-globulin (IVIG).[7] In the absence of controlled studies, case reports and small series have been used for insight in the management of MAS. Treatment with high-dose steroids is effective in most patients. Immunosuppressants may cause a reduction in mortality in patients where RHS was precipitated by an underlying autoimmune process. It has been reported that cyclosporine or etoposide would be effective in steroid-refractory cases. Etanercept has been reported as an alternative for RHS patients refractory to steroids, cyclosporine-A, and IVIG therapy.[8]

The similarity in presentations and the high frequency of RHS in patients with AOSD have prompted experts to consider these conditions as the two ends of the spectrum, with classic AOSD being the mild form and RHS with multiorgan involvement the most severe, life-threatening one. A common pathogenetic link, that is, IL18, a pivotal AOSD cytokine, has been suggested in a recent study. A study of 20 patients, with 21 separate hemophagocytic episodes meeting the International Histiocyte Society criteria, showed that serum IL-18 concentrations were significantly higher in the affected population when compared to healthy controls.[9] In addition, investigators observed an imbalance between IL-18 and IL-18-binding peptide (BP is IL18's natural inhibitor), where concentrations of IL-18BP were insufficient to bind the entire amount of circulating IL-18. A paradoxical decrease of natural killer (NK) cell numbers and cytotoxic functions in secondary RHS was also observed. Based on this study, the authors proposed the potential use of exogenous recombinant IL-18BP, in addition to traditional therapy, for the treatment of severe cases of RHS.

14.3
Severe Destructive Arthritis

The evolution of AOSD from the acute syndrome, where often systemic complaints such as fever and rash predominate, into the chronic articular pattern is a negative prognostic sign. There is less of a chance for spontaneous remission, and the associated polyarthritis can be destructive if left untreated and lead to increased morbidity and disability. Fortunately, in most cases of AOSD, polyarthritis methotrexate (MTX), with or without small doses of oral corticosteroids, can be very effective in controlling the symptoms and preventing radiographic progression.[10] However, MTX refractoriness has been frequently documented and alternative therapies have been sought. In the prebiologic era, alternative DMARDs were tried, alone or in combination. In a small series where cyclosporin-A was tried, remission in 66% of cases and improvement in the other 33% were reported.[11] Sulfasalazine should be avoided in treatment of AOSD as multiple studies proved low efficacy and high drug toxicity (60% vs. 15% of other drugs) related to treatment with sulfasalazine.[12] CD34-selected autologous peripheral blood stem cell transplantation was attempted in some cases of refractory disease and prolonged remission was achieved after transplantation.[13] Other less studied agents include hydrochloroquine, gold, penicillamin, leflunomide, azathioprine, tacrolimus, and cyclophosphamide. Recent advances in the immunopathogenesis of AOSD and the availability of biologic DMARDs for the treatment of RA has led to their off-label use in refractory AOSD with variable success. In particular, pro-inflammatory cytokines such as TNFα, IL-1, and IL-6 were targeted.

The first group of biologic agents clinically used was the TNF-α inhibitors. Multiple case reports and small series suggested that infliximab, etanercept, and adalimumab may have a role in refractory cases.[1] In an observational series of 12 patients, addition of etanercept to the pre-study regimens of prednisone, MTX, and NSAIDs leads to an improvement in the number of tender and swollen joints count higher than 63%.[14] A European study of eight patients attempted to evaluate the long-term outcome of patients treated with infliximab (a monoclonal chimeric anti-TNF antibody) after the failure of treatments with corticosteroids and DMARDs: The clinical and serological responses improved rapidly in seven out of eight patients, and five of them went into long-term remission even after discontinuation of therapy.[10,15]

IL-1 inhibition has emerged as an even more promising therapeutic strategy, based on our understanding of the role of the NALP-3 inflammasome and IL-1 in inflammation and anakinra; a recombinant competitive IL-1 receptor antagonist has recently emerged as a promising new therapeutic option.[16] In 2008, Lequerre et al.[17] reported 20 cases of SoJIA and 15 cases of AOSD treated with anakinra. Seventy-three percent of the cases of AOSD demonstrated prompt and dramatic improvement in their arthritis and disease activity markers, while allowing for a dramatic decrease of the administered corticosteroid dose.

IL-6 represents an important inflammatory cytokine involved in the pathogenesis of AODS, and it may be a promising target, especially with the development of anti-human IL-6 receptor monoclonal antibody tocilizumab.[17] A case of refractory AOSD successfully treated with rituximab (chimeric anti CD-20 monoclonal antibody) has also been described.[18]

14.4
Cardiac Complications

AOSD commonly involves the pericardium, although the presence of pericarditis in Still's disease does not seem to negatively affect prognosis in the absence of tamponade, since it is usually mild or even asymptomatic. Nonetheless, the clinician should keep in mind that adults with known cardiac involvement may be at a higher risk of developing cardiac decompensation, especially in the acute systemic subgroup of AOSD. Pouchot et al. described series of 23 cases of pericarditis in their 62 cases of AOSD (37%), 3 of which developed tamponade.[19]

The optimal treatment for AOSD-associated pericarditis has not been defined due to the rarity of its occurrence and the lack of controlled studies. Individual approach should be used in treatment of patients with pericarditis and cardiac tamponade. In cases of mild pericarditis, NSAIDs alone may suffice. Systemic use of steroids remains controversial. Lietman and Bywaters[20] in their series of patients with pericarditis did not demonstrate efficacy of steroids in altering the course of pericarditis. However, steroids may be useful in the presence of massive effusion, evidence of cardiac compromise, or progression of effusions not responding to NSAIDs. Drainage of pericardial fluid remains the cornerstone of therapy in the presence of significant cardiac compromise.

Myocardial involvement in adult-onset Still's disease is reportedly low, although likely to be underdiagnosed. Data concerning the clinical course of Sill's myocarditis are lacking, and there is no clear recommendation for the follow-up of myocardial function in similar conditions. Usually Still's disease–related myocarditis has rapid onset and readily responds to prompt corticosteroid treatment, resulting in quick normalization of myocardial function. Regular follow-up of myocardial function is recommended even if clinical symptoms and inflammatory markers have normalized.

14.5
Pulmonary Complications

In contrast to other autoimmune systemic diseases, little attention has been paid to the pulmonary complications of AOSD. Most common pulmonary manifestations of AOSD include pleurisy, acute and chronic pneumonitis, diaphragmatic dysfunction, and drug-induced lung disease.[21] While most cases with acute pneumonitis respond favorably to systemic corticosteroids, there are rare instances where these abnormalities progress to severe respiratory failure requiring mechanical ventilation, pulse corticosteroids, and/or aggressive immunosuppressive therapy. The most characteristic paradigm of such severe life-threatening complication with significant morbidity and mortality would be the adult respiratory distress syndrome (ARDS). ARDS development has been reported in several patients with AOSD, often complicated by multiorgan involvement and disseminated intravascular coagulation (DIC).[22,23]

More recently, Sari et al. presented a case of chronic AOSD complicated with diffuse alveolar hemorrhage (DAH) during an acute flare of the disease.[24] It is not known whether the association between AOSD and DAH is coincidental or whether there is a common pathophysiologic link.

14.6
Hepatic Involvement

Liver dysfunction in AOSD has been well described, ranging from asymptomatic liver function test (LFT) abnormalities to overt liver failure. Andres et al. retrospectively reviewed data from 17 patients with AOSD and found abnormalities in liver biochemistry in 76% of the subjects.[25] However, it is often difficult to differentiate liver dysfunction due to AOSD per se from drug-induced liver dysfunction, since most of the reported cases occurred during treatment with potentially hepatotoxic drugs. Recently, Chen et al. described high levels of soluble intercellular adhesion molecule 1 (sICAM-1) in patients with active untreated AOSD and proposed that elevated serum sICAM-1 level may be a predictor of liver dysfunction in AOSD. Moreover, serum sICAM-1 levels significantly correlated with disease activity and serum ferritin levels which have also been utilized to monitor disease activity in adult Still's.[26] In any case, close monitoring of LFTs is warranted in AOSD patients, especially early in the disease course, since it often parallels disease activity and abnormalities have been shown to respond to successful treatment.

Fulminant hepatitis or hepatic failure is extremely rare, and most of the reported cases occurred during treatment with hepatotoxic drugs.[27-29] Experimental and clinical data suggest a critical role for cytokines in the development of fulminant hepatic failure. Sekiyana et al. have observed higher serum levels of IL-1β and a significantly reduced ratio of IL-1Ra to IL-1β (IL-1Ra/IL-1β) in patients with fulminant hepatic failure who subsequently died when compared with survivors.[30] In 2007, Mylona et al. presented a case of fulminant hepatic failure in AOSD that was successfully treated with anakinra, a recombinant interleukin-1 receptor antagonist (IL-1Ra), which also supports a possible role for IL-1 inhibition in fulminant hepatic failure.[31]

Autoimmune hepatitis (AIH) is a rare complication of AOSD. In 2010, Liu et al.[32] reported a refractory case of AIH during an AOSD relapse, successfully treated with plasma exchange after other treatment options were exhausted. After five plasmapheresis sessions, autoantibody titers were normalized, as well as serum IgG, LDH, and serum ferritin. Furthermore, leukocytosis and LFT abnormalities resolved. This case was in sharp contrast to other AIH cases, reported by the same authors that had fatal outcomes after treatment with systemic corticosteroids and intravenous immunoglobulin alone. Therefore, AIH may be an indicator for poor prognosis in AOSD, and plasma exchange therapy should be considered, especially in severe cases of liver injury, in combination with high-dose corticosteroids and other immunomodulatory treatments.

Lastly, in exceptionally rare cases, AOSD liver involvement can present with very atypical features. In 2009, Sari et al.[33] presented a case of hepatomegaly in AOSD where liver biopsy histology revealed a ground-glass like hepatocyte inclusion. Ground-glass hepatocytes (GGH) are live cells with a glassy-granular, eosinophilic cytoplasm on light microscopy.[34] GGH represents a histological hallmark of chronic Hepatitis B virus (HBV) infection and is an occasional finding in some noninfectious chronic inflammatory hepatopathies. In such cases, LFTs continue to rise, despite active treatment, with AST levels occasionally exceeding 1,000 IU/L in the absence of viral infection. GGH are revealed on biopsy along with signs of steatohepatitis, and it is unclear at present time whether this finding represents hepatocyte adaptation or injury.[35]

14.7
Oculomotor Disorders

In rare cases, AOSD patients may develop periodic horizontal micro-saccadic oscillations and rapid clockwise torsional eye movements followed by counterclockwise torsional drifts. It has been hypothesized that saccadic burst neurons, excitatory burst neurons

(EBN), and inhibitory burst neurons (IBN) comprise a reciprocally innervated premotor circuit. The neuron membranes contain ion channels that are important for the rebound increase in neural firing after transient external inhibition—post-inhibitory rebound (PIR).[36] Inflammation may alter the fine balance between EBNs and IBNs and produce clinical symptoms.

In 2009, Shaikh et al presented such a case with bursts of horizontal saccadic oscillations, without intersaccadic intervals, and clockwise rapid torsional eye movement that had the same peak velocity–amplitude relationship as torsional quick phases of nystagmus. They suggested that this could be attributed to an immune-mediated alteration in the midbrain neurons of the reciprocally innervated premotor circuit. In such patients, medications that reduce central excitability—for example, antiepileptics such as levetiracetam, gabapentine, and clonazepam—might be useful.

14.8
Leukocytoclastic Vasculitis

Leukocytoclastic vasculitis is characterized by angiocentric segmental inflammation, fibrinoid necrosis, and a neutrophilic infiltrate around the vessel walls with erythrocyte extravasation. Leukocytoclastic vasculitis has been observed in Henoch–Schonlein purpura, Wegener's granulomatosis, and microscopic polyangiitis; however, it had not, until recently, been reported in AOSD.[37] In 2009, Hidekatsu Yanai et al. described a case of AOSD with atypical rash, which skin biopsy revealed to be due to leukocytoclastic vasculitis. Elevated blood vWF - Von Willebrand factor and VEGF - Vascular Endotelial Growth Factor levels in given AOSD patient suggest a potential association between AOSD and vasculitis. Immunologic testing with a negative PR3-proteinase 3 and MPO-ANCA is Myeloperoxidase- Anti-neutrophil cytoplasmic antibodies help rule out Wegener's granulomatosis or microscopic polyangiitis, respectively, in cases of atypical Still's rash.

14.9
Renal Involvement

Recently, Babacan et al.[38] presented a case of AOSD-associated membranous glomerulonephritis successfully treated with Infliximab. Notably, the same patient also suffered from a severe inflammatory polyarthritis, unresponsive to high-dose steroids and DMARDs for a period of 5 years.

Glomerulonephritis (GN) is a rare complication of AOSD. However, its importance for prognosis and therapy is such that it should be considered in the presence of proteinuria. Thonhofer et al. described a case of mesangio-proliferative immunocomplex-based GN accompanied by proteinuria in 2006.[39] While GN has been reported at other instances as the cause of proteinuria,[40,41] other AOSD-associated complications such as collapsing glomerulopathy[42] and thrombotic microangiopathy,[43] however rare, cannot be excluded

Table 14.4 Comparison of amyloidosis in patients with AOSD

First author	Age of disease onset/sex	Number of years before amyloidosis onset	Drug therapy for renal amyloidosis
Fautrel[44]	32/M	ND	PD, MTX
Rivera[45]	26/M	16	PD, AZA
Hashimoto[46]	25/F, 26/M	ND, ND	PD, PD
Ishii[47]	32/F	7	PD, CTX
Bambery[48]	36/F	8	Steroid, dialysis
Wendling[49]	57/F	4	ND
Vingeron[50]	23/F, 27/F	1.5, 4	PD, dialysis both cases
Harrington[51]	26/F	30	PD, COL

ND non- described, *PD* prednisone, *MTX* methotrexate, *AZA* azathioprine, *CTX* cyclophosphamide, *COL* colchicine

and should be ruled out. A hypothesis by Elkon in 1982 that a smoldering vasculitis, mediated by non-necrotizing immune complexes, may support the hypothesis that GN is part of the disease. The possibility of a more active renal process can be supported by the significant decrease in proteinuria after anti-inflammatory treatment. In general, aggressive immunosuppression is recommended in patients with proliferative forms of GN, with a high histological score for active lesions and a low score for chronic lesions. Biologic agents, such as TNF-α blockers, have been suggested as an alternative in AOSD-associated GN refractory to standard immunosuppressants.[14]

Amyloidosis may be a more common AOSD-related renal complication leading to proteinuria and has been described in several case reports and series. (Table 14.4) It can develop as soon as 18 months or as late as 30 years after the diagnosis of AOSD with an incidence of 4.7–14.3%.[44] The majority of the patients developing renal amyloidosis will require treatment with systemic corticosteroids and/or cytotoxic agents.[44,52] In severe cases complicated with renal failure, treatment with hemodialysis in addition to prednisone therapy was administered with good outcomes.[48,51] In new era of biologics, better control of the underlying chronic inflammation by judicious use of these potent medications may prevent the appearance of amyloidosis and/or improve its management.

14.10
Conclusion

AOSD is a rare, auto-inflammatory systemic disorder with significant phenotypic variability that often makes diagnosis difficult. The majority of the cases can be readily managed after proper diagnosis. However, the disease has been associated with rare but serious complications that are associated with significant morbidity and, even, mortality.

The clinician should be aware of such complications and be able to recognize them and refer appropriately for specialized care. Significant advances in our understanding of the disease pathophysiology and the recent availability of targeted biologic treatments have enhanced our ability to intervene therapeutically.

References

1. Kontzias A, Efthimiou P. Adult-onset Still's disease: pathogenesis, clinical manifestations and therapeutic advances. *Drugs*. 2008;68(3):319-337.
2. Yamaguchi M et al. Preliminary criteria for classification of adult Still's disease. *J Rheumatol*. 1992;19(3):424-430.
3. Fautrel B et al. Proposal for a new set of classification criteria for adult-onset still disease. *Med (Baltimore)*. 2002;81(3):194-200.
4. Arlet JB et al. Reactive haemophagocytic syndrome in adult-onset Still's disease: a report of six patients and a review of the literature. *Ann Rheum Dis*. 2006;65(12):1596-1601.
5. Emmenegger U et al. Haemophagocytic syndromes in adults: current concepts and challenges ahead. *Swiss Med Wkly*. 2005;135(21–22):299-314.
6. Karras A, Hermine O. Hemophagocytic syndrome. *Rev Méd Interne*. 2002;23(9):768-778.
7. Henter JI et al. Treatment of hemophagocytic lymphohistiocytosis with HLH-94 immuno-chemotherapy and bone marrow transplantation. *Blood*. 2002;100(7):2367-2373.
8. Makay B et al. Etanercept for therapy-resistant macrophage activation syndrome. *Pediatr Blood Cancer*. 2008;50(2):419-421.
9. Mazodier K et al. Severe imbalance of IL-18/IL-18BP in patients with secondary hemophago-cytic syndrome. *Blood*. 2005;106(10):3483-3489.
10. Efthimiou P, Paik PK, Bielory L. Diagnosis and management of adult onset Still's disease. *Ann Rheum Dis*. 2006;65(5):564-572.
11. Marchesoni A et al. Cyclosporin A in the treatment of adult onset Still's disease. *J Rheumatol*. 1997;24(8):1582-1587.
12. Jung JH et al. High toxicity of sulfasalazine in adult-onset Still's disease. *Clin Exp Rheumatol*. 2000;18(2):245-248.
13. Lanza F et al. Prolonged remission state of refractory adult onset Still's disease following CD34-selected autologous peripheral blood stem cell transplantation. *Bone Marrow Transplant*. 2000;25(12):1307-1310.
14. Husni ME et al. Etanercept in the treatment of adult patients with Still's disease. *Arthritis Rheum*. 2002;46(5):1171-1176.
15. Dechant C et al. Longterm outcome of TNF blockade in adult-onset Still's disease. *Dtsch Med Wochenschr*. 2004;129(23):1308-1312.
16. Fitzgerald AA et al. Rapid responses to anakinra in patients with refractory adult-onset Still's disease. *Arthritis Rheum*. 2005;52(6):1794-1803.
17. Lequerre T et al. Interleukin-1 receptor antagonist (anakinra) treatment in patients with systemic-onset juvenile idiopathic arthritis or adult onset Still disease: preliminary experience in France. *Ann Rheum Dis*. 2008;67(3):302-308.
18. Ahmadi-Simab K et al. Successful treatment of refractory adult onset Still's disease with rituximab. *Ann Rheum Dis*. 2006;65(8):1117-1118.
19. Pouchot J, Vinceneux P. Usefulness of closed needle biopsy of sacroiliac joint in pyogenic sacroiliitis. *J Rheumatol*. 1991;18(12):1944-1945.
20. Lietman PS, Bywaters EG. Pericarditis in juvenile rheumatoid arthritis. *Pediatrics*. 1963;32:855-860.

21. Cheema GS, Quismorio FP Jr. Pulmonary involvement in adult-onset Still's disease. *Curr Opin Pulm Med.* 1999;5(5):305-309.

22. Gibbs CJ et al. Disseminated intravascular coagulation in adult-onset Still's disease with neurological, respiratory and hepatic sequelae. *Br J Hosp Med.* 1993;50(5):278-279.

23. Pedersen JE. ARDS–associated with adult Still's disease. *Intensive Care Med.* 1991; 17(6):372.

24. Sari I et al. A case of adult-onset Still's disease complicated with diffuse alveolar hemorrhage. *J Korean Med Sci.* 2009;24(1):155-157.

25. Andres E et al. Retrospective monocentric study of 17 patients with adult Still's disease, with special focus on liver abnormalities. *Hepatogastroenterology.* 2003;50(49):192-195.

26. Chen DY et al. Association of intercellular adhesion molecule-1 with clinical manifestations and interleukin-18 in patients with active, untreated adult-onset Still's disease. *Arthritis Rheum.* 2005;53(3):320-327.

27. McFarlane M, Harth M, Wall WJ. Liver transplant in adult Still's disease. *J Rheumatol.* 1997;24(10):2038-2041.

28. Dino O et al. Fulminant hepatic failure in adult onset Still's disease. *J Rheumatol.* 1996;23(4):784-785.

29. Ott SJ et al. Liver failure in adult Still's disease during corticosteroid treatment. *Eur J Gastroenterol Hepatol.* 2003;15(1):87-90.

30. Sekiyama KD, Yoshiba M, Thomson AW. Circulating proinflammatory cytokines (IL-1 beta, TNF-alpha, and IL-6) and IL-1 receptor antagonist (IL-1Ra) in fulminant hepatic failure and acute hepatitis. *Clin Exp Immunol.* 1994;98(1):71-77.

31. Mylona E et al. Acute hepatitis in adult Still's disease during corticosteroid treatment successfully treated with anakinra. *Clin Rheumatol.* 2008;27(5):659-661.

32. Liu LL et al. A case report of successful treatment with plasma exchange for adult-onset Still's disease with autoimmune hepatitis. *J Clin Apher* 2010;25(4):235.

33. Sari A et al. Ground-glass-like hepatocellular inclusions in the course of adult-onset Still's disease. *Mod Rheumatol.* 2010;20(1):90-92.

34. Cohen C. "Ground-glass" hepatocytes. *S Afr Med J.* 1975;49(34):1401-1403.

35. Wisell J et al. Glycogen pseudoground glass change in hepatocytes. *Am J Surg Pathol.* 2006;30(9):1085-1090.

36. Perez-Reyes E. Molecular physiology of low-voltage-activated t-type calcium channels. *Physiol Rev.* 2003;83(1):117-161.

37. Yanai H et al. Myositis, vasculitis, hepatic dysfunction in adult-onset Still's disease. *Case Report Med.* 2009;2009:504897.

38. Babacan T et al. Successful treatment of refractory adult Still's disease and membranous glomerulonephritis with infliximab. *Clin Rheumatol.* 2010;29:223-226.

39. Thonhofer R et al. Decrease of proteinuria in a patient with adult-onset Still's disease and glomerulonephritis after anti-TNFalpha therapy. *Scand J Rheumatol.* 2006;35(6):485-488.

40. Ohta A et al. Adult Still's disease: review of 228 cases from the literature. *J Rheumatol.* 1987;14(6):1139-1146.

41. Wendling D, Hory B, Blanc D. Adult Still's disease and mesangial glomerulonephritis. Report of two cases. *Clin Rheumatol.* 1990;9(1):95-99.

42. Kumar S, Sheaff M, Yaqoob M. Collapsing glomerulopathy in adult still's disease. *Am J Kidney Dis.* 2004;43(5):e4-e10.

43. Quemeneur T et al. Thrombotic microangiopathy in adult Still's disease. *Scand J Rheumatol.* 2005;34(5):399-403.

44. Fautrel B et al. Corticosteroid sparing effect of low dose methotrexate treatment in adult Still's disease. *J Rheumatol.* 1999;26(2):373-378.

45. Rivera F et al. Vascular renal AA amyloidosis in adult Still's disease. *Nephrol Dial Transplant.* 1997;12(8):1714-1716.

46. Hashimoto M et al. Clinical studies on 14 cases of adult-onset Still's disease. *Nihon Rinsho Meneki Gakkai Kaishi*. 1995;18(1):45-52.

47. Ishii T et al. Systemic amyloidosis in a patient with adult onset Still's disease. *Intern Med*. 1993;32(1):50-52.

48. Bambery P et al. Adult onset Still's disease: clinical experience with 18 patients over 15 years in northern India. *Ann Rheum Dis*. 1992;51(4):529-532.

49. Wendling D et al. Adult onset Still's disease and related renal amyloidosis. *Ann Rheum Dis*. 1991;50(4):257-259.

50. Vigneron AM et al. [Amyloidosis in adult Still's disease. Apropos of 2 cases]. *Ann Med Interne (Paris)*. 1986;137(5):406-408.

51. Harrington TM, Moran JJ, Davis DE. Amyloidosis in adult onset Still's disease. *J Rheumatol*. 1981;8(5):833-836.

52. Gertz MA, Kyle RA. Amyloidosis: prognosis and treatment. *Semin Arthritis Rheum*. 1994; 24(2):124-138.

Managing Acute and Complex Dermatological Situations

15

Eduardo Fonseca and Rosa M. Fernández-Torres

Abstract Cutaneous manifestations are almost always present in systemic autoimmune diseases. Identification of these manifestations is essential to establish an adequate diagnosis and treatment, especially in situations that may be indicative of a life-threatening condition or result in permanent sequelae.

Lupus erythematosus is an example of disease with a great variety of cutaneous manifestations, ranging from lesions suggestive of only cutaneous or mild systemic involvement (chronic and subacute cutaneous lupus erythematosus) to lesions indicative of more severe systemic involvement (acute malar rash).

Dermatomyositis initially presents with skin lesions in a high percentage of cases, some of which are pathognomonic of the disease, as Gottron's papules or heliotrope rash, and may suggest an underlying neoplasm.

Panniculitis may be secondary to a wide variety of systemic diseases, including infections, drugs, and autoimmune and metabolic disorders. In these cases, histopathological examination is usually needed to clarify the diagnosis.

In other cases, the most challenging aspect of the disease is its treatment, for example, calcinosis in juvenile dermatomyositis, digital ulcers in scleroderma, or severe Raynaud's phenomenon.

In this chapter, we review some cutaneous manifestation that may be helpful in the diagnosis of autoimmune diseases and sometimes indicative of systemic involvement or of a worse prognosis. Furthermore, differential diagnosis of diseases that may present with similar cutaneous manifestations and treatment of complex dermatological situations is discussed.

Keywords Dermatomyositis • Digital ulcers • Facial rash • Kikuchi–Fujimoto disease • Lupus erythematosus • Panniculitis • Purpura • Raynaud • Scleroderma • Ulcers • Vasculitis

E. Fonseca (✉)
Department of Dermatology, Hospital Universitario de La Coruña,
Xubias de Arriba 84, La Coruña 15006, Spain
e-mail: eduardo.fonseca.capdevila@sergas.es

M.A. Khamashta and M. Ramos-Casals (eds.), *Autoimmune Diseases*,
DOI: 10.1007/978-0-85729-358-9_15, © Springer-Verlag London Limited 2011

The accurate identification and management of cutaneous manifestations is absolutely essential to establish an adequate diagnosis and prognostic in patients with autoimmune diseases as well as to indicate the most convenient therapy. The dependence of factors as the morphologic diagnostic and the low incidence and high variability of some of these disorders makes the dermatological aspects one of the most wide and challenging of the autoimmune diseases.

15.1
Facial Rash

Skin involvement occurs in 70–85% of all patients with lupus erythematosus (LE) and may be one of its most refractory manifestations. Skin disease may be classified into two broad categories: LE-specific, which demonstrate interface dermatitis on histopathological examination, and nonspecific-LE, which may appear on other situations. LE-specific skin manifestations may be classified into three types: acute cutaneous LE (ACLE), subacute cutaneous LE (SCLE), and chronic cutaneous LE (CCLE).[1]

ACLE may present with the classic butterfly rash from which the term lupus erythematosus was coined. It is commonly the first manifestation of systemic lupus erythematosus (SLE) and may precede the onset of systemic involvement or coincide with exacerbation of the systemic disease.

The butterfly rash is characterized by erythema and edema, sometimes with fine scale, involving the malar areas and the bridge of the nose and sparing the nasolabial folds (Fig. 15.1). Patients with malar rash often have a positive lupus band test. Antinuclear antibodies (ANA) are present in more than 80% of patients with SLE, and anti-ds-DNA antibodies are generally demonstrable in patients with renal affectation. Anti-Sm antibodies are specific for SLE and are usually detected in patients with pulmonary fibrosis and nervous system and renal involvement, correlating with a poor

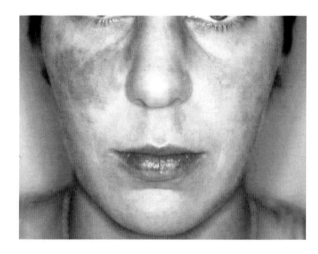

Fig. 15.1 Typical butterfly rash of acute cutaneous lupus erythematosus with erythema and edema over the malar area and the nasal bridge

Table 15.1 Differential diagnosis of facial rash

Acute cutaneous lupus erythematosus
Rosacea
Contact dermatitis
Photodermatitis
Seborrheic dermatitis
Atopic dermatitis
Dermatomyositis
Pseudodermatomyositis (Still's disease, hydroxyurea)
Erysipelas/cellulitis
Angioedema
Facial tinea

prognosis.[2] The main causes of malar rash to be considered in the differential diagnosis are listed in Table 15.1.

Treatment of patients with ACLE depends on the severity of the systemic disease, which is usually controlled with corticosteroids and other immunosuppressive drugs. The standard therapy for skin involvement consists of sunscreens, topical corticosteroids, and antimalarials. Several immunosuppressive drugs have been tried with variable success for resistant lesions, including thalidomide, methotrexate, azatioprine, and mycophenolate mofetil.[3]

Dermatomyositis may present with skin manifestations in 30–40% of adults and in 95% of children. Some cutaneous signs are highly specific of this disease, such as heliotrope rash and Gottron's papules. Heliotrope rash is a violaceus to erythematous rash, with or without edema, involving periorbital skin. Gottron's papules are located over bony prominences, mainly the interphalangeal joints. Other cutaneous manifestations are characteristic but not pathognomonic of dermatomyositis, such as malar erythema, generalized rash or edema, poikiloderma in a photosensitive distribution and cuticular changes.[4]

Sometimes, dermatomyositis lesions may be difficult to distinguish form LE. It may help differentiate both that hand dermatomyositis lesions occur more over bony prominences and are frequently accompanied by severe pruritus, while LE lesions are most often located between the knuckles and are usually asymptomatic.[4] Dermatomyositis may also present with the typical rash but without muscle weakness or laboratory evidence of muscle involvement for years after appearance of skin lesions. This condition is known as *amyopathic dermatomyositis* or *dermatomyositis sine myositis* and represents 2–18% of cases.[5]

Cutaneous manifestations of dermatomyositis are one of the most challenging and resistant manifestations of the disease. They may precede the development of myopathy and may persist despite the improvement of muscular symptoms after treatment.

Oral corticosteroids (usually oral prednisone 0.5–1.5 mg/kg in a single daily dose) are the initial agents for treatment, especially for muscular manifestations. Methotrexate is the first-line adjuvant therapy in cases recalcitrant to steroids, usually in a dosage of 7.5–10 mg/week, increasing by 2.5 mg/week up to a total of 25 mg/week. Hydroxychloroquine may reduce the rash resistant to steroids and other therapies.

Other adjuvant therapies include azathioprine, cyclophosphamide, cyclosporine, mycophenolate mofetil, rituximab, intravenous immunoglobulins, and tumor necrosis factor (TNF)-α antagonists.[6]

15.2
Subacute Cutaneous Lupus Erythematosus

SCLE skin lesions may be of two types: annular and papulosquamous. Annular lesions are characterized by erythematous rings with central clearing (Fig. 15.2), while papulosquamous lesions are characterized by plaques and papules with scale. Both types can coexist in about 10% of patients[7] and are usually distributed on sun-exposed areas. They may cause pigmentary changes and telangiectasia but not dermal atrophy or scarring.[7]

The risk of systemic involvement in patients with SCLE is approximately 10%, although around of a half meet criteria to be classified as SLE.[8] Therefore, in most of these patients, the disease is limited to the skin and the prognosis is relatively benign. There are often serological abnormalities, especially anti-SSA/Ro antibodies (70–90%) and anti-SSB/La antibodies (35%) and 40–50% of patients have arthralgias or arthritis, but other systemic manifestations, such as serositis, central nervous system or renal disease, are very uncommon.[9]

SCLE has been described in association with other conditions as Sjögren syndrome,[10] idiopathic thrombocytopenic purpura,[11] urticarial vasculitis, other cutaneous vasculitic syndromes, and deficiency of complement components.[12]

The main diseases that should be differentiated from SCLE are listed in Table 15.2.

Standard SCLE management includes photoprotective measures and topical corticosteroids. Topical tacrolimus and pimecrolimus have also been reported to be useful. Intralesional injections of corticosteroids may be effective in lesions refractory to topical therapy.

When the disease is not controlled with local treatment, antimalarial drugs are the first-line therapy, usually hydroxychloroquine (5–6.5 mg/kg/day) that appears to produce less retinal toxicity than chloroquine (3.5 mg/kg/day). Hydroxychloroquine and chloroquine should not be used together because of the higher risk of retinopathy but, if they are not effective separately, each of them may be used together with quinacrine.

Systemic corticosteroids are generally reserved for life-threatening systemic manifestations, but it may be useful, at dosages of 0.5–1 mg/kg/day, to control active phases of skin lesions or in patients unresponsive to antimalarials. The combination of prednisone

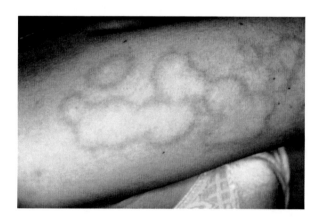

Fig. 15.2 Annular lesions of subacute cutaneous lupus erythematosus with central clearing and erythematous border

Table 15.2 Differential diagnosis of subacute cutaneous lupus erythematosus

Annular forms
Psoriasis
Erythema annular centrifugum
Other annular erythemas
Erythema multiforme
Lichen planus
Dermatophytosis
Granuloma annulare
Syphilis
Leprosy
Sarcoidosis
Papulosquamous forms
Psoriasis
Polymorphous light eruption
Dermatophytosis
Syphilis
Pityriasis rosea
Lichen planus
Parapsoriasis/mycosis fungoides

(0.5–1 mg/kg/day) and antimalarials for 2–3 weeks may achieve a faster resolution. However, because of systemic side effects, long-term steroid treatment is not recommended, especially in skin-limited forms.[13]

Some patients who failed to respond to conventional therapy have proved to be responsive to thalidomide, dapsone, retinoids, oral gold, or clofazimine.

Thalidomide is usually started at a dosage of 50–100 mg daily and then reduced to the lowest effective dose (often 25 mg given twice a week). Improvement is generally observed after 2 weeks with the maximum benefit occurring within 3 months. However, relapse occurs in up to 70% of patients, so low-dose maintenance therapy is often necessary. Thalidomide use is limited by its serious side effects, mainly embryopathy and polyneuropathy.[14]

Oral gold may be effective for cutaneous LE. Complete remission occurs in approximately 15% and a partial response in about two-thirds of patients. It is usually begun at a dose of 3 mg/day and, after a week that can be raised to twice daily, if there are no adverse events.

Isotretinoin and acitretin have been useful in patients refractory to conventional therapy, especially in hypertrophic CCLE or lesions located on palms and soles.

Immunosuppressive drugs, such as azathioprine, methotrexate, mycophenolate mofetil cyclophosphamide, or cyclosporine, are limited to patients unresponsive to other therapies.[15]

Anti-TNF-α agents as infliximab, adalimumab, and etanercept have proved to be effective in cutaneous LE. However, they have also been related to development of drug-induced SCLE and SLE, so randomized-controlled studies are needed to demonstrate their security and effectiveness.[16]

High-dose intravenous immunoglobulin (1 g/kg/day for two consecutive days monthly) and rituximab have been employed for severe, resistant ACLE and SCLE cases that failed to respond to first-, second- and third-line therapies.[17,18]

15.3
Toxic Epidermal Necrolysis-Like Acute Cutaneous Lupus Erythematosus

Toxic epidermal necrolysis (TEN)-like ACLE is a new term introduced to describe cases of SLE with clinical and histopathological skin features similar to drug-induced classical TEN (Fig. 15.3), but without some characteristic features of TEN, as systemic involvement and history of recent drug ingestion.[19]

These patients share a TEN-like histopathology and varying degrees of systemic involvement resulting from SLE, including lupus nephritis, hematological abnormalities, and low complement levels. All patients for whom data are available had positive ANA and a significant part of them had anti-SSA/Ro antibodies, suggesting they could be a serologic marker for this subset of LE.[19,20]

The main causes of vesicles and/or blisters are listed in Table 15.3 and should be taken into account for differential diagnosis.[21]

Treatment for TEN-like LE is controversial as it is based on isolated case reports, most of which were responsive to systemic corticosteroids. Unresponsive cases have been

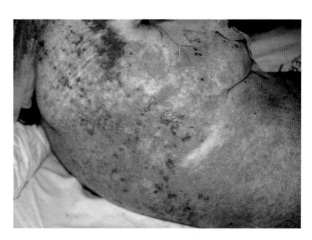

Fig. 15.3 Erythema, bullae, and erosions affecting almost the entire body surface in a patient with toxic epidermal necrolysis-like cutaneous lupus erythematosus

Table 15.3 Diseases that can present with vesicles and/or blisters

Porphyrias	Renal failure
Herpetiform dermatitis	Gianotti–Crosti syndrome
IgA lineal dermatitis	Herpes
Pemphigus	(simples/chickenpox/zoster)
Paraneoplastic pemphigus	Staphylococcal scalded skin syndrome
Pemphigoid	Toxic shock syndrome
Epidermolysis bullosa acquisita	Erythema multiforme
Subcorneal pustulous dermatosis	Toxic epidermal necrolysis
Collagenosis	Hypozincemia
Vasculitis	Glucagonoma syndrome
Diabetes	Toxicoderma
Coma	Insect bites

treated with corticosteroids in combination with intravenous immunoglobulin 0.75 g–1 g/kg/day for 3–5 days.[22] Given the possibility of similar pathogenetic pathways in TEN and TEN-like LE, plasmapheresis is a promising option in refractory cases.[23]

15.4
Kikuchi–Fujimoto Disease (KFD)

KFD is a benign form of histiocytic necrotizing lymphadenitis (HNL) that usually affects young women and presents with lymphadenopathy involving mainly posterior cervical lymph nodes.

Sometimes fever, weight loss, nausea, vomiting, diarrhea, upper respiratory symptoms, chills, night sweating, myalgias, arthralgias, and hepatosplenomegaly may be present. Laboratory tests can reveal mild leukopenia, anemia, erythrocyte sedimentation rate elevation, and atypical peripheral blood lymphocytes (15–30%).[24]

Skin lesions have been reported in 30% of patients with KFD (Fig. 15.4), including urticarial, morbilliform, rubella-like or drug-eruption-like rashes, acneiform eruptions, facial erythema, generalized erythema and papules, plaques and nodules, leukocytoclastic vasculitis, erythema multiforme, papulopustules, eyelid or lip edema, and oral ulcers. Face and upper trunk are their most common localizations.[25]

The diagnosis is based on lymph node histology, which shows irregular paracortical areas of coagulative necrosis with abundant karyorrhectic debris and histiocytes at the margin of the necrotic areas.

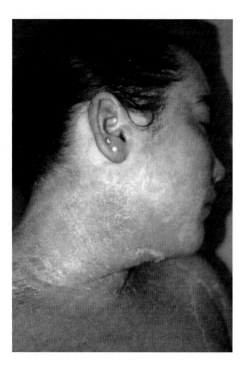

Fig. 15.4 Erythematoedematous rash affecting face, neck, and upper trunk in a patient with Kikuchi–Fujimoto disease

Although association with mixed connective tissue disease, polymyositis, antiphospholipid syndrome, Still's, and Sjögren diseases has been reported, the main systemic associated disease is SLE. HNL may occur in patients with preexisting SLE, may coexist or may evolve into SLE. The high frequency of flares of lupus activity with the onset of KFD and the simultaneous occurrence of both diseases indicate that they are not independent events.[26]

Although the precise relation between KFD and SLE is still unclear, interface dermatitis in skin biopsy could be a histopathological marker of evolution into SLE, and therefore, it might help predict the clinical outcome of KFD.[27]

KFD is typically self-limiting within 1–4 months, but recurrence has been reported in 3–4% of cases. There is no specific treatment, and because of the self-limiting course, only symptomatic measures are recommended. The use of corticosteroids has been proposed in severe extranodal or generalized forms, but its efficacy is uncertain. There is an anecdotal report of resolution with oral minocycline.[28]

Serious morbidities have been reported, including myocarditis, aseptic meningitis, and cerebellar ataxia, and in a few cases, outcome was fatal. A regular follow-up for several years is needed to rule out the development of SLE.

15.5
Neonatal Lupus Erythematosus (NLE)

NLE is a multiorganic disease of the newborn caused by transplacental transmitted autoantibodies, particularly anti-SSA/Ro (90%) and/or anti-SSB/La (50%), from their mothers who frequently suffer SLE, Sjögren's syndrome, or other connective tissue diseases.

Clinical manifestations involve skin (50%), heart (50%), and less frequently, liver (20–40%) and the hematological system (10–20%). About 10% of patients have both heart and skin manifestations.[29]

The noncardiac manifestations are transient, clearing within the first 6 months of life, when maternal autoantibodies disappear from the neonatal circulation.

Cutaneous manifestations are clinically and histopathologically similar to SCLE. They typically present as erythematous, scaling, and annular plaques, mainly on sun-exposed areas and resolve after several months with hypopigmentation, epidermal atrophy, and telangiectasia (Fig. 15.5). A second type of cutaneous lesion occurring in a minority of children is persistent telangiectasia.

The most serious and irreversible clinical feature is congenital complete heart block which has a significant mortality (10–30%) and morbidity (22–71%). It is usually detectable in utero as arrhythmia or bradycardia during the second trimester of pregnancy.[30]

Hematological findings consist of thrombocytopenia and hepatic involvement usually presents as cholestasis with abnormal bilirubin levels and mild increased aminopherase levels, although fulminant liver failure has been reported.[31]

Diagnosis is based on clinical findings in a newborn whose mother has anti-SSA/Ro, anti-SSB/La or in some cases anti-U$_1$RNP. Although there is no specific autoantibody profile to predict outcome, it has been suggested that high titers of anti-SSA/Ro antibodies are more frequently associated with congenital heart block or skin manifestations.[32]

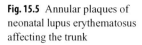

Fig. 15.5 Annular plaques of neonatal lupus erythematosus affecting the trunk

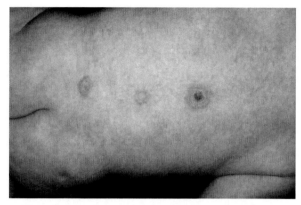

Photoprotective measures and occasionally topical corticosteroids are the mainstay of therapy for skin lesions. Serious liver and hematological disease may be treated with systemic corticosteroids, although its efficacy has not been established. Congenital heart block often requires pacemaker implantation. Some studies have suggested the use of dexamethasone for mothers with positive autoantibodies to minimize the risk of NLE. Intravenous immunoglobulin is being evaluated as a potential prophylactic approach in mothers who have previously had an affected child.[33] Long-term prognosis is unknown. Although there are some cases of NLE developing into SLE, there seems no significant increased risk for developing autoimmune diseases later in life. For women who already have a child with NLE, the estimate risk of having another affected one is about 25%.[34]

15.6
Urticarial Vasculitis

Urticarial vasculitis is a small vessel vasculitis presenting with urticarial-type lesions that usually last for more than 24 h and are characterized by pain or burning rather than pruritus.

The spectrum of clinical manifestations varies from mild symptoms to serious systemic disease affecting gastrointestinal, pulmonary, renal, cardiac, and central nervous systems. Urticaria vasculitis is associated with a wide variety of systemic diseases, infections, and drugs (Table 15.4).

Hypocomplementemia is observed in many patients correlating with systemic involvement and a high prevalence of autoantibodies to endothelial cells.

Demonstration of leukocytoclastic vasculitis in a skin biopsy of an active lesion remains the gold standard for diagnosing urticarial vasculitis[35] although similar features can be observed in common chronic urticaria.

Treatment depends on the severity of the disease and the underlying cause, if identified. Antihistamines are the mainstay for patients with only cutaneous manifestations, often combined with other agents, including systemic corticosteroids, indomethacin, colchicine, dapsone, and hydroxychloroquine.

Table 15.4 Causes and associations of urticarial vasculitis

Idiopathic
Connective tissue diseases
Systemic lupus erythematosus
Sjögren's syndrome
Immune abnormalities
Serum sickness
IgM monoclonal gammopathy (Schnitzler's syndrome)
IgG gammopathy (paraproteinemia)
IgD, IgA gammopathy
Cryoglobulinemia
C3, C4 deficiency, C3 nephritic factor activity
Infections
Hepatitis A, B, and C virus
Mycoplasma pneumoniae
Hematologic diseases
Leukemia
Lymphoma
Myeloma
Polycythemia rubra vera
Idiopathic thrombocytopenia purpura
Drugs
Diltiazem, potassium iodide, cimetidine, procarbazine, fluoxetine, paroxetine, butylhydroxytoluene, butylated hydroxyanisole, methotrexate, etanercept, procainamide, centrally acting appetite suppressants (dexfenfluramine), cocaine, Bacille-Guérin vaccine
Physical causes (cold, ultraviolet light, exercise)
Other:
Inflammatory bowel disease, amyloidosis (Muckle Wells syndrome), Cogan's syndrome, Jaccoud's syndrome, pregnancy, malignancy

In cases of severe systemic disease, corticosteroids may have additional benefit when combined with other immunosuppressants, such as azathioprine, dapsone, cyclophosphamide, cyclosporine, and mycophenolate mofetil. Interferon-α (IFN-α) has proved to be effective to treat urticarial vasculitis associated with hepatitis C virus infection.[35,36]

The course of urticarial vasculitis is unpredictable, and patients may develop new lesions from weeks to years. The major causes of morbidity and mortality are chronic obstructive pulmonary disease and laryngeal edema.

15.7
Panniculitis

Panniculitis is an inflammatory reaction of the subcutaneous adipose tissue that may be secondary to a wide variety of systemic diseases, infections, drugs, and other causes (Table 15.5).

Table 15.5 Causes of panniculitis

Erythema nodosum
  Idiopathic (up to 55%), streptococcal infection, tuberculosis, salmonellosis, yersiniosis, histoplasmosis, cutaneous mycosis, cat scratch disease, sarcoidosis, Crohn disease, ulcerous colitis, Behçet disease, lymphoma, carcinoma, pregnancy, toxics, drugs
Erythema nodosum leprosum
Nodular vasculitis (erythema induratum of Bazin)
  Tuberculin hyperergia, tuberculosis, hepatitis C virus infection
Thrombophlebitis migrans
  Neoplasms, Behçet disease, Buerger disease, Hodgkin lymphoma, mieloma, syphilis, rickettsiosis, coagulation factors deficit
Subcutaneous fact infection
  Bacteria, mycobacteria, fungi
Parasitosis
Subcutaneous fat necrosis
  Pancreatitis, pancreatic tumors
α_1-antitrypsin deficiency
Necrobiosis lipoidica and annular granuloma
  Diabetes, thyroid diseases
Lupus erythematosus
Scleroderma
Myositis/dermatomyositis
Cytophagic panniculitis
  Viral and bacterial infections, lymphomas, hereditary causes
Rheumatoid nodules
Hyperuricemia (gout panniculitis)
Sarcoidosis
Lymphomas
Perniosis
Factitial panniculitis

15.7.1
Lupus Panniculitis (LP)

LP or lupus erythematosus profundus is a chronic inflammatory reaction of the subcutaneous fat occurring in 2–3% of patients with LE. Conversely, between 10% and 50% of patients with LP might develop SLE.

It typically presents as multiple, firm, mobile, often painful nodules involving the arms, face, buttocks, leg, breast (lupus mastitis), abdomen, back, and neck (Fig. 15.6).

Most patients have no systemic disease, although arthralgias, Raynaud's phenomenon, and rarely, renal or neurologic disease may occur.

ANA are often demonstrated at low titers, and they might indicate a high probability of systemic involvement.[37] Other possible laboratory findings include lymphopenia, anemia, low complement levels, false-positive syphilis serology, positive rheumatoid factor, and elevated erythrocyte sedimentation rate.[38]

The histopathology of LP is characteristic, and clinical and histological findings are usually enough to establish the diagnosis. It is mostly lymphocytic lobular panniculitis,

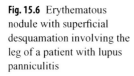
Fig. 15.6 Erythematous nodule with superficial desquamation involving the leg of a patient with lupus panniculitis

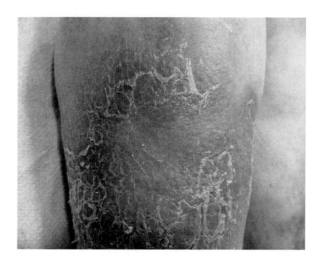

and lymphocytic vasculitis and hyaline fat necrosis are considered highly specific findings. Direct immunofluorescence shows deposits of immunoglobulins (IgG, IgM, IgA) and complement at the basement membrane and sometimes around the blood vessels.[37]

LP may be clinically and histologically very similar to subcutaneous T-cell lymphoma (SCTCL). Some findings considered typical of SCTCL such as lymphoid atypia and rimming of the adipocytes by lymphocytes have also been described in LP, so some authors believe that there is a spectrum of lymphoid dyscrasia encompassing LP, an intermediate entity called indeterminate lymphocytic lobular panniculitis (ILLP), and SCTCL. Patients with LP and atypical lymphocytes in the skin biopsy should be followed up for the development of T-cell lymphomas.[39]

The nodules of LP are persistent, difficult to treat, and may often become painful and ulcerative. LP tends to follow a chronic course with recurrences and remissions leading to characteristic atrophic and depressed scars.

Antimalarials are the initial treatment as in other subsets of cutaneous LE. About two-thirds of patients treated with antimalarials show some improvement, but the relapse rate is high when they are discontinued or tapered, so treatment for several months to years may be required.[40] Corticosteroid may be used in patients with more extensive, symptomatic disease or having systemic involvement, at doses ranging from 15 to 100 mg daily.

Other authors prefer combined therapy with systemic corticosteroids (prednisone 0.5 mg/kg/day) and antimalarial drugs (hydroxychloroquine 5–6.5 mg/kg/day or chloroquine 3.5 mg/kg/day). The corticosteroids are gradually tapered as the lesions subside, and the antimalarial is continued for 6–12 months to maintain remission. Other suggested treatments include potent topical steroids (0.05% clobetasol propionate) under occlusion with a hydrocolloid dressing or intralesional injections of triamcinolone (5 mg/ml). However, intralesional steroids are often ineffective and may exacerbate the atrophic process.

There are several case reports, mainly in Japanese patients, successfully treated with dapsone.[41,42] The initial dose was 25–75 mg/daily, and remission was obtained between 1 and 8 weeks. Although maintenance therapy and long-term follow-up were not reported, no recurrence was described.

Success with azathioprine, cyclosporin, and thalidomide has been described in anecdotal case reports. More recently, intravenous immunoglobulin and rituximab have been successfully used in isolated cases refractory to conventional therapies.[40]

Surgery should be avoided whenever possible as it can exacerbate the disease. However, it may be attempted when all other modalities have failed and lesions cause significant disability.

15.7.2
Panniculitis in Dermatomyositis

Panniculitis is less frequent in dermatomyositis than in LE and scleroderma. It may be associated with other skin manifestations or may appear as the only cutaneous manifestation, making the diagnosis more difficult.

Histopathological findings are similar to those of LP. Panniculitic lesions respond to systemic treatment of dermatomyositis, mainly to systemic corticosteroids alone or in combination with methotrexate, cyclosporine, or intravenous immunoglobulin.[43]

15.7.3
Panniculitis in Scleroderma

Scleroderma may also affect the subcutaneous adipose tissue without involvement of the epidermis. Lesions present as subcutaneous nodules located on the shoulders, arms, and trunk, which usually heal with dermal atrophy. Histopathological examination shows marked thickening of the septa of adipose tissue which is replaced by fibrous tissue. Inflammatory infiltrate may be observed in the earlier stages of the disease and consists of aggregations of lymphocytes and plasma cells.

15.7.4
Eosinophilic Fasciitis

Is a rare disease characterized by progressive skin thickening and generally considered as a variant of scleroderma. Patients usually show swelling and cutaneous thickening involving the extremities that can progress to *peau d'orange*, hyperpigmentation, and induration. Extracutaneous manifestations include joint contractures, arthritis, restrictive lung disease, and pleural effusions. Laboratory examinations show elevated erythrocyte sedimentation rate, peripheral eosinophilia, and hypergammaglobulinemia. Histopathological examination reveals thickening of the dermis due to collagen deposition with lymphocytic and eosinophilic infiltrate on the fascia. Differential diagnosis should be made with other causes of sclerodermiform changes (Table 15.6).

Prognosis is usually good, and spontaneous remission occurs in about one-third of patients. Systemic corticosteroids are the mainstay of therapy, especially in the early

Table 15.6 Main sclerodermiform diseases

Scleroderma
Eosinophilic fasciitis
Dermatomyositis
Rheumatoid arthritis
Lupus erythematosus
Overlap syndromes
Raynaud's syndrome
Dupuytren's disease
Porphyrias
Chronic edema
Chronic scurvy
Carcinoid syndrome
Werner's syndrome
Graft-versus-host disease
Toxic oil syndrome
Eosinophilia-myalgia syndrome
Polyvinyl chloride exposure
Nephrogenic systemic fibrosis
Mucinosis
Diffuse myxedema
Pretibial myxedema
Lichen myxedematosus
Scleredema
Scleromyxedema (papular mucinosis)
Phenylketonuria
Acrodermatitis atrophicans (Borrelia infection)
Drug-induced sclerodermiform syndromes
Cutaneous T-cell lymphoma
Progeroid syndromes

stages. Other therapies used for non-responding patients or as steroid-sparing agents include hydroxychloroquine, photochemotherapy, methotrexate, D-penicillamine, azathioprine, cimetidine, and anti-TNF-α.[44]

15.7.5
Erythema Nodosum (EN)

EN is the most common type of panniculitis. The typical eruption consists of symmetrical, tender, erythematous nodules, usually located on the lower extremities, although they may also involve other areas, mainly the ankles, the lower parts of the thighs, and the forearms. They have a contusiform-like color evolution from bright red to brownish-yellow, and it is not uncommon to observe nodules in different stages of evolution. Systemic symptoms, such as fever, malaise and arthralgias, may also be present.

EN may be idiopathic or associated with a wide variety of infections, drugs, and systemic diseases, whose incidence varies depending on the geographic origin of the series. Streptococcal infections are the most common cause in children, whereas other infections, drugs, sarcoidosis, and autoimmune and inflammatory processes are more frequent in adults.[45]

Histopathological examination shows a mostly septal lymphocytic panniculitis without vasculitis. Although it characteristically affects the septal component of the adipose tissue, there is often involvement of the lobule, especially in older lesions. In early stages, inflammatory infiltrate may be composed of neutrophils, but they are soon replaced by lymphocytes and histiocytes. A histopathologic hallmark of EN are the Miescher's radial granulomas, which are septal collections of histiocytes surrounding a cleft-like space. However, they may be seen in other diseases as Sweet's syndrome, necrobiosis lipoidica, and nodular vasculitis.[46]

Treatment of EN should be directed to the underlying cause, if identified. General measures include rest, and nonsteroidal anti-inflammatory drugs, such as indomethacin (100–150 mg/day) or naproxen (500 mg/day). For recurrent or persistent lesions, oral potassium iodide prepared as a supersaturated solution in a dosage of 400–900 mg daily for 1 month has proved to be useful.

Systemic corticosteroids (1 mg/kg/day) may be a therapeutic option if underlying infection or malignancy has been excluded. Steroids in combination with hydroxychloroquine, cyclosporine, or thalidomide have been used to treat inflammatory bowel disease associated to EN.

EN-like lesions occur in one-third of patients with Behçet's disease. Lesions are mostly seen in females, usually on the lower extremities, although the buttocks, arms, neck, and face may also be involved. They are not ulcerated and generally resolve within 2–3 weeks, sometimes with residual pigmentation. Although they are similar to EN secondary to other systemic diseases, they may be differentiated by its microscopic findings characterized by neutrophilic vascular reaction or vasculitis in the dermis and subcutaneous fat and perivascular lymphocytic dermal inflammation. Colchicine has been proposed as treatment.[46,47]

15.8
Cutaneous Purpura

Purpura may be a cutaneous manifestation of numerous systemic diseases (Table 15.7).

15.9
Cutaneous Ulcers

There are a great number of processes that may cause cutaneous ulcers (Table 15.8). Mucous and digital ulcers will be discussed separately as they have different causes and treatment.

Table 15.7 Causes of purpura

Vasculitis	Connective tissue diseases
Hypersensitivity vasculitis	Erythematous lupus
Schönlein-Henoch purpura	Scleroderma
Lymphocytic vasculitis	Dermatomyositis
Polyarteritis nodosa	Rheumatoid arthritis
Wegener's granulomatosis	Sjögren syndrome
Allergic granulomatosis	Overlap syndromes
Giant cell arteritis	Embolism
Obliterating endarteritis	Chronic hepatopathy
Antiphospholipid syndrome	Amyloidosis
Sepsis	Hyperthyroidism
Thrombocytopenia /thrombocytopathy	Hypothyroidism
Coagulopathy	Renal failure
Disseminated intravascular coagulopathy	Cushing syndrome
Calciphylaxis	Whipple disease
Cryoagglutinins	Scurvy
Cryoglobulinemia	C and S protein deficiency
Senile purpura (Bateman's purpura)	Vitamin K deficiency
Neoplasms	Factitious purpura
Waldenström macroglobulinemia	Psychogenic purpura
Marfan syndrome	Trauma
Ehlers–Danlos syndrome	Abuse
Pseudoxanthoma elasticum	Drugs and toxics
Venous insufficiency	

Table 15.8 Causes of cutaneous ulcers

Ulcerous colitis	Mycobacteriosis
Crohn disease	Leishmaniasis
Diabetes	Syphilis
Lupus erythematosus	Chancroid
Raynaud syndrome/scleroderma	Herpes simplex/zoster
Antiphospholipid syndrome	Cytomegalovirus
Arterial hypertension	Deep mycosis
Vasculitis	Osteomyelitis
Cryoglobulinemia	Amyloidosis
Embolism/ischemia	Werner syndrome
Thrombocytosis/polycythemia	Graft-versus-host disease
Disseminated intravascular coagulopathy	Anemia
C and S protein deficiency	Calcinosis
Buerger disease	Calciphylaxis
Arterio-venous anastomosis	Peripheral neuropathies
Venous insufficiency	Syringomyelia
Neoplasms/metastasis	Spinal dysraphism/spinal cord injuries
Gangrenous pyoderma	Radiodermatitis
Bacterial sepsis	Drugs/toxics
Ecthyma gangrenosum	Factitious ulcers
Gangrene/necrotizing fasciitis	Prolidase deficiency

15.9.1
Antiphospholipid Syndrome (APS)

APS is a multisystem disorder of hypercoagulation in which venous or arterial thrombosis, obstetric complications, thrombocytopenia, and circulating antiphospholipid antibodies are the most characteristic findings.

Cutaneous findings are extremely common in APS and, although they are not diagnostic criteria due to their lack of specificity, they may be the first manifestation of the disease and may help establish the diagnosis. In a large retrospective study, 40% of APS patients with skin manifestations developed other multisystemic thrombotic phenomena, highlighting the importance of skin for diagnosis and as a marker of systemic involvement.[48]

Livedo reticularis is the most common cutaneous lesion in APS, which has been associated with a greater frequency of arterial thrombosis, heart valve disease, arterial hypertension, and Raynaud's phenomenon.

Skin ulcers are the third most common cutaneous manifestation in APS (Fig. 15.7), after livedo reticularis and superficial thrombophlebitis. They are usually painful and located on the legs. They may be postphlebitic, secondary to skin necrosis, atrophie blanche lesions or secondary to livedoid vasculitis. Other skin manifestations include large ulcerative lesions, pyoderma gangrenosum-like or similar to pseudo-Kaposi's sarcoma, distal cutaneous ischemia, superficial thrombophlebitis, porcelain-white scars, thrombocytopenic purpura, dermatographism, chronic urticaria, acrocyanosis, and alopecia.[48,49]

Histopathological features of skin lesions may not be diagnostic but may provide important clues to consider the possibility of APS. The most characteristic findings are noninflammatory thrombosed vessels, which may be accompanied by capillary proliferation in the subpapillary dermis, endarteritis obliterans, dermal hemorrhage, and hemosiderin deposition.[48]

Antiplatelet therapy, such as low-dose aspirin (75 mg/day), is usually the first-line treatment for mild dermatological manifestations. Hydroxychloroquine has also antiplatelet effects and can reduce the risk of thrombosis in SLE patients and animal models of APS.[50]

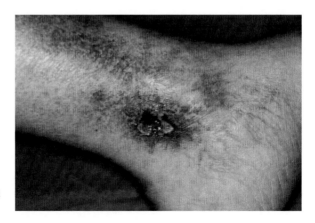

Fig. 15.7 Vasculitic ulcer in a patient with antiphospholipid syndrome

15.9.2
Calcinosis

Is a frequent complication of connective tissue diseases, mostly of childhood-onset dermatomyositis, being uncommon in adult-onset disease. It occurs in 40% of cases of juvenile dermatomyositis, correlating with skin disease severity, vasculopathy, and delay in therapy. The most common complications are ulceration with drainage of calcareous material, secondary infection, and joint contractures, causing significant disability. Calcinosis also occurs in about 25% of scleroderma and 17% of SLE patients.

No definitive medical therapy is available. However, several therapies, such as aluminum hydroxide, warfarin, colchicine, bisphosphonates, diltiazem, minocycline, probenecid, intralesional corticosteroids, surgery, and carbon dioxide laser, have been used with variable success.[51] Spontaneous regression may occur.

15.9.3
Vasculitis

Superficial ulcerations and cutaneous infarction may be a presentation of vasculitis in SLE and other connective tissue diseases, such as rheumatoid arthritis, dermatomyositis, and Sjögren syndrome. Cutaneous vasculitis is found in 10–20% of SLE patients and may lead to a variety of skin lesions, including palpable purpura, petechiae, papulonodular or bullous lesions, urticaria, and livedo reticularis.

Cutaneous vasculitis often occurs together with flares of systemic disease. So, in the presence of any of these cutaneous lesions, associated visceral vasculitis should be ruled out.[52]

Management includes general measures as avoiding sunlight, analgesia, and ulcer protection against injuries and infection. Patients may be treated depending on multiorgan involvement with systemic corticosteroids alone or in combination with other immunosuppressive drugs (cyclophosphamide, azathioprine, methotrexate, or mycophenolate mofetil).

15.9.4
Behçet's Disease

Behçet's disease cause cutaneous ulcerations in about 3% of patients, especially in children. They have tendency to recurrence and to heal with scarring. Common locations include legs, axillae, breast, interdigital skin of the foot, inguinal region, and neck.[47] Treatment will be discussed in the section of orogenital ulcers.

15.10
Digital Ulcers

Digital ulcers affect up to a half of patients with systemic sclerosis during the course of the disease. They are painful necrotic lesions located at the distal tips of digits or overlying bony prominences. Lesions located on distal tips result mainly from ischemic injury, while those located over joints are more related to repetitive trauma; so these ulcers are thought to be less responsive to vasodilating therapies than ulcers located on distal digits. Recurrent ischemic injury, microtrauma, and poor blood flow result in reduced healing, scarring, and digital tuft reabsorption, and leading to functional disability, gangrene, or amputation.

Potential risk factors for the development of digital ulcers in patients with systemic scleroderma have been identified as male sex, pulmonary arterial hypertension, esophagus involvement, anti-Scl 70 antibodies, young age at onset of Raynaud's phenomenon, and elevated erythrocyte sedimentation rate.[53]

Management of digital ulcers is difficult. Patients must minimize trauma and avoid cold and emotional stimuli as well as vasoconstrictors, such as nicotine and sympathomimetics. Topical hydrocolloid and occlusive dressing induce ulcer healing, reduce pain, and provide protection from trauma.

Digital ulcers are extremely painful; so analgesics are usually required. Multiple courses of oral antibiotics are often necessary to treat infection.

Several vasodilating drugs have been used with variable success to treat digital ulcers in systemic sclerosis. Nifedipine, a calcium-channel blocker, has proved to decrease the number of digital ulcers in a small study comparing oral nifedipine with intravenous iloprost.[54]

Iloprost is a prostacyclin analog that has demonstrated efficacy in the healing of digital ulcers, in decreasing the frequency and severity of Raynaud's phenomenon, and in preventing the development of new ulcers. In patients with severe systemic sclerosis and digital ischemia, it is parenterally administered at a dosage of 2 ng/kg/min, infused for 6 h/day, for 5 days. Their disadvantages are the high cost and the need of intravenous administration.

Bosentan is an endothelin receptor antagonist that has showed to promote ulcer healing in small studies. Two large studies showed no significant effects on ulcer healing, although there was a significant effect on the prevention of new ulcers (decreased the number of new ulcers 30–48%), specially in patients with severe disease.[55,56]

Sildenafil is a phosphodiesterase-5 inhibitor that induces vasodilatation by increasing nitric oxide levels. Several reports have demonstrated its efficacy on treating digital ulcers.

Antiplatelet and anticoagulant therapies as well as other agents to maintain vascular integrity such as statins and N-acetylcysteine need further evaluation to determine their efficacy in the treatment of digital ulcers.

Surgical procedures may be considered in severe and refractory ulcers. They include microsurgical revascularization of the hand, digital arterial reconstruction, and peripheral or digital sympathectomy. However, these techniques are invasive and recurrences have been documented in up to one-third of patients, so they should be reserved for those refractory to medical therapies.[57]

15.11
Genital Ulcers/Oral Ulcers

Oral and genital ulcers are among the most important manifestations of Behçet's disease and are essential for the diagnosis (Table 15.9).[58] Together with skin manifestations, eyes, central nervous system, joints, and gastrointestinal tract are usually involved.

Table 15.9 Criteria for diagnosis of Behçet's disease. International study group criteria for the diagnosis of Behçet's disease

Recurrent oral ulceration
Minor aphthous, major aphthous, or herpetiform ulceration observed by physician or patient, which have recurred at least three times in a 12-month period

And two of the following
Recurrent genital ulceration
Aphthous ulceration or scarring, observed by physician or patient

Eye lesions
Anterior uveitis, posterior uveitis, or cells in vitreous on slit lamp examination; or retinal vasculitis observed by ophthalmologist

Skin lesions
Erythema nodosum observed by physician or patient, pseudofolliculitis or papulopustular lesions; or acneiform nodules observed by the physician in post-adolescent patients not on corticosteroid treatment

Positive pathergy test
Read by physician at 24–48 h

Source: Reprinted from International Study Group for Behçet's Disease[58]. Copyright 1990, with permission from Elsevier

Oral ulcers are usually the first sign of the disease and may precede the onset of systemic manifestations by years. They are usually located on the tongue, lips, soft palate, and gingival and buccal mucosa and often occur at sites of local trauma.[47] They are classified as

- Minor ulcers: Superficial ulcers with a diameter of 2–6 mm, surrounded by and erythematous halo and healing without scarring.
- Major ulcers: They are deeper, more painful, and persistent and may leave scars after healing.
- Herpetiform ulcers: Recurrent crops of small and painful ulcers, which may become confluent.

Genital ulcers occur in 72–94% of patients with Behçet's disease. They are similar to oral ulcers, but tend to be deeper and leave scars. They are usually located on the vulva, vagina, and cervix in women and on the scrotum and prepuce in men. Other cutaneous manifestations that are part of the diagnostic criteria include EN-like lesions and papulopustular eruptions. Less frequently, Sweet-like lesions, pyoderma gangrenosum-like lesions, erythema multiforme-like lesions, palpable purpura, subungual infarctions, hemorrhagic bullae, and extragenital ulcerations may be present.[59] Other causes of oral and genital ulcers that should be considered in the differential diagnosis of Behçet's disease are listed in Table 15.10.

No standard therapy has been established for mucocutaneous manifestations of Behçet's disease, and a wide number of agents have been employed with variable outcome.[47,59] Topical corticosteroids are widely used, especially in early stages. They can reduce pain severity and promote ulcer healing. Triamcinolone acetonide cream 0.1% in Orabase is one of the most used formulations. For patients with multiple oral ulcers, corticosteroid

Table 15.10 Causes of oral and genital ulcers

Oral ulcers	Genital ulcers
Aphthous stomatitis	Allergic reactions
Allergic reactions	Adverse drug reactions
Behçet disease	Behçet disease
Adverse drug reactions	Herpes simplex
Herpes simplex	Syphilis
Epstein–Barr virus	Epstein–Barr virus
Bacterial infections	Chancroid
Syphilis	Granuloma inguinale
Mycosis	Lymphogranuloma venereum
Reiter's syndrome	Amebiasis
Systemic lupus erythematosus	Reiter's syndrome
Kikuchi–Fujimoto disease	Crohn disease
Erythema multiforme	Erythema multiforme
Lichen planus	Lichen planus
Pemphigus	Pemphigus
Mucosal pemphigoid	Tumor
Necrotizing ulcerative gingivitis	Factitial
Oral cancer	Trauma
Trauma	

tablets dissolved in water or elixir formulations may be easier to apply. Potent topical corticosteroids are also effective in genital ulcers, although long-term use may lead to skin atrophy. Major oral or genital ulcers can be treated by triamcinolone 5–10 mg/ml injection to the base of the lesion.

Other topical measures include antiseptics (chlorhexidine 1–2%), anesthetics (lidocaine 2–5%), anti-inflammatory agents (benzydamine, diclofenac 3%), and tetracycline mouthwash (250 mg capsule dissolved in 5 ml of water). Topical sucralfate suspension (1 g/5 ml) proved to be effective for oral and genital ulceration due to the formation of a protective barrier.

Systemic treatment is required in severe or recalcitrant mucocutaneous lesions. Systemic corticosteroids are effective in all mucocutaneous manifestations, alone or in combination with other drugs. However, due to possible side effects, long-term use should be avoided. Prednisone 1 mg/kg/day for 1–2 weeks and then tapering the dosage gradually over 4 weeks has been recommended.

Thalidomide (50–300 mg/day) is highly effective for orogenital ulceration and follicular lesions, but it should be reserved for patients resistant to other options, because of the risk of teratogenicity and polyneuropathy. Furthermore, discontinuation of the treatment results in recurrence; so a maintenance treatment with 50 mg/day to 50 mg twice a week is required.

Colchicine (0.5–2 mg/day orally) and dapsone (100–150 mg/day orally) are effective for oral and genital ulcers and other cutaneous manifestations of the disease.

Other agents, as azathioprine (2.5 mg/kg), cyclosporine (5–10 mg/kg/day), and methotrexate (7.5–20 mg/kg/week), have been found to be an effective choice for orogenital ulcers. However, they should be reserved for severe cases because of possible adverse events.

Fig. 15.8 Ulcers in the hard palate in a patient with systemic lupus erythematosus

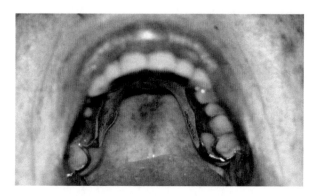

IFN-α-2a significantly decreases pain and duration of oral and genital ulcers. The recommended regimen is a high dose of IFN-α-2a (9 million units/3 times/week) for 3 months followed by a low maintenance dose (3 million units/3 times/week).

Recent trials of two anti-TNF-α inhibitors, infliximab and etanercept, have showed promising results in recalcitrant oral and genital ulcers, besides ocular and gastrointestinal symptoms. However, further studies are needed to establish their effectiveness.

Behçet's disease has a variable and recurrent clinical course with a gradual reduction in severity with the passage of time. Blindness and neurological manifestations are the major causes of morbidity.

Oral ulcers are included among the American College of Rheumatology criteria for SLE. They have been considered as a sign of vasculitis, and therefore, they would be histopathologically nonspecific and a marker of active systemic disease (Fig. 15.8).

15.12
Severe Raynaud

Raynaud's phenomenon is a painful cycle of color changes (pallor, hyperemia, and return to normality) in response to cold and emotional stimuli. It affects mainly the digits, but may appear in the nose, ears, and occasionally be associated with migraine and chest pain.

It may be primary, without an identifiable cause, or secondary to an underlying disease (Table 15.11), mainly systemic sclerosis (present in more than 95% of patients, often as the initial manifestation) or other connective tissue diseases as SLE, rheumatoid arthritis, and polymyositis.

There are some findings that allow suspecting a secondary cause, such as asymmetrical involvement of the digits, new-onset Raynaud at age older than 40 years, or nailfold capillaroscopy abnormalities with enlarged capillaries. In these patients, ANA and other test to exclude a connective tissue disease should be performed.[60]

Complications in primary Raynaud are extremely rare. In secondary Raynaud, especially to scleroderma, complications include digital ulcers, digital tuft reabsorption, ischemia of the digits, infection, and autoamputation. Anti-endothelial cell antibodies are associated with severe Raynaud, digital ulcers, gangrene, and pulmonary hypertension.

Table 15.11 Causes of secondary Raynaud's phenomenon

Connective tissue diseases
Scleroderma
Systemic lupus erythematosus
Dermatomyositis and polymyositis
Rheumatoid arthritis
Mixed connective tissue disease
Sjögren syndrome
Primary biliary cirrhosis

Endocrine causes
  Hypothyroidism
  Pheochromocytoma
  Carcinoid syndrome
  Diabetes mellitus
  Vascular causes
  Tromboangitis obliterans
  Atheroma
  Peripheral embolism
  Vasculitides (giant-cell arteritis, Takayasu)

Hematological causes
  Cryoglobulinemia
  Cryofibrinogenemia
  Cold agglutinin disease
  Paraproteinemia
  Polycythemia
  Protein C, S and antithrombin III deficiency
  Factor V Leiden
  Myeloproliferative and lymphoproliferative disorders

Neoplasms
Infections
  Hepatitis B and C
  Mycoplasma
  Parvovirus B19
  Helicobacter pylori

Traumatism
  Vibration injury
  Repetitive stress injury (pianists, typists, etc.)

Drugs
  Beta-adrenergic blockers
  Clonidine
  Ergot derivates, methysergide
  Cancer chemotherapy (bleomycin, vinblastine, cisplatin, tegafur)
  Cyclosporine
  Bromocriptine
  Interferons α and β
  Vinyl polychloride
  Fluorescein
  Cocaine, nicotine

Treatment is similar in some aspects to that of digital ulcers in the setting of sclero-derma. Patients should avoid exposure to cold and vasoconstrictor drugs. Calcium-channel blockers are the most common used drugs, usually at higher dosages than for hypertension (up to 60 mg of nifedipine or 20 mg of amlodipine). Nitrate derivates, α-adrenergic antag-onists, prostaglandins, endothelin receptor antagonists, and phosphodiesterase inhibitors have also been effective in severe Raynaud refractory to calcium-channel blockers. The selective serotonin reuptake inhibitor fluoxetine and the angiotensin II receptor antagonist losartan proved to decrease the frequency and severity of crisis, especially in patients with primary Raynaud.[60] Surgical procedures are rarely used due to the risk of morbidities and high rate of recurrences.

References

1. Gillian JN, Sontheimer RD. Distinctive cutaneous subsets in the spectrum of lupus erythema-tosus. *J Am Acad Dermatol.* 1981;4:471-475.
2. Walling HW, Sontheimer RD. Cutaneous lupus erythematosus: issues in diagnosis and treat-ment. *Am J Clin Dermatol.* 2009;10:365-381.
3. Sticherling M, Bonsmann G, Kuhn A. Diagnostic approach and treatment of cutaneous lupus erythematosus. *J Dtsch Dermatol Ges.* 2008;6:48-59.
4. Santmyire-Rosenberger B, Dugan EM. Skin involvement in dermatomyositis. *Curr Opin Rheumatol.* 2003;15:714-722.
5. El-Azhary RA, Pakzad SY. Amyopathic dermatomyositis: retrospective review of 37 cases. *J Am Acad Dermatol.* 2002;46:560-565.
6. Quain RD, Werth V. Management of cutaneous dermatomyositis. Current therapeutic options. *Am J Clin Dermatol.* 2006;7:341-351.
7. Sontheimer RD, Thomas JR, Gillian JN. Subacute cutaneous lupus erythematosus: a cutane-ous marker for a distinct lupus erythematosus subset. *Arch Dermatol.* 1979;115:1409-1415.
8. Cohen MR, Crosby D. Systemic disease in subacute cutaneous lupus erythematosus: a con-trolled comparison with systemic lupus erytethematosus. *J Rheumatol.* 1994;21:1665-1669.
9. Parodi A, Caproni M, Cardinali C, et al. Clinical, histological and immunopathological features of 58 patients with subacute cutaneous lupus erythematosus: a review by the Italian Group of Immunodermatology. *Dermatology.* 2000;200:6-10.
10. Watanabe T, Tsuchida T, Ito Y, et al. Annular erythema associated with lupus erythematosus/Sjögren's syndrome. *J Am Acad Dermatol.* 1997;36:214-218.
11. Unal I, Ceylan C, Ozdemir F, et al. ITP as an initial manifestation of subacute cutaneous lupus erythematosus. *Int J Dermatol.* 2005;32:727-730.
12. Berti S, Moretti S, Lucin C, et al. Urticarial vasculitis and subacute cutaneous lupus erythema-tosus. *Lupus.* 2005;14:489-492.
13. Callen JP. Cutaneous lupus erythematosus: a personal approach to management. *Australas J Dermatol.* 2006;47:13-27.
14. Briani C, Zara G, Rondinone R, et al. Positive and negative effects of thalidomide on refrac-tory cutaneous lupus erythematosus. *Autoimmunity.* 2005;38:549-555.
15. Callen JP. Management of "refractory" skin disease in patients with lupus erythematosus. *Best Pract Res Clin Rheumatol.* 2005;19:767-784.
16. Fautrel B, Foltz V, Frances C, et al. Regression of subacute cutaneous lupus erythematosus in a patient with rheumatoid arthritis treated with a biologic tumor necrosis factor alpha-blocking agent. *Arthritis Rheum.* 2002;46:1408-1409.

17. Goodfield M, Davison K, Bowden K. Intravenous immunoglobulin (IVIg) for therapy-resistant cutaneous lupus erythematosus (LE). *J Dermatol Treat*. 2004;15:46-50.
18. Kieu V, O'Brien T, Yap LM, et al. Refractory subacute cutaneous lupus erythematosus ssssuccessfully treated with rituximab. *Australas J Dermatol*. 2009;50:202-206.
19. Ting W, Stone NS, Racila D, Scofield RH, Sontheimer RD. Toxic epidermal necrolysis-like acute cutaneous lupus erythematosus and the spectrum of the acute syndrome of apoptotic pan-epidermoloysis (ASAP): a case report, concept, review and proposal for new classification of lupus erythematosus vesiculobullous skin lesions. *Lupus*. 2004;13:941-50.
20. Paradela S, Martínez-Gómez W, Fernández-Jorge B, et al. Toxic epidermal necrolysis-like acute cutaneous lupus erythematosus. *Lupus*. 2007;16:741-745.
21. Fonseca Capdevila E. Manifestaciones cutáneas de enfermedades sistémicas. In: Rozman C, ed. *Medicina Interna Farreras-Rozman*. 15th ed. Madrid: Harcourt; 2004:1319-1328.
22. Mandelcorn R, Shear NH. Lupus-associated toxic epidermal necrolysis: a novel manifestation of lupus? *J Am Acad Dermatol*. 2003;48:525-529.
23. Simsek I, Cinar M, Erdem H, Pay S, Meric C, Dinc A. Efficacy of plasmapheresis in the treatment of refractory toxic epidermal necrolysis-like acute cutaneous lupus erythematosus. *Lupus*. 2008;17:605-606.
24. Dorfman RF, Berry GJ. Kikuchi's histiocytic necrotizing lymphadenitis: an analysis of 108 cases with emphasis on differential diagnosis. *Semin Diagn Pathol*. 1988;5:329-345.
25. Yen HR, Lin PY, Chuang WY, Chang ML, Chiu CH. Skin manifestations of Kikuchi-Fujimoto disease: case report and review. *Eur J Pediatr*. 2004;163:210-213.
26. Santana A, Lessa B, Galrao L, Lima I, Santiago M. Kikuchi-Fujimoto's disease associated with systemic lupus erythematosus: case report and review of the literature. *Clin Rheumatol*. 2005;24:60-63.
27. Paradela S, Lorenzo J, Martínez-Gómez W, Yebra-Pimentel T, Valbuena L, Fonseca E. Interface dermatitis in skin lesions of Kikuchi-Fujimoto's disease: a histopathological marker of evolution into systemic lupus erythematosus? *Lupus*. 2008;17:1127-1135.
28. Takada K, Suzuki K, Hidaka T, et al. Immediate remission obtained by minocycline in a patient with histiocytic necrotizing lymphadenitis. *Intern Med*. 2001;40:1055-1058.
29. Fonseca E, Contreras F, García-Frías E, Carrascosa MC. Neonatal lupus erythematosus with multisystem organ involvement preceding cutaneous lesions. *Lupus*. 1991;1(1):49-50.
30. Brucato A, Franceschini F, Buyon JP. Neonatal lupus: long term outcomes of mothers and children and recurrence rate. *Clin Exp Rheumatol*. 1997;15:467-473.
31. Lee LA, Sokol RJ, Buyon JP. Hepatobiliary disease in neonatal lupus: prevalence and clinical characteristics in cases enrolled in a national registry. *Pediatrics*. 2002; 109(1):E11.
32. Izmirly PM, Llanos C, Lee LA, Askanase A, Kim MY, Buyon JP. Cutaneous manifestations of neonatal lupus and risk for subsequent congenital heart block. *Arthritis Rheum*. 2010;62(4): 1153-1157.
33. Shinohara K, Miyagawa S, Fujita T, Aono T, Kidoguchi K. Neonatal lupus erythematosus: results of maternal corticosteroid therapy. *Obstet Gynecol*. 1999;93(6):952-957.
34. Buyon JP, Clancy RM, Friedman DM. Cardiac manifestations of neonatal lupus erythematosus: guidelines to management, integrating clues from the bench and bedside. *Nat Clin Pract Rheumatol*. 2009;5(3):139-148.
35. Davis M, Brewer JD. Urticarial vasculitis and hypocomplementemic urticarial vasculitis syndrome. *Immunol Allergy Clin N Am*. 2004;24:183-213.
36. Kobza Black N. Urticarial vasculitis. *Clin Dermatol*. 1999;17:565-569.
37. Pei-Ling P, Hoon Tan S, Tan T. Lupus erythematosus panniculitis: a clinicopathologic study. *Int J Dermatol*. 2002;41:488-490.
38. Martens P, Moder KG, Ahmed I. Lupus panniculitis: clinical perspectives form a case series. *J Rheumatol*. 1999;26:68-72.

39. Magro MC, Crowson AN, Kovatich AJ, Burns F. Lupus profundus, indeterminate lympho-cytic lobular panniculitis and subcutaneous T-cell lymphoma: a spectrum of subcuticular T-cell lymphoid dyscrasia. *J Cutan Pathol.* 2001;28:235-247.

40. Fabbri P, Cardinali C, Giomi B, Caproni M. Cutaneous lupus erythematosus. Diagnosis and management. *Am J Clin Dermatol.* 2003;4(7):449-465.

41. Ujiie H, Shimizu T, Ito M, Arita K, Shimizu H. Lupus erythematosus profundus successfully treated with dapsone: review of the literature. *Arch Dermatol.* 2006;142:399-401.

42. Fernández-Torres R, Sacristán F, Del Pozo J, et al. Lupus mastitis, a mimicker of erysipela-toides breast carcinoma. *J Am Acad Dermatol.* 2009;60(6):1074-1076.

43. Solans R, Cortés J, Selva A, et al. Panniculitis: a cutaneous manifestation of dermatomyosis-tis. *J Am Acad Dermatol.* 2002;46:S148-S150.

44. Bischoff L, Derk CT. Eosinophilic fasciitis: demographics, disease pattern and response to treatment: report of 12 cases and review of the literature. *Int J Dermatol.* 2008;47:29-35.

45. Schwartz RA, Nervi SJ. Erythema nodosum: a sign of systemic disease. *Am Fam Physician.* 2007;75:695-700.

46. Mana J, Marcoval J. Erythema nodosum. *Clin Dermatol.* 2007;25:288-294.

47. Marshall SE. Behçet's disease. *Best Pract Res Clin Rheumatol.* 2004;18:291-311.

48. Alegre VA, Gastineau DA, Winkelmann RK. Skin lesions associated with circulating lupus anticoagulant. *Br J Dermatol.* 1989;120:419-429.

49. Kriseman YL, Nash JW, Hsu S. Criteria for the diagnosis of antiphosholipid syndrome in patients presenting with dermatologic symptoms. *J Am Acad Dermatol.* 2007;57:112-115.

50. Asherson RA, Frances C, Iaccarino L, et al. The antiphospholipid antibody syndrome: diag-nosis, skin manifestations and current therapy. *Clin Exp Rheumatol.* 2006;24:S46-S51.

51. Boulman N, Slobodin G, Rozenbaum M. Calcinosis in rheumatic diseases. *Semin Arthritis Rheum.* 2005;34:805-812.

52. Ramos-Casals M, Nardi N, Lagrutta M, et al. Vasculitis in systemic lupus erythematosus. Prevalence and clinical characteristics in 670 patients. *Medicine.* 2006;85:95-104.

53. Sunderkötter C, Herrgott I, Brückner C, Moinzadeh P, et al. Comparison of patients with and without digital ulcers in systemic sclerosis: detection of possible risk factors. *Br J Dermatol.* 2009;160:835-843.

54. Rademarker M, Cooke ED, Almond NE, et al. Comparison of intravenous infusions of ilo-prost and oral nifedipine in treatment of Raynaud's phenomenon in patients with systemic sclerosis: a double blind randomised study. *Br Med J.* 1989;298:561-564.

55. Horn JH, Mayes M, Matucci-Cerinic M, et al. Digital ulcers in systemic sclerosis: prevention by treatment with bosentan, an oral endothelin receptor antagonists. *Arthritis Rheum.* 2004;50:3985-3993.

56. Seibold JR, Matucci-Cerinic M, Denton CP, et al. Bosentan reduces the number of new digital ulcers in patients with systemic sclerosis. *Ann Rheum Dis.* 2006;65(supp II):90.

57. Bogoch E, Gross D. Surgery of the hand in patients with systemic sclerosis: outcomes and considerations. *J Rheumatol.* 2005;32:642-648.

58. International Study Group for Behçet's Disease. Criteria for diagnosis of Behçet's disease. *Lancet.* 1990;335:1078-1080.

59. Alpsoy E, Zouboulis CC, Ehrlich GE. Mucocutaneous lesions of Behçet's disease. *Yonsei Med J.* 2007;48:573-585.

60. Pope JE. The diagnosis and treatment of Raynaud's phenomenon. A practical approach. *Drugs.* 2007;67:517-525.

Life-Threatening Autoimmune Hematological Disorders

16

Emmanuel Andrès, Helen Fothergill, and Mustapha Mecili

Abstract Autoimmune hematological disorders include all conditions in which blood components are attacked by the immune system. The autoimmune cytopenias are a typical example, including: autoimmune thrombocytopenic purpura, autoimmune hemolytic anemia, Evans syndrome, and autoimmune neutropenia. Other autoimmune hematological disorders include acquired thrombotic thrombocytopenic purpura which is linked to the presence of anti-ADAMTS 13 autoantibodies, and acquired hemophilia – due to the presence of anticoagulation factor antibodies. All these conditions are characterized by their acute onset and often need urgent medical attention. This chapter addresses the clinical, diagnostic, and treatment options of hematological autoimmune disorders in the emergency setting.

Keywords Acquired hemophilia • Anticoagulation factor autoantibodies • Autoimmune cytopenia • Autoimmune hemolytic anemia • Autoimmune neutropenia • Autoimmune thrombocytopenic purpura • Autoimmune thrombotic thrombocytopenic purpura • Autoimmunity • Emergency • Immune thrombocytopenia • Life-threatening disorders

16.1
Introduction

Autoimmune hematological disorders include all conditions in which blood components are attacked by the immune system – notably certain factors of hemostasis. Their sudden onset, potential seriousness, and unpredictable nature necessitate quick and efficient

E. Andrès (✉)
Service de Médecine Interne, Diabète et Maladies Métaboliques,
Clinique Médicale B, Hôpital Civil, Hôpitaux Universitaires de Strasbourg,
Strasbourg Cedex, France
e-mail: emmanuel.andres@chru-strasbourg.fr

M.A. Khamashta and M. Ramos-Casals (eds.), *Autoimmune Diseases*,
DOI: 10.1007/978-0-85729-358-9_16, © Springer-Verlag London Limited 2011

management in the acute stages. Furthermore, the treatment initiated must take account of the wide range of etiologies responsible for these disorders. Thus, practitioners are often confronted with both diagnostic and therapeutic dilemmas.[1, 2]

This chapter reviews the practical aspects in the emergency management of autoimmune thrombocytopenic purpura, autoimmune hemolytic anemia, autoimmune neutropenia, autoimmune thrombotic thrombocytopenic purpura, and certain autoimmune coagulation abnormalities.

16.2
Autoimmune Thrombocytopenic Purpura (AITP) or Immune Thrombocytopenia

This term, which has replaced the old name "idiopathic thrombocytopenic purpura," illustrates recent advances in the understanding of the etiology behind AITP.[3] Indeed, this condition is caused by destruction of autologous platelets (or megakaryocytic precursor cells) by the body's immune system, and is the most frequent cause of thrombocytopenia due to decreased platelet survival.

Acute AITP (more frequent in children) must be distinguished from chronic AITP (more frequent in adults). During AITP, serious complications are essentially clinical, and are related to the occurrence, or risk of occurrence, of a potentially life-threatening hemorrhage.[3-6]

16.2.1
Positive Diagnosis of AITP

AITP is a diagnosis of exclusion. It is based on the confirmation of thrombocytopenia (platelet count <150 × 10⁹/l; currently defined as a platelet count <100 x 109/l in the new consensual definition of ITP) that is not due to impaired platelet production and which cannot be explained by other causes of decreased platelet survival.[3, 4]

On a clinical level, its main symptom is purpura – or more specifically flat and diffuse purpuric lesions, which are often associated with mucosal bleeding (epistaxis, gingivorrhagia, menorrhagia, etc.). Due to the absence of infiltration and necrotic features, a disorder of platelet origin is a more likely cause than one of vascular origin. Intra-articular bleeds and soft tissue hemorrhages are rare. In the absence of symptoms, thrombocytopenia is the most common condition leading to the diagnosis of an AITP.

In clinical practice, thrombocytopenia is confirmed by taking a full blood count. Bone marrow aspirate is the gold standard for ascertaining the origin of this type of thrombocytopenia, but its routine performance has been questioned in recent years. Current guidelines recommend carrying out a bone marrow aspirate only in patients: (a) over 60 years of age; (b) in the case of abnormalities found on the peripheral blood film; (c) other cytopenias detected in the full blood count; or (d) in the case of a poor response to first-line treatment, with an indication for splenectomy.[5]

16.2.2
Differential Diagnosis of AITP in the Emergency Setting

In the emergency setting, the main differential diagnoses for hemorrhagic purpura are septic purpura, notably *purpura fulminans*, and acute leucosis. These disorders, particularly the infections, can be excluded after clinical assessment and baseline investigations have been performed such as a full blood count.[7] From a laboratory perspective, "false thrombocytopenia" must be ruled out by performing a peripheral blood smear or collecting a blood sample into a citrate tube. It should be noted that false thrombocytopenias are observed in approximately 0.1% of patients, due to natural and physiological anti-GPIIbIIIa antibodies.[8]

On confirmation of thrombocytopenia and its origin, the differential diagnoses for AITP must be excluded, such as the other causes of decreased platelet survival. In the emergency setting sepsis, drug-induced thrombocytopenia, viruses (particularly HBV, HCV, and HIV), and consumption disorders (thrombotic microangiopathy and disseminated intravascular coagulation) must first be ruled out. Other differential diagnoses include acute disseminated systemic lupus erythematosus (ADLE), Evans syndrome, lymphoproliferative disorders, hypersplenism, and myelodysplasia.

In pregnant women, HELLP syndrome (Hemolysis, Elevated Liver function tests, Low Platelet count), thrombotic thrombocytopenic purpura, and gestational thrombocytopenia are other potential differential diagnoses.[6, 9, 10] If the patient has traveled in malaria-endemic regions, malaria must also be considered (as well as airport-contracted malaria).

Furthermore, Common Variable Immunodeficiency (CVID) associated with certain forms of AITP must be excluded, as this influences the treatment choice.

16.2.3
Criteria for Assessing the Severity of AITP

The severity of AITP is mainly due to the potential, unpredictable nature of potential hemorrhages. Concerning signs must be sought in all patients with thrombocytopenia, especially if the platelet count is lower than $30–50 \times 10^9/l$. These include oral hemorrhagic bullae, conjunctival or retinal hemorrhages on fundal examination, overt or occult visceral hemorrhages, headaches or visual disturbances which may be indicative of intracranial or retinal bleeding, as well as signs of haemodynamic instability due to profuse hemorrhages. Khellaf et al. have proposed a score designed to objectively assess the risk of hemorrhage. This score is made up of seven parameters: age, cutaneous and mucosal hemorrhages, as well as digestive, urinary, gynecological, and cerebromeningeal bleeds. According to the authors, a hemorrhagic score above 8 is indicative of an emergency situation, requiring prompt initiation of treatment.[7, 11]

With respect to laboratory tests, it is currently accepted that in the case of platelet counts exceeding $30–50 \times 10^9/l$, bleeding risk is minimal, and that in case of platelet counts above $10 \times 10^9/l$, *serious* bleeding risk is "minor" (between 1% and 5% at 10 years).[12, 13] Furthermore, given equal platelet count values, risk of hemorrhage seems to be lower in thrombocytopenia due to decreased platelet survival than for thrombocytopenia due to impaired platelet production. This may be accounted for by the flow of young, giant, and hyperfunctional platelets into peripheral blood.[14]

16.2.4
Management of AITP in the Emergency Setting

Treatment of life-threatening AITP aims to quickly restore the platelet count to acceptable levels, hence avoiding serious hemorrhages ($>50 \times 10^9/l$). If bleeding does occur, all patients should be hospitalized immediately, particularly if one or several clinical signs of severity coexist (cf. previous paragraph). Hospital admission is strongly advised when the platelet count is lower than $10 \times 10^9/l$.[15]

Platelet transfusion, which is rather ineffective given the peripheral mechanism of this type of thrombocytopenia, may be necessary in association with other treatments in cases of severe hemorrhage or in preparation for surgical intervention. Corticosteroid therapy and intravenous immunoglobulins (IVIg) are the treatments of choice in the acute setting. Corticosteroids may be administered as an intravenous bolus of methyl-prednisolone at a dose of 15 mg/kg/day during days 1–3, with a maximum daily dose of 1 g. Treatment is then continued with oral prednisone equivalents at a dose of 1 mg/kg/day. IVIg are given at a dose of 0.4 g/kg/day for 5 days or 1 g/kg/day for 2 days. The second regimen seems more effective and appropriate in the emergency setting. Of note, the main studies comparing corticosteroids with IVIg did not show any superiority of one drug category over the other, neither did they show any advantages of prescribing corticosteroids with IVIg over corticosteroids or IVIg alone (apart from an earlier rise in platelet count).[1, 6, 14-16] As a second-line treatment, splenectomy may be necessary in the long-term, when hemorrhages prove medically uncontrollable and life-threatening.[17] Rituximab (Mabthera®) seems to display a rather delayed efficacy, rendering it inappropriate for use in the emergency setting. However, insufficient data is not yet available and further studies are ongoing, which should provide a basis for drawing definitive conclusions.[18, 19] The same applies to thrombopoietin receptor agonists (romiplostim and eltrombopag).

16.3
Autoimmune Hemolytic Aaemia (AIHA)

Autoimmune hemolytic anemia (AIHA) is the most common extracorpuscular hemolytic anemia. AIHAs are related to the presence of autoantibodies directed against components of the erythrocyte membrane. The prevalence of AIHAs is estimated at 1–3 per 100,000 inhabitants, being less common than AITP. The thermal optimum of reactivity allows us to distinguish warm antibody AIHAs (the most frequent form, mostly of the IgG type) from cold antibody AIHAs (of the IgM type), which have a completely different etiological and therapeutic profile (cf. next paragraph).[20-22]

The combination of both AIHA and AITP points to the diagnosis of Evans syndrome, which is mainly caused by ADLE and lymphoproliferative syndromes in adults. In children, this syndrome is mainly observed in congenital cases of defective lymphocyte apoptosis due to an autoimmune lymphoproliferative disorder (Canale Smith syndrome). The acute management of Evans syndrome does not differ from that used when each cytopenia occurs independently.[1]

16.3.1
Positive Diagnosis of AIHA

The usual clinical presentations of AIHA include those of an anemia i.e., pallor, tachycardia, polypnea, asthenia, and excessive fatigability under stress, with those of hemolysis including jaundice, dark urine, and splenomegaly. In the emergency setting, AIHAs most often present as acute intravascular hemolysis, in which jaundice and splenomegaly may be absent, while fever, hemoglobinuria, acute lumbalgia, renal insufficiency, and hemodynamic instability may predominant – the latter possibly leading to hypovolemic shock. Such a clinical picture is much more common in cold antibody AIHAs. In the presence of an acrosyndrome and when a hemolytic crisis is triggered by cold exposure, a cold antibody AIHA must be considered. In secondary AIHAs, the clinical presentation may be dominated by clinical signs of the primary condition, such as arthralgia and cutaneous signs (*vespertilio*, photosensitivity, etc.) as observed in cases of ADLE.[1, 20, 23-25]

The definitive diagnosis of AIHA is based upon confirmation of hemolysis as well as detection of autoantibodies. Hemolytic anemia should be suspected if the following signs are present: acute-onset anemia (hemoglobin < 120 g/l), normocytosis or macrocytosis (mean erythrocyte cell volume > 100 fl), reticulocytosis (reticulocyte count > 120,000/mm³), hyperbilirubinemia with a predominance of unconjugated bilirubin, raised LDH levels and decreased haptoglobin (the most constant sign). In addition, thrombocytosis and hyperleukocytosis may also be observed. Peripheral blood film may be useful, as this examination is likely to provide additional indicators of hemolysis and its cause. In 30% of cases, reticulopenia is observed initially, and if it persists, causes of impaired platelet production or reticulocyte hemolysis should be considered.[26, 27]

A direct Coombs' test is the gold standard examination for diagnosing AIHA. Using specific antiglobulins, this test allows detection of antibodies and/or complement fraction fragments fixed on red cell surfaces. Most often, IgG immunoglobulins are detected, and more rarely, IgA or IgM immunoglobulins. A direct Coombs' test may be performed at a temperature of either 4°C or 37°C. Low antibody density (<200 antibody molecules per red cell) may result in false-negative results, whereas false-positive test results may be linked to a transfusion history, foetomaternal incompatibility, or nonspecific immunoglobulin adsorption in the case of monoclonal or polyclonal gammopathy. In the case of a positive direct Coombs' test with complement alone, the presence of cold agglutinins must be sought for. Further diagnostic tests include the Elution test and indirect Coombs' test. An Elution test (which is not essential for diagnosis) is performed by removing antibodies from the red cell surface membrane and bringing them into contact with a specific erythrocyte panel, thus enabling their identification and classification. Alternatively, the indirect Coombs' test may be used. This can be carried out at different temperatures, and circulating autoantibodies are detected and identified using a control erythrocyte panel.[1, 20, 28-30]

16.3.2
Differential Diagnosis of AIHA in the Emergency Setting

Depending on whether cold or warm antibodies are identified, the causes of AIHA vary. Predominant etiologies of warm antibody AIHAs include: ADLE, certain viruses,

Table 16.1 Main causes, laboratory findings and recommended management steps in hemolytic anemia (AHAI)

	Warm antibody AIHA	Cold antibody AIHA
Incidence	+++	+
Direct Coombs' test	Positive (IgG, IgG+complement, IgA)	Positive (isolated complement or IgM+complement)
Elution test	Positive (IgG)	Nonreactive
Indirect Coomb's test	Positive (IgG)	Positive (high levels IgM at 30°C)
Context	Adult	Child or adult
Etiologies	Drugs, acute disseminated lupus erythematosus, lymphoproliferative disorders, viruses	Donath-Landsteiner hemoglobinuria in children and infectious diseases (EBV, CMV, *Mycoplasma* sp.), cold agglutinin disease (other lymphoproliferative disorders)
Investigations in emergency setting	Blood count and blood smears, lymphocyte phenotype, bone marrow examination, B and C virus serology, HIV serology, antinuclear antibodies, thoracic X-ray, abdominal ultrasound?	Blood count and blood smears, lymphocyte phenotype, serum protein electrophoresis, bone marrow examination, EBV and CMV serology, Mycoplasma serology, chest X-ray
Treatment in emergency setting	Symptomatic (red cell transfusions) and treatment of underlying cause, steroids (oral or intravenous), intravenous immunoglobulin, rituximab, splenectomy, immunosuppressive agents	Symptomatic (red cells transfusions) and treatment of underlying cause, rituximab, plasmapheresis

and lymphoproliferative disorders. The main causes of cold antibody anemia include: Mycoplasma, Cytomegalovirus, and EBV infections (in transient adult AIHAs) and biphasic hemolysin (Donath-Landsteiner) in young children, as well as lymphoproliferative disorders. In the acute setting, clinical history and examination as well as baseline investigations are essential for ascertaining the etiology and diagnosis.[20, 31, 32] The main causes of AIHAs as well as laboratory findings and recommended management steps are summarized in Table 16.1. In all cases, DIC must be excluded as a matter of routine.

16.3.3
Differential Diagnosis of Hemolytic Anemia the Emergency Setting

In the emergency setting, all other causes of acute anemia must be differentiated from AIHA. Severe active hemorrhage can easily be ruled out. Patient history and clinical examination may reveal signs in favor of sepsis, toxin, or allergy-mediated immune hemolysis. Based on the results of the full blood count and blood film, the differential diagnosis must include other conditions potentially associated with spherocytosis, e.g., inherited microspherocytosis, Wilson's disease, and, in particular, septic hemolytic anemia caused by *Clostridium perfringens*. When considering infectious causes, babesioses must be excluded. Examination of the blood film allows the physician to exclude hemolysis, and the percentage of schistocytes also needs to be assessed to rule out thrombotic microangiopathy. Finally, patient's age and personal/family history plays a significant role in the diagnosis of an acute episode of constitutional hemolytic anemia. It should also be noted that all causes leading to jaundice with fever, notably those conditions where jaundice is the predominant feature, should also be considered in the differential diagnosis.[1, 20, 31, 33]

16.3.4
Criteria for Assessing the Severity of AIHA

Once AIHA has been diagnosed in the acute stage, its degree of severity must be assessed. The extent of the anemia, the clinical condition of the patient, and acute onset generally mean that prompt therapeutic intervention is required – particularly in elderly patients or patients with underlying organic diseases (cardiac insufficiency, ischemic cardiopathy, etc.).

Certain etiologies such as HIV, ADLE, and lymphoproliferative disorders are likely to result in a worse prognosis due to their systemic effects in conjunction with AIHA, or due to complications, which arise from opportunistic infections in states of immunodeficiency.[20, 34]

16.3.5
Management of AIHA in the Emergency Setting

Clinically, if the anemia is poorly tolerated, urgent treatment is required. Oxygen therapy is generally necessary, particularly if signs of hypoxia are observed. Although careful attention to hydration status and avoidance of intravascular volume depletion are necessary (particularly in cases of hemodynamic instability), frequent administration of large volumes of crystalloid should be avoided, due to the risk of hemodilution. Hemofiltration may be required in cases of anuria secondary to acute hemolysis.[1, 20, 35] The indication for blood transfusion must be carefully considered, particularly in AIHA cases with complement alone, as the transfused red blood cells are extremely fragile due to the active hemolytic process. Moreover, alloantibody test results may be falsely negative because of the presence of masking autoantibodies. In AIHAs, transfusion is only considered in combination with other treatments, for example, in cases of severe, poorly tolerated acute anemia.[1, 36, 37] A summary of the main therapeutic principles for AIHAs is given in Table 16.1.[27, 38]

Maintenance treatment depends on the type of AIHA. For warm antibody AIHAs, corticosteroid therapy in the form of methylprednisolone pulse therapy at a dose of 15 mg/kg/

day for 3 days is administered as emergency treatment. Thereafter, oral prednisone at a dose of 1 or 1.5 mg/kg/day is given. Splenectomy and other immunosuppressant medications, notably rituximab (Mabthera®), are indicated should there be any resistance to corticosteroids.[1, 27, 31, 39, 40] Polyvalent immunoglobulins are far less effective than for AITP treatment. Since plasmapheresis has a targeted action on plasma, its efficacy is much lower in warm antibody AIHAs where hemolysis is chiefly interstitial, than in cold agglutinin disease, where hemolysis is mostly intravascular.[41, 42] In the acute setting, the additional use of simple treatments must not be underestimated, and patients should be supplemented with folate (vitamin B9), iron, and if necessary, vitamin B12 to promote medullary regeneration. In cases of treatment failure and in the absence of a reticulocytosis, infection with parvovirus B19 must be excluded.

Avoiding cold exposure is an obvious but necessary measure in the treatment of cold antibody AIHAs. By using this measure alone, acute hemolytic crises can be prevented in moderate cases of AIHA, thus reducing the need for transfusions. In severe cases, cold avoidance is necessary but not sufficient. In this instance, corticosteroids are rarely effective, or may even be ineffective, and splenectomy is of little use as erythrocytes are destroyed in the liver and not in the spleen. Rituximab has been used in the treatment of AIHAs, resulting in responses ranging from 40% to 100%. It appears to be less effective in warm antibody AIHAs than in cold agglutinin disease – for which it is considered to be a first-line treatment. Plasmapheresis, which shows good efficacy as a "rescue solution," is rarely used as first-line treatment.[40-44] In most cases, post-infectious hemolysis resolves spontaneously, and treatment is essentially symptomatic.[45, 46]

16.4
Autoimmune Neutropenia (AIN)

Autoimmune neutropenia (AIN) is characterized by immune-mediated quantitative and/or qualitative polynuclear neutrophil alterations, resulting in an increased susceptibility to infections. In children, AIN is most often a primary, benign, transient condition, whereas in adults, AIN is usually chronic, comprising idiopathic and secondary forms.[47, 48]

16.4.1
Diagnosis and Etiology of AIN

A positive diagnosis of AIN is based on the detection of neutropenia (neutrophil count $< 1.5 \times 10^9$/l) and the presence of antibodies directed against polynuclear neutrophils.

Irrespective of its cause, neutropenia generally results in increased susceptibility to infections, the severity and frequency of which are directly proportional to the extent and duration of neutropenia.[48] Agranulocytosis is the most severe cause, with a polynuclear neutrophil count less than 0.5×10^9/l. Other factors may influence the clinical severity, such as the acute onset of the condition and the etiology behind it, which is likely to affect the availability and mobilization capacity of granulocyte progenitor medullary reserves.[47, 48]

Antibodies directed against polynuclear neutrophils can be detected using several techniques. The most widely accepted methods include the agglutination test and the direct and indirect granulocyte immunofluorescence tests. Although the MAIGA (Monoclonal Antibody-specific Immobilization of Granulocyte Antigen) technique has recently been proposed in order to avoid problems with false-positive results as observed with the two first methods, it is rarely used in routine practice. Due to low antibody titers and low antibody avidity, the sensitivity of the above three techniques is largely compromised, and does not exceed 45%. In cases of strong clinical suspicion, repetition of the tests may be required.[47, 48]

In the emergency setting, it is important to exclude causes of AIN which require immediate, specific management – such as AIN caused by certain medications, viral infections such as HIV, proliferative syndromes including large granular lymphocytic leukemia (LGL), and certain systemic conditions, particularly rheumatoid arthritis with Felty's syndrome.[47, 48]

16.4.2
Differential Diagnosis of AIN in the Emergency Setting

In the emergency setting, the main differential diagnoses for AIN are severe bacterial infections, notably septicemia or typhoid, brucellosis, and tuberculosis. In children, congenital neutropenia must be ruled out. In adults, the history, clinical setting, and baseline investigations allow the physician to exclude potential causes such as infections, (even simple viral infections), drug intake, hypersplenism, vitamin deficiency, and hematological or systemic diseases, e.g., collagen disorders.[48] The main causes of neutropenia in adults are summarized in Table 16.2. Clinicians must keep in mind the possibility of late onset neutropenia related to rituximab use (3–12 months after rituximab administration). Finally, when an infection and neutropenia coexist, the distinction between an infection secondary to neutropenia and a post-infectious neutropenia may prove difficult in the acute setting.[47]

Table 16.2 Main causes of neutropenia in adults

- *Normal variations*: ethnic and familial neutropenia
- *Splenic sequestration*: cirrhosis and portal hypertension (alcoholism), Gaucher's disease
- *Nutritional deficiencies*: cobalamin and folate deficiencies, copper deficiency, cachexia (Kwashiorkor)
- *Infectious:* bacterial (typhoid fever, brucellosis, tuberculosis, Rickettsia, severe sepsis), viral (Epstein–Barr virus, cytomegalovirus, human immunodeficiency virus, hepatitis virus, rubella, parvovirus B19), protozoal and fungal (histoplasmosis, leishmaniasis, malaria…)
- *Immune neutropenia*: isolated autoimmune neutropenia, collagen vascular autoimmune disease (systemic lupus erythematosus, rheumatoid arthritis or Felty's syndrome), T γ-δ lymphocytosis
- *Hematological disease*: myelodysplasia, pure white blood cell aplasia and red cell aplasia, Marchiafava-Micheli disease
- *Primary congenital or chronic neutropenia* (familial and nonfamilial cyclic neutropenia…)

16.4.3
Criteria for Assessing the Severity of AIN

The concern in neutropenic patients is related to the presence of infection, notably its severity, speed of progression, and particular clinical profile.[47, 48] Indeed, the clinical presentations of these infections are often atypical, with few inflammatory signs as the formation of pus is rendered impossible by the lack of neutrophils. As a result, any fever in a neutropenic patient must be considered to be of infectious origin, and must be treated as a medical emergency, requiring rapid administration of empirical antibiotic therapy (most often broad-spectrum antibiotics) after having taken microbiology specimens (blood culture, urine culture, etc.). However, a thorough history and full clinical examination are essential for detecting any signs of severe sepsis or septic shock, as well as possible entry sites such as gingivitis, oropharyngeal or cutaneous cellulites (including the extremely serious perineal cellulitis).[49]

16.4.4
Management of AIN in the Emergency Setting

It is essential to assess and treat severe infections by using broad-spectrum parenteral, preferably bactericidal, antibiotics.

Corticosteroids and IVIG have been successfully used in approximately 50% of cases as maintenance therapy for certain AINs.[47, 50] Since their onset of action takes 1–2 weeks, hematopoietic growth factors, such as the Granulocyte-Colony Stimulating Factor (G-CSF), are of particular interest and currently considered as the first-line treatment in AINs.[47, 51] The G-CSF starting dose is usually 5–10 µg/kg/day, administered subcutaneously over 3 days. Thereafter, administration frequency and dose are based on the response to treatment.[47] Of note is that pegylated G-CSF is currently not recommended for this indication.

16.5
Autoimmune Thrombotic Thrombocytopenic Purpura (TTP)

Thrombotic thrombocytopenic purpura (TTP), or Moschowitz syndrome, is due to congenital or acquired deficiency of a metalloprotease (ADAMTS 13) belonging to the A Disintegrin and Metalloproteinase with Thrombospondin-I motifs category A Disintegrin and Metalloprotease with Thrombo-Spondin (ADAMTS) protease family. This enzyme is responsible for cleaving high-molecular-weight multimers (HMWM) of von Willebrand factor (VWF), a potent inducer of platelet adhesion. Accumulation of HMWM, secondary to ADAMTS 13 deficiency, leads to diffuse microthrombi formation in small vessels resulting in cytopenia of mechanical origin, diffuse visceral pain, and multiple organ failure. In 90% of cases, acquired TTP is related to the presence of anti-ADAMTS 13 autoantibodies, and in 30% of patients, its clinical course is characterized by a succession of relapses and remissions.[52, 53]

16.5.1
Differential Diagnosis and Etiology of TTP in the Emergency Setting

For the diagnosis of an acquired TTP relapse, thrombotic microangiopathy must first be identified using clinical and biological investigations, and then confirmed by the presence of ADAMTS 13 deficiency (Fig. 16.1).

Hemolytic anemia of mechanical origin, thrombocytopenia, fever, renal involvement, and a fluctuating neurological deficit are the five main abnormalities indicative of thrombotic microangiopathy.[52, 53] The presence of schistocytes on the peripheral blood film is the disease hallmark, enabling the physician to confirm thrombotic microangiopathy by demonstrating the mechanical origin of the hemolysis.

Low ADAMTS 13 levels are indicative of TTP, allowing exclusion of other causes of thrombotic microangiopathy, notably hemolytic-uremic syndrome (due to bacteria such as *E. coli* OH157, etc.) and related thrombotic microangiopathies such as malignant hypertension and HELLP syndrome. Catastrophic antiphospholipid syndrome (CAPS) and scleroderma renal crisis presenting as a thrombotic microangiopathy are other conditions that must be differentiated from TTP. It should be noted that vitamin B12 deficiency may also present with signs mimicking a thrombotic microangiopathy, which spontaneously resolve following vitamin supplementation.[54, 55]

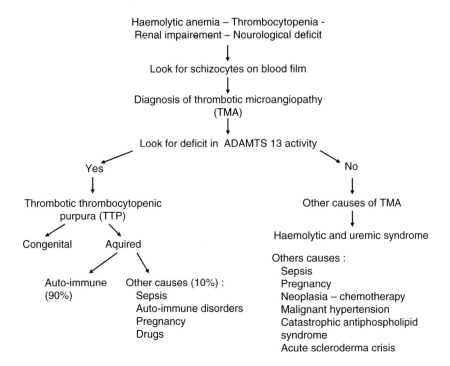

Fig. 16.1 Differential diagnosis and etiology of TTP in the emergency setting

Regarding the etiology, when TTP occurs in a young child, a congenital origin must first be considered. Acquired TTP is autoimmune in 90% of cases. Other etiologies include pregnancy, drug ingestion, neoplasia, infections, and autoimmune diseases such as lupic disease (ADLE). Anti-ADAMTS 13 antibody titers are useful for the diagnosis and post-treatment monitoring.[52-55]

16.5.2
Treatment of TTP in the Emergency Setting

TTP is a medical emergency. Based on plasma exchange, the treatment aims to provide the patient with large amounts of fresh frozen plasma by using the solvent/detergent method, which does not alter ADAMTS-13 activity.[52-55] In the acute setting, the usual plasma exchange regimen consists of 40–60 ml of plasma/kg/day. This quantity may be doubled in severe cases. Plasmapheresis has to be continued until laboratory investigations return to within the normal range, in particular the platelet count. ADAMTS-13 activity and autoantibody titer kinetics may be used for monitoring purposes.

The use of platelet antiaggregating agents is still highly controversial as no efficacy has been shown so far. Corticosteroid therapy, at a dose of 1 mg/kg/day, is often combined with plasmapheresis.[52, 54, 55] Furthermore, platelet transfusions are strictly contraindicated, unlike red blood cell transfusions, which may be used.[56] Immunoglobulins seem to be ineffective and may even be harmful.[57] In contrast, rituximab appears to be a particularly promising therapeutic option, and its use should be considered, even in the initial treatment phase of TTP.[52-56]

16.6
Anticoagulation Factor Autoantibodies, Using Factor VIII as an Example

This rare condition, associated with severe hemophilia-like symptoms, must be considered if non-traumatic or minor traumatic bleeding occurs in a patient without any previous bleeding history, as well as in the case of isolated activated clotting time prolongation.[58, 59] Autoantibodies may target several coagulation factors. Anti-factor VIII antibodies are the most common, and can be found in particular physiological conditions such as advanced age and postpartum, or specific diseases such as ADLE, lymphoproliferative disorders, prostate tumors and after administration of certain drugs.[58, 59]

Diagnosis is based on the identification of factor VIII deficiency related to the presence of factor VIII inhibitor antibodies, detected using the Bethesda assay.

In addition to treating the underlying cause, management in the acute stage consists of controlling hemorrhages and reducing factor VIII deficiency. This can be achieved by administering desmopressin, which stimulates the release of factor VIII, or by administering recombinant factor VIII or recombinant factor VII, all resulting in the conversion of factor X into activated factor X, in the absence of factor VIII. According to the most recent consensus, the use of eptacog alfa (Novoseven®) is recommended. Immunosuppression induced by the combination of prednisone/cyclophosphamide may also be considered in order to slow down the autoimmune process, as well as rituximab. Lastly, it should be highlighted that immunoglobulins and plasmapheresis are also effective treatment options.[60]

References

1. Suarez F, Ghez D, Delarue R, Hermine O. Cytopénies auto-immunes périphériques. *Réanimation*. 2005;14:587-593.
2. Habibi B, Salmon Ch. Auto-immunité en hématologie. *Rev Fr Allergol*. 1974;14:277-279.
3. Viallard JF. Prise en charge diagnostique et thérapeutique du purpura thrombopénique idiopathique. *Rev Méd Interne*. 2009;30:9-12.
4. Godeau B, Provan D, Bussel J. Immune thrombocytopenic purpura in adults. *Curr Opin Hematol*. 2007;14:535-556.
5. Cines DB, Blanchette VS. Immune thrombocytopenic purpura. *N Engl J Med*. 2002;346: 995-1008.
6. Guidelines for the investigation and management of idiopathic thrombocytopenic purpura in adults, children and in pregnancy. *Br J Haematol* 2003;120:574-596.
7. Andrès E, Zimmer J, Affenberger S, Grosu D, Maloisel F. Traitement du purpura thrombopénique idiopathique de l'adulte: expérience personnelle et revue de la littérature. *Méd Thér*. 2005;11:167-175.
8. Vicari A, Banfi G, Bonini PA. EDTA-dependent pseudothrombocytopaenia. A 12-month epidemiological study. *Scand J Clin Lab Invest*. 1988;48:537-542.
9. Federici L, Serraj K, Maloisel F, Andrès E. Thrombopénie et grossesse: du diagnostic étiologique à la prise en charge thérapeutique. *Presse Méd*. 2008;37:1299-1307.
10. Kessler I, Lancet M, Borenstein R, Berrebi A, Mogilner BM. The obstetrical management of patients with immunologic thrombocytopenic purpura. *Int J Gynaecol Obstet*. 1982;20:23-28.
11. Khellaf M, Michel M, Schaeffer A, Bierling P, Godeau B. Assessment of a therapeutic strategy for adults with severe autoimmune thrombocytopenic purpura based on a bleeding score rather than platelet count. *Haematologica*. 2005;90:829-832.
12. Portielje JE, Westendorp RG, Kluin-Nelemans HC, Brand A. Morbidity and mortality in adults with idiopathic thrombocytopenic purpura. *Blood*. 2001;97:2549-2554.
13. Daou S, Federici L, Zimmer J, Maloisel F, Serraj K, Andrès E. Idiopathic thrombocytopenic purpura in elderly patients: a study of 47 cases from a single reference center. *Eur J Intern Med*. 2008;19:447-451.
14. George JN, Woolf SH, Raskob GE, et al. Idiopathic thrombocytopenic purpura: a practice guideline developed by explicit methods for the American Society of Hematology. *Blood*. 1996;88:3-40.
15. Cines DB, Bussel JB, McMillan RB, Zehnder JL. Congenital and acquired thrombocytopenia. *Hematology Am Soc Hematol Educ Program*. 2004;1:390-406.
16. Godeau B, Chevret S, Varet B, et al. Intravenous immunoglobulin or high-dose methylprednisolone, with or without oral prednisone, for adults with untreated severe autoimmune thrombocytopenic purpura. A randomised, multicentre trial. *Lancet*. 2002;359:23-9.
17. Cines D, Bussel JB. How I treat idiopathic thrombocytopenic purpura (ITP). *Blood*. 2005;106:2244-2251.
18. Stasi R, Pagano A, Stipa E, Amadori S. Rituximab chimeric anti-CD20 monoclonal antibody treatment for adults with chronic idiopathic thrombocytopenic purpura. *Blood*. 2001;98:952-957.
19. Arnold DM, Dentali F, Crowther MA, et al. Systematic review: efficacy and safety of rituximab for adults with idiopathic thrombocytopenic purpura. *Ann Intern Med*. 2007;146:25-33.

20. Philippe P. Diagnostic et prise en charge de l'anémie hémolytique auto-immune. *Presse Méd.* 2007;36:1959-1969.

21. Rochant H. Anémies hémolytiques auto-immunes. *Rev Prat.* 2001;51:1534-1541.

22. Sokol RJ, Booker DJ, Stamps R. The pathology of auto-immune haemolytic anaemia. *J Clin Pathol.* 1992;45:1047-1052.

23. Rosse WF, Hillmen P, Schreiber AD. Immune-mediated hemolytic anemia. *Hematology Am Soc Hematol Educ Program.* 2004;1:48-62.

24. Pirofsky B. Clinical aspects of auto-immune haemolytic anemia. *Semin Hematol.* 1976;13: 251-265.

25. Philippe P, Ruivard M, Fouilhoux AC, Colombier L, Tous les membres de l' Association pour le développement de la Médecine Interne en Auvergne. Analyse de la prise en charge diagnostique et thérapeutique de l'anémie hémolytique auto-immune (à propos de 66 cas). *Rev Med Intern.* 1996;17:55.

26. Conley CL, Lippman SM, Ness PM, Petz LD, Branch DR, Gallagher MT. Autoimmune hemolytic anemia with reticulocytopenia and erythroid marrow. *N Engl J Med.* 1982;306:281-286.

27. King KE, Ness PM. Treatment of autoimmune hemolytic anemia. *Semin Hematol.* 2005;42: 131-136.

28. Pérel Y, Aladjidi N, Jeanne M. Prise en charge d'une anémie hémolytique auto-immune à la phase aiguë. *Arch Pediatr.* 2006;13:514-517.

29. Hoffman PC. Immune hemolytic anemia-selected topics. *Hematology Am Soc Hematol Educ Program.* 2009:80-86.

30. Michel M. Caractéristiques des anémies hémolytiques auto-immunes à anticorps 'chauds' et du syndrome d'Evans de l'adulte. *Presse Méd.* 2008;37:1309-1318.

31. Packman CH. Hemolytic anemia due to warm autoantibodies. *Blood Rev.* 2008;22:17-31.

32. Berentsen S, Ulvestad E, Langholm R, et al. Primary chronic cold agglutinin disease: a population based clinical study of 86 patients. *Haematologica.* 2006;91:460-466.

33. Genty I, Michel M, Hermine O, Schaeffer A, Godeau B, Rochant H. Caractéristiques des anémies hémolytiques auto-immunes de l'adulte: analyse rétrospective d'une série de 83 patients. *Rev Méd Interne.* 2002;23:901-909.

34. Roth S, Obrecht V, Putetto M, Miniconi Z, Chaillou-Opitz S, Pesce A. Anémies du sujet âgé: expérience d'un service de gériatrie et recommandations. *Rev Méd Interne.* 2009;30:S111.

35. Heinrich B, Schrembs I, Brudler O, Bangerter M. Anemia: from symptoms to diagnosis and therapy. *MMW Fortschr Med.* 2009;151:31-35.

36. Petz LD. "Least incompatible" units for transfusion in auto-immune hemolytic anemia: should we eliminate this meanigless term? A commentary for clinicians and transfusion medicine professionals. *Transfusion.* 2003;43:1503-1507.

37. Garratty G, Petz LD. Approaches to selecting blood for transfusion to patients with autoimmune hemolytic anemia. *Transfusion.* 2002;42:1390-1392.

38. Hall RI. The utility of hemoglobin based oxygen carriers (HBOC) – can animal studies help? *Can J Anaesth.* 2005;52:895-898.

39. Atkinson JP, Schreiber AD, Frank MM. Effects of corticosteroids and splenectomy on the immune clearance and destruction of erythrocytes. *J Clin Invest.* 1973;52:1509-1517.

40. Zecca M, Nobili B, Ramenghi U, Perrotta S, Amendola G, Rosito P. Rituximab for the treatment of refractory autoimmune hemolytic anemia in children. *Blood.* 2003;101:3857-3861.

41. Narat S, Gandla J, Hoffbrand AV, Hughes RG, Mehta AB. Rituximab in the treatment of refractory autoimmune cytopenias in adults. *Haematologica.* 2005;90:1273-1274.

42. Shanafelt TD, Madueme HL, Wolf RC, Tefferi A. Rituximab for immune cytopenia in adults: idiopathic thrombocytopenic purpura, autoimmune hemolytic anemia, and Evans syndrome. *Mayo Clin Proc.* 2003;78:1340-1346.

43. Quartier P, Brethon B, Philippet P, Landman-Parker J, Le Deist F, Fischer A. Treatment of childhood autoimmune haemolytic anaemia with rituximab. *Lancet.* 2001;358:1511-1513.

44. Taaning EB, Klausen TW, Birgens H. Rituximab in chronic cold agglutinin disease: a prospective study of 20 patients. *Leuk Lymphoma*. 2006;47:253-260.
45. Flores G, Cunningham-Rundles C, Newland AC, Bussel JB. Efficacy of intravenous immunoglobulin in the treatment of autoimmune hemolytic anemia: results in 73 patients. *Am J Hematol*. 1993;44:237-242.
46. McLeod BC. Evidence based therapeutic apheresis in autoimmune and other hemolytic anemias. *Curr Opin Hematol*. 2007;14:647-654.
47. Capsonil F, Sarzi-Puttini P, Zanella A. Primary and secondary autoimmune neutropenia. *Arthritis Res Ther*. 2005;7:208-214.
48. Bux J, Behrens G, Jaeger G, WelteBlood K. Diagnosis and clinical course of autoimmune neutropenia in infancy: analysis of 240 cases. *Blood*. 1998;91:181-186.
49. Andrès E, Maloisel F. Idiosyncratic drug-induced agranulocytosis or acute neutropenia. *Curr Opin Hematol*. 2008;15:15-21.
50. Donadieu J, Fenneteau O. Neutropénies constitutionnelles et acquises. *EMC-Hématologie*. 2007;4:10-34.
51. Taniguchi S, Shibuya T, Harada M, Niho Y. Decreased levels of myeloid progenitor cells associated with long-term administration of recombinant human granulocyte-stimulating factor in patients with autoimmune neutropenia. *Br J Haematol*. 1993;83:384-387.
52. Schleinitz N, Poullin P, Camoinc L, et al. Le purpura thrombotique thrombocytopénique acquis de l'adulte: actualités. *Rev Méd Interne*. 2008;29:794-800.
53. Verbeke L, Delforge M, Dierickx D. Current insight into thrombotic thrombocytopenic purpura. *Blood Coagul Fibrinolysis*. 2010;21:3-10.
54. Kwaan HC. Thrombotic thrombocytopenic purpura: a diagnostic and therapeutic challenge. *Semin Thromb Hemost*. 2005;31:615-624.
55. Coppo P, Vernant JP, Veyradier A, et al. Bussel A pour le Réseau d'étude des microangiopathies thrombotiques de l'adulte. Purpura thrombotique thrombocytopénique et autres syndromes de microangiopathie thrombotique. *EMC-Hématologie*. 2005;2:14-34.
56. Moake J. Thrombotic thrombocytopenia purpura (TTP) and other thrombotic microangiopathies. *Best Pract Res Clin Haematol*. 2009;22:567-576.
57. Scully MA, Machin SJ. Berend Houwen memorial lecture: ISLH Las Vegas May 2009: the pathogenesis and management of thrombotic microangiopathies. *Int J Lab Hematol*. 2009; 31:268-276.
58. Cohen AJ, Kessler CM. Acquired inhibitors. *Baillières Clin Haematol*. 1996;9:331-354.
59. Levesque H, Borg JY, Bossi P, Goudemand J, Guillet B, Cabane J. L'hémophilie acquise: approches diagnostiques et thérapeutiques actuelles. *Rev Méd Interne*. 2001;22:854-866.
60. Huth-Kühne A, Baudo F, Collins P, et al. International recommendations on the diagnosis and treatment of patients with acquired hemophilia A. *Haematologica*. 2009;94:566-575.

Autoimmune Ear, Nose, and Throat Emergencies

17

Aharon Kessel, Zahava Vadasz, and Elias Toubi

Abstract The involvement of the ear-nose-and-throat (ENT) in many autoimmune diseases such as systemic lupus erythematosus or in anti-neutrophil-cytoplasmic antibody (ANCA)–related vasculitis should be brought into greater attention.

Sudden or rapidly progressive sensorineural hearing loss was reported extensively in both primary and secondary antiphospholipid syndrome, and frequently as a presenting symptom. Ear or nose involvement was also described in ANCA-related vasculitis, especially the inner ear in Wegener's granulomatosis. Relapsing polychondritis frequently presents with external ear inflammation, nasal chondritis, and laryngotracheal damage.

This review gives special attention to early diagnosis and therapy, mainly when ENT involvement is considered an emergency. In such cases, aggressive immunosuppressive therapy ought to be initiated early to minimize inflammatory destruction.

Keywords ANCA • Antiphospholipid antibodies • Autoimmunity • ENT • Polychondritis

17.1
Autoimmunity and ENT

Systemic autoimmune diseases such as systemic lupus erythematosus (SLE), rheumatoid arthritis (RA), and systemic sclerosis (SSc) are characterized by involving almost all organs and systems. Thus, it is more than reasonable to look for ear-nose-and-throat (ENT) involvement in these diseases. ENT damages in both SLE and RA patients have been occasionally reported, being presented as sensorineural hearing loss (SNHL), tinnitus, and vertigo.

A support for the assumption that SNHL is autoimmune in part was derived from a seminal study by McCabe,[1] in which immunosuppressive therapy with corticosteroids

A. Kessel(✉)
Division of Clinical Immunology and Allergy, Bnai-Zion Medical Center,
affiliated with the Technion Faculty of Medicine, Golomb str. 47, 31048 Haifa, Israel
e-mail: aharon.kessel@b-zion.org.il

M.A. Khamashta and M. Ramos-Casals (eds.), *Autoimmune Diseases*,
DOI: 10.1007/978-0-85729-358-9_17, © Springer-Verlag London Limited 2011

and cyclophosphamide improved rapidly progressive SNHL (PSNHL). In later studies, it was shown that autoimmune SNHL (ASNHL) is mediated by inner ear–specific autoreactive T cells. However, other studies provided evidences of a humoral-mediated (autoantibody) response against inner ear antigens.[2,3]

Autoimmunity in patients with PSNHL was later supported by the following:

1. Disease-related autoantibodies, such as anti-dsDNA, antithyroid (ATA), anticardiolipin antibodies (aCL), and rheumatoid factor (RF), were detected in sera of these patients.[4]
2. Many trials have shown that prompt administration of corticosteroids and/or methotrexate double the likelihood of hearing recovery.[5]
3. Inner ear damage has been developed in animal models following immunization with heterologous cochlear antigens and immune adjuvant.[6]
4. Inner ear pathology was documented to be part of the SLE-like phenomena, known to develop spontaneously in the MRL-lpr/lpr mice.[7]

Many studies reported on the occurrence of SNHL in patients with SLE. These studies pointed to the fact that in SLE, audiovestibular disturbances (affecting mainly the middle and higher frequencies and also vertigo) are more prevalent than previously thought.[8] The involvement of SNHL and conductive hearing loss in patients with RA was suggested to be a result of systemic inflammation and tissue injury. In these studies, the frequency of SNHL in patients with RA was much higher than in normal controls (36.1% vs 13.9%; $p < 0.01$).[9] In a recent study, inner ear involvement was recorded as well in patients with SSc and presented by tinnitus in 50%, hyperacusis in 40%, and hearing loss in 40%.[10] All this supports the notion that inner ear involvement should be looked for when autoimmune diseases are followed.

Looking into the autoantigens' origin in ASNHL, many specific antigens were proposed as playing a role in this organ-specific autoimmune disease. In an attempt to identify the main target antigens for autoantibodies reactive against guinea pig inner ear proteins, sera from 110 patients with a clinical diagnosis of either PSNHL, Meniere's disease (MD), or other etiologies of hearing loss were screened by Western blot technique. Forty-four percent of the patients' sera had antibodies to several inner ear proteins, of which the 30-, 42- and 68-kDa proteins were found the most reactive. These proteins were demonstrated to be the major peripheral myelin protein PO and the beta-actin protein, respectively, while sequence analysis indicated that the 68-kDa protein was novel. Autoantibodies to PO were reported in additional studies that occurred in association with progressive ASNHL. Clinical data and audiometric results indicated that a progressive hearing loss was more frequently recorded in patients in the anti-PO antibody-positive group (82% [14/17]) than in those in the anti-PO antibody-negative group (35% [6/17]) ($p < 0.005$).[11]

In order to determine the role of self-antigens in the pathogenesis of SNHL, antibody responses to the inner ear-specific proteins, cochlin, beta-tectorin, and also the nonspecific heat shock protein 70 (HSP 70), were analyzed by a Western blot assay to assess IgG antibody responses to the recombinant human HSP 70. In this study, of 58 patient samples analyzed, 19 tested positive to the HSP 70, eight to cochlin, and one to beta-tectorin, giving a prevalence of 33%, 14%, and 2%, respectively. The study pointed to the additive value of assessing anti-cochlin antibodies in these patients.[12]

The role of these antibodies in the development of ASNHL was repeatedly shown by others. Mathews et al.[13] presented a series of patients with clinically suspected autoimmune hearing loss in whom the presence of antibodies against bovine heat shock protein 70 (one of the many cross-reacting proteins against the inner ear in these patients) was a marker for the response to steroid treatment.

When ENT involvement is discussed, one should mention in addition to the above, the possibility of its involvement in antiphospholipid syndrome both in secondary and primary. In vasculitis, namely the anti-neutrophil-cytoplasmic antibody (ANCA) related one, ENT involvement was reported to be one among other symptoms and in some cases even a selective presenting symptom. The ear and nose are target organs in diseases such as polychondritis and Cogan's syndrome. In this chapter, we discuss ENT involvement and in some cases even emergencies in the above medical situations.

17.2
Sudden Sensorineural Hearing Loss (SSNHL)

SSNHL is a frustrating entity appearing usually unilaterally but in some cases bilateral as well. It is frequently associated with tinnitus and vertigo leading to high disability. In most cases, it is idiopathic, but causes such as infections, vascular events, and immune-mediated inflammation are proposed. Of all emergencies, vascular events and malignancies should be urgently taken care of.

In a recent study, the issue of SNHL was extensively searched in the literature of the last 4 decades. The etiology of SSNHL remains unknown in most cases (71%). However, viral infections were thought to be the cause in 12.6%, trauma in 4.2%, vascular events in 2.8%, neoplastic in 2.3%, and other causes in 7.1%. Thus, establishment of a direct causal link between SSNHL and all these etiologies remains elusive.[14]

In another study, 8.7% of all studied individuals (1,423 with SSNHL and 5,692 controls) had strokes during the 5-year follow-up period. After adjusting for other factors, the hazard of stroke during the 5-year follow-up period was 1.64 times greater for SSNHL patients than for a control group.[15] This is why a link between SSNHL and antiphospholipid syndrome is proposed and is well investigated.

Small vessel occlusions are frequently described to be a part of the vascular manifestations of the antiphospholipid syndrome (APS) involving glomerular, cutaneous, retinal, and inner ear microcirculation. In some of these, such as in sudden hearing loss or retinal occlusions, microthrombosis remains unproven by biopsies or imaging.[16] The frustrating entity of sudden sensorineural hearing loss (SSNHL) affects both males and females between the age 30 and 60 years; it is presented as unilateral in 80% of cases and as bilateral in the remainder. This emergency though mostly idiopathic is extensively reported to be a part of, or in some cases, a presenting symptom of the antiphospholipid syndrome (APS). Thus, it is recommended that patients presenting with SSNHL are investigated for evidence of antiphospholipid antibodies.[17]

The presence of aCL in the sera of patients with SNHL was first reported in 1997. Low-to-moderate positive aCL to one or both IgG/IgM isotypes were found in 8/30 (27%)

patients, whereas none were detected in healthy controls.[18] In 1998, Heller et al. studied the incidence and clinical relevance of antibodies to phospholipids in patients with sudden deafness ($n=55$) and progressive inner ear hearing loss ($n=80$). Antiphospholipids antibodies were demonstrated in 49% of the patients with sudden hearing loss and 50% of the patients with progressive hearing loss.[19] Both of these studies reported on the association between SSNHL and the existence of aCL, but they did not investigate their persistency over time. Whereas autoimmune aCL are of persistent character and mostly seen in conjunction with anti-β_2-glycoprotein-I antibodies (anti-β_2-GP1), transient aCL, in the absence of anti-β_2-GP1 was reported to be the result of viral infections.

Later, we assessed 51 patients who met the diagnostic criteria of SNHL in an extended study. We found low-to-moderate positive titers of aCL in 16 patients (31%) compared with 2 (6%) in the healthy controls. Six patients (12%, all aCL positive) were also positive for anti-β_2-GP1. Three months later, positive aCL persisted in seven (14%) patients, four of whom were also positive for anti-β_2-GP1. This was consistent with the knowledge that anti-β_2-GP1 antibodies are more specifically associated with thromboembolism, thus considering some cases of SSNHL to be part of primary APS.[20] Mouadeb et al. investigated the possible association between antiphospholipid antibodies and SNHL of unknown origin in a cohort of 168 patients. Forty-two patients (25%) had at least one elevated antiphospholipid antibody marker. Twenty patients had two or more positive test results. Of the 42 patients, 64% ($n=27$) met the diagnostic criteria for MD, and the remainder were diagnosed with idiopathic SSNHL. Within this group of patients, 24 patients (57%) had unilateral hearing loss, and 18 (44%) had bilateral hearing loss. These data further support the hypothesis that antiphospholipid antibodies are involved in the pathogenesis of some forms of inner ear dysfunction, presumably by causing microthrombosis in the labyrinthine vasculature.[21]

The incidence of SSNHL being a presenting emergency of the primary APS (PAPS) is yet to be defined. However, during the last few years, many case reports on this issue were published. In one of these, a 46-year-old man with PAPS developed a sudden onset of hearing loss and tinnitus in the right ear, following the discontinuation of warfarin usage. Electronystagmography displayed multiple central signs and bilateral canal paresis, while a vestibular-evoked myogenic potential test revealed bilateral delayed responses. Three days after re-treatment with warfarin, audiometry recovery of right-sided hearing was documented.[22] In support with this, other case reports strengthened the association between the occurrence of SSNHL and PAPS mentioning in some the development of even bilateral hearing loss.[23] SSNHL has been also reported to be one of the symptoms complicating autoimmune diseases with antiphospholipid antibodies (secondary APS).

In this setting, SSNHL in the right ear was reported in a young woman with SLE in whom aCL was positive as well.[24] In a recent study, 71 patients with mixed connective tissue disease were investigated for the frequency of SNHL. Out of 71 patients, 33 (46.4%) had SSNHL. This was recorded to occur in association with positive aCL compared to patients without SNHL ($p<0.001$).[25]

Antiphospholipid antibodies may activate endothelial cells within the cochlear circulation, directly or by inducing the formation of free radicals that cause damage to the endothelium. These upregulated endothelial cells would initiate local microthrombus formation and subsequent ischemia to the inner ear. In these cases, treatment is directed toward preventing thromboembolic events. Of these medications, only warfarin has been shown to be beneficial in achieving antithrombotic effect. However, it is also accepted that steroid therapy, in addition to its anti-inflammatory effect, may also protect neural tissues from ischemic injury, stabilize the vascular endothelium, and restore the blood–brain barrier to normal. Though anticoagulant therapy was reported to be useful in some patients with SSNHL, it cannot become a routine regimen in the absence of histological or imaging tools to demonstrate microthrombosis in the inner ear of patients with SSNHL. Thus, feature studies should establish clear standard approaches regarding the need to start with anticoagulation therapy in patients who were admitted with SSNHL.

17.3
ENT Emergencies in ANCA-Related Vasculitis

The vasculitides are a heterogeneous group of relatively uncommon diseases characterized by inflammatory cell infiltration and necrosis of blood vessel walls. ANCA-associated systemic vasculitides, including Wegener's granulomatosis (WG), Churg–Strauss syndrome (CSS), and microscopic polyangiitis (MPA), are mostly systemic but are rarely presented with selective organ damage. By involving small vessels, the nose and ear are target sites that should be looked for in ANCA-related vasculitis. Here, we focus on this involvement, pointing especially to ENT-emergencies in these diseases.

17.3.1
Wegener's Granulomatosis

Wegener's granulomatosis is a rare, multisystem disease involving in most patients face sinuses and the lungs. Kidneys are involved frequently together with the lungs, but in some cases, glomerulonephritis is a presenting symptom. Aiming to assess the prevalence of ENT involvement in WG, 199 patients were studied. In this study, 63% of patients initially presented with ENT-related symptoms. In most of them, the final diagnosis was late by 1 month. Undertreatment of ENT symptoms is a possible consequence of this, highlighting the need for awareness in thinking of WG in the ENT community.[26]

Nasal and paranasal sinuses involvement, are the most common affected sites, usually insidiously presented with nasal obstruction and chronic recurrent infections. Bloody or mucopurulent discharge, crusting, and nasal obstruction are also frequent manifestations. Pain over the face and nasal bridge occurs due to inflammation over the bony prominences or the sign of sinusitis.[27] In cases of inadequate treatment, saddle nose deformities can occur due to collapse of the nasal septum (Fig. 17.1). The disease process can also damage areas such as the maxillary ostia, erosion of the turbinates and, less commonly, damage to the soft palate. Nasal damage may lead to inflammation of the tear duct as well as conductive hearing loss. In rare cases, erosion of the hard palate can occur.

The second most common affected ENT site in WG is the ears. Hearing loss was reported to develop in 30% of patients, occurring mostly with other systemic symptoms that are

Fig. 17.1 Saddle nose deformity due to collapse of the nasal septum

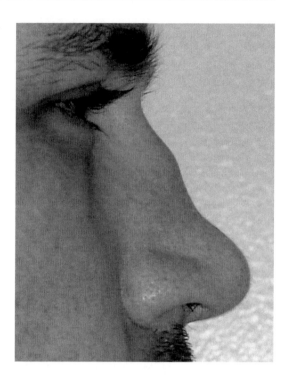

related to vasculitis.[28] Hearing loss, however, although uncommon, was reported to be a presenting symptom in WG. Since biopsy specimens are not available, awareness is crucial and C-ANCA (positive in most of these cases) should be looked for.[29] Hearing loss and tinnitus are frequently associated with otitis media (OM), and therefore, WG should be included in the differential diagnosis when atypical inflammation of the ear is presented.[30] Symptoms such as SNHL, vertigo, tympanic membrane perforation, and otorrhoea accompanied in some cases with facial nerve palsy are also not common but are all reported in the literature.[31] The oral cavity, hypopharynx, and larynx are the least commonly affected areas of the head and neck, but have characteristic presentations that are almost pathognomonic. Gingival inflammation and bleeding and deep painless mucosal ulcers are rare features of WG. However, the presence of a single ulcer in the hard palate surrounded by petechiae is suspicious of WG. The traditional description of gingival hyperplasia due to WG is strawberry gums, which is hyperplastic gingivitis with red–purple edematous interdental papillae diffusely covered with petechiae. Histological analysis is helpful in arriving to a diagnosis, but not always specific, so a combination of clinical assessment by a specialist and serological markers together with histological information form the mainstay of diagnosis. Involvement of the major salivary glands is rare and usually occurs early in the disease.[32,33]

In the larynx, WG manifests itself as subglottic stenosis, in 10–25% of patients, presenting with dyspnea on exertion and stridor or with voice changes and rarely, could be asymptomatic. The stenosis results from circumferential inflammation, edema, and fibrosis. It can be an anterior web or ring-like causing severe airway narrowing. Subglottic stenosis often occurs or progresses independently of features of active WG. The diagnosis is made by using flow-volume spirometry, and imaging technique as CT; however, a tissue biopsy is required for definite diagnosis.[34,35]

Measuring ANCA levels is of high diagnostic importance in patients with a clinical picture suggestive of vasculitis (e.g., unexplained sensorineural hearing loss) and with raised inflammatory markers. The expected result would be a cytoplasmic distribution on immunofluorescence and elevated proteinase-3 binding by ELISA.[36] Imaging in the acute setting can be used to exclude other diagnoses such as malignancy. CT scans is important for confirming bony destruction, bony thickening, and sclerosing osteitis. MRI scans can identify granulomas in the head and neck area as low-density masses in T1 and T2 sequences that exhibit heterogeneous enhancement with gadolinium.[37]

Currently, the standard of treatment for vasculitis affecting the ENT is cyclophosph-amide and corticosteroids until remission is achieved, followed by a less toxic immuno-suppressant such as azathioprine.[38] In cases limited to ENT involvement, methotrexate and corticosteroids have proven useful in achieving remission with the obvious advantage of avoiding exposure to cyclophosphamide.[39] Co-trimoxazole is advocated to prevent relapses in patients who are carriers of *Staphylococcus aureus*. Other treatments consist of relieving symptoms and treating concurrent infections. These include antibiotic drops for the ears in case of otitis externa or otitis media with a tympanic perforation, and oral antibiotics in the case of sinusitis. In some reports, it was demonstrated that topical treatments such as ste-roids and nasal irrigation are widespread, but their efficacy is questionable.If there is a middle ear effusion, grommets may be indicated. There is no long-term data from the use of grommets, particularly regarding prevention of damage. Mastoidectomies do not appear to benefit patients in terms of long-term hearing or decreased discharge in the presence of disease activity. Subglottic stenosis in the acute phase may respond to immunosuppres-sion, although many of these patients will require surgical intervention. These include dila-tations with balloons or bougies, laser or diathermy. In the acute phase, intralesional steroids have proven useful, especially in patients who develop subglottic stenosis in the absence of other features of active disease, allowing reducing the treatment-related toxicity. Currently, tracheostomies and stents are seldom used due to the effectiveness of immuno-suppression and success of repeated endoscopic procedures.[40]

17.3.2
Churg–Strauss Syndrome (CSS)

Churg–Strauss syndrome is a rare multisystem autoimmune disease characterized by diffuse eosinophilic infiltration and necrotizing vasculitis. Ear, nose, and throat involve-ment is common in CSS, usually manifesting as allergic rhinitis and chronic rhinosinusitis with or without polyps. The awareness of otolaryngologists is crucial in making an early diagnosis of ENT-CSS.

When patients with long-lasting asthma require additive therapies, the option of having CSS should be raised. This option is supported by the finding of high IgE levels, raised blood eosinophilia, and increased ESR. Non-fixed parenchymal abnormalities (infiltrates, nodules) in chest radiographic studies, peripheral neuropathy at electromyography, and ANCA positivity are highly characteristic for making a definite diagnosis.

When ENT manifestations were assessed in 21 well-defined CSS patients, the following was recorded: Of the 21 patients, 13 (61.9%) had ENT involvement at asthma onset and 8 (38%) during follow-up. The most common ENT manifestations were allergic rhinitis in nine (42.8%) patients and nasal polyposis in 16 (76.1%). Three (14.2%) patients developed chronic rhinosinusitis without polyps, three (14.2%) had nasal crusting, one (4.7%) serous otitis media, one (4.7%) purulent otitis media, two (9.5%) PSNHL, and one (4.7%) unilateral facial palsy.[41]

The involvement of ears in the course of CSS is reported to be in the range of 20% of patients. Possible otological manifestations include secretive otitis media, chronic ear drainage, and progressive SNHL, most of them occurred during the advanced phases of CSS. In another case report, otological involvement was characterized by dense aural discharge and granulomatous eosinophilic infiltrates in the mastoid and middle ear in association with SSNHL.[42,43] Although the exact mechanism of SNHL associated with CSS is unknown, it is believed to be the result of vasculitis of the internal auditory artery and the development of ischemia of the cranial nerve.

Of all laboratory findings, the most important are leukocytosis with marked eosinophilia (>10% eosinophils), elevated serum IgE levels, and high acute phase reactant levels. ANCA (mostly P-ANCA), though not specific, is a frequent finding and of high additive value in diagnosis. Tissue biopsy, although not obligatory for a definite diagnosis of CSS, should be obtained whenever possible in order to document histopathologic features of vasculitis or extravascular granulomas. Three major histological features are suggestive of CSS: necrotizing vasculitis, extravascular necrotizing granulomas, and tissue eosinophilia.[44]

Patients with active disease are treated with oral prednisone (1 mg/kg/day) proceeded by an intravenous methylprednisolone bolus of 1 g for 3 consecutive days, and cyclophosphamide (1.5–2 mg/kg/day), as induction treatment. Patients who experienced remission, maintenance therapy consisted of low doses of oral prednisone combined with immunosuppressive drugs (cyclophosphamide or methotrexate) for at least 1 year after remission.

17.3.3
Microscopic Polyangiitis (MPA)

MPA could present with upper airway symptoms, which resembles those of WG. Progressive ear disease – presented as sensorineural or conductive or mixed hearing loss – could represent the first manifestation of the disease. In such cases, the finding of myeloperoxidase-associated antineutrophil cytoplasmic antibody (MPO-ANCA) positive titers is a useful diagnostic marker.[45] The treatment of the disease is similar to the treatment which was mentioned above for WG or CSS.

17.4
Relapsing Polychondritis

Relapsing polychondritis (RP) is a rare, autoimmune condition characterized by recurrent inflammation of the cartilaginous structures of the external ear, nose, peripheral joints, larynx, and tracheobronchial tree, leading to destruction of cartilage and other connective tissues. Inflammation of other proteoglycan-rich structures, such as the eyes, heart, blood vessels, inner ear, and kidneys, may also be present. Its annual incidence is estimated to be about 3 per million. The average patient age at diagnosis is between 40 and 60 years, and both sexes are equally affected, with no familial tendency. It is believed that autoantibodies to cartilage components specifically IgG antibodies to type II collagen, which is restricted to and is the predominant collagen of cartilage, can be detected in one-half of patients, with titers corresponding to disease activity.[46,47]

Criteria for the diagnosis, as suggested by McAdams and colleagues, include three or more of the following clinical features:

1. Bilateral auricular chondritis
2. Nasal chondritis
3. Respiratory tract chondritis
4. Non-erosive seronegative inflammatory polyarthritis
5. Ocular inflammation (conjunctivitis, keratitis, scleritis/episcleritis, uveitis)
6. Cochlear and/or vestibular dysfunction (conductive hearing loss, tinnitus, and/or vertigo)
7. Compatible histological features in a cartilage biopsy specimen[48]

The diagnosis of the disease can also be based on the modified diagnostic criteria proposed by Michet et al.[49] Histopathologic studies reveal cartilage destruction with loss of basophilic staining and islands of lymphocytic infiltration. Subsequently, fragmentation of cartilage occurs with replacement by fibrous tissue.[50] The most frequent rheumatologic disorder associated with RP is systemic vasculitis followed by rheumatoid arthritis, systemic lupus erythematosis, and Sjögren syndrome.[48] Respiratory tract involvement is seen in 14–38% of patients with RP at presentation and in 48–67% throughout the course of the disease.[48,49] The mortality due to respiratory involvement reportedly accounts for up to 50% of the deaths from this disorder.[48,51] Tracheobronchomalacia (TBM), due to loss of the supportive cartilaginous scaffolding of the upper respiratory airways, can be seen as chronic sequelae of RP due to recurrent inflammation.[52] Respiratory compromise stemming from fixed airway obstruction or hyperdynamic collapse may cause significant morbidity and mortality.[48] Laryngotracheal involvement may initially manifest as recurrent cough, hoarseness, dyspnea, and anterior neck pain; stridor and wheezing may also be observed. The obstruction is due to edema, vocal cord palsy, and fixed subglottic or bronchial stenosis. In spite of aggressive medical therapy, in some patients, this may suddenly exacerbate to dynamic airway collapse necessitating the need for emergency tracheostomy, which may not be fully palliative due to frequent obstruction and malacia of more distal airways beyond the tracheotomy site.[53] Airway complications, including laryngeal collapse and tracheal stenosis, occur late in the disease course and can be fatal.[54] Therefore, whenever RP is diagnosed, aggressive immunosuppressive therapy ought to be initiated early to minimize the inflammatory destruction of cartilage that leads to life-threatening airway collapse.

The external ear inflammation is the most common feature of RP; it appears in up to 83% of the patients and could be present for days or weeks. The onset may be acute or subacute, and the affected auricles present a diffuse violaceous, erythematous appearance

Fig. 17.2 External diffuse violaceous
erythematous inflammation of
the ear

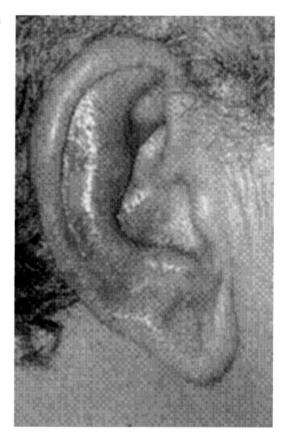

with sparing of the non-cartilaginous ear lobes (Fig. 17.2). Other otological feature may include secretory otitis media due to involvement of the Eustachian tube cartilage. Sensorineural or mixed hearing loss, bilateral or unilateral, is also known as a feature of RP that may occur suddenly or progress over the weeks. It can become more serious when it encroaches on the external auditory meatus, compromise hearing, and can affect the retro auricular soft tissue. Direct damage of the eighth nerve by "vasculitis" (internal auditory artery) may occur leading to ataxia, vertigo, nausea, and vomiting due to involvement of the vestibular portion can.[55-58]

Glucocorticoids, although have been disappointing in some cases, are the therapeutic choice for reducing the inflammatory process in patients with RP. Therefore, immuno-suppressants such as cyclophosphamide, azathioprine, cyclosporine, mycophenolate mofetil, and anti-tumor necrosis factor (anti-TNF) have been used for severe manifestations of refractory RP with varying degrees of efficacy. Other drugs, including nonsteroidal anti-inflammatory drugs, dapsone, and colchicine, have been proposed for mild cases. In case reports, plasmapheresis, anti-CD4 monoclonal antibodies, and autologous stem cell transplantation have also been suggested as an alternative treatment.[46]

17.5
Cogan's Syndrome

The earliest description of nonsyphilitic keratitis coexisting with vestibuloauditory disturbances, namely hearing loss and dizziness, was published by Morgan and Baumgarther in
1934.[59] In 1945, David Cogan, an ophthalmologist, described four patients with the same
symptoms and classified this entity as "Cogan's syndrome" (CS).[60] Fifteen years later,
Cody and Williams emphasized the systemic manifestations of this syndrome. Several
authors divide CS into typical and atypical varieties based on the type of ocular inflammation present. Typical CS manifests primarily with interstitial keratitis, whereas atypical CS
may exhibit scleritis, choroiditis ortenonitis, in addition to or instead of interstitial keratitis. Atypical CS is usually associated with systemic inflammatory vascular disease and
carries a less favorable prognosis than typical CS.[61,62]

The most common systemic features described in CS include: headache, arthralgia,
arthritis, myalgia, abdominal pain, vasculitis, aortic sclerosis, aortitis, and general features
such as fever and weight loss.[63] No laboratory or radiographic test is diagnostic of CS.
Although the cause of CS is unknown, an autoimmune-mediated cellular or humoral
process has been postulated by previous reports. This opinion has been supported by the
findings of antibodies against inner ear and corneal tissue, along with the presence of
a lymphocytic and plasma cell infiltrate in the cornea and inner ear.[64-66] The association of
CS with vasculitis and its response to corticosteroids and immunosuppressive drugs
support the notion of CS being an immune-mediated condition.

In a large series of 60 patients following CS throughout a half century at the Mayo
Clinic, the most otolaryngologic manifestations were hearing loss in all patients, 90% had
vertigo, 80% had tinnitus, 53% had ataxia, and 25% of the patients had oscillopsia. Hearing
loss was noted in both ears at some point in every patient. On examination, 20% of patients
had spontaneous and/or gaze-induced nystagmus sometime during the disease. A total of
46 out of 60 patients underwent formal vestibular function testing, of which 43 (93%) had
abnormal results. Many patients experienced symptoms of vestibulopathy that lasted for
days or weeks from the time of onset without resolution that frequently required hospitalization and/or rehabilitation. In almost 50% of the patients in this study, the presenting
syndrome was sudden hearing loss.[63]

Emergency admission to the ENT department includes patients with the classical audiovestibular presentation of CS; a sudden onset of nausea, vomiting, tinnitus, vertigo, and hearing
loss, usually bilateral.[62] Hearing loss may initially fluctuate with repeated attacks but generally
progresses to irreversible, bilateral deafness in 50–85% of patients.[63,67] Usually, the hearing
loss in CS is classified as sensorineural, preferentially affecting medium to high frequencies,
although a mechanical component has also been reported.[68] These manifestations and visual
symptoms usually occur either concurrently or sequentially within a few weeks to
months. Rarely, few years may separate the visual and audiovestibular manifestations.[63]
At the onset of audiovestibular dysfunction, rapid initiation of high-dose corticosteroids
(1–1.5 mg/kg of prednisone daily) is recommended. If there is no response after 2 weeks,
the steroids are rapidly tapered. Many reports have documented resolution of the hearing
loss with a similar regimen, but no controlled studies have been done. If hearing improves,

steroids are tapered slowly and continued for 2–6 months. In a 5-year follow-up, 95% of untreated patients had permanent hearing loss, while 55% of patients who were treated with systemic steroids within 2 weeks of initial hearing loss had hearing improvement, compared to only 8% of patients who were treated after 2 weeks.[62,69]

Other pharmacological therapies which were used in some of the patients in the Mayo Clinc series were methotrexate, cyclophosphamide, azathioprine, and infrequently, entanercept, ethambutol, hydroxychloroquine sulfate, and intravenous immunoglobulins. Even though half of the patients ended with profound hearing loss and eight patients underwent cochlear implantation.[63]

17.6
Summary

ENT is one of the many organs that are involved in various autoimmune inflammatory diseases namely, APS, SLE, ANCA-related vasculitis, and Cogan's syndrome. When ENT involvement is the only presenting symptom of these diseases, a delay in the diagnosis and therapy may cause serious organ damage. Thus, awareness of specialists of all disciplines is required in order to prevent the development of these emergencies and make a proper diagnosis on time.

References

1. McCabe BF. Autoimmune sensorineural hearing loss. *Ann Otol Rhinol Laryngol*. 1979;88: 585-589.
2. Baek MJ, Park HM, Johnson JM, et al. Increased frequencies of cochlin-specific T cells in patients with autoimmune sensorineural hearing loss. *J Immunol*. 2006;177(6):4203-4210.
3. Loveman DM, de Comarmond C, Cepero R, et al. Autoimmune sensorineural hearing loss: clinical course and treatment outcome. *Semin Arthritis Rheum*. 2004;34:538-543.
4. Bovo R, Ciorba A, Martini A. The diagnosis of autoimmune inner ear disease: evidence and critical pitfalls. *Eur Arch Otorhinolaryngol*. 2009;266(1):37-40.
5. Matteson EL, Fabry DA, Strome SE, et al. Autoimmune inner ear disease: diagnostic and therapeutic approaches in a multidisciplinary setting. *J Am Acad Audiol*. 2003;14:225-230.
6. Solares CA, Hughes GB, Tuohy VK. Autoimmune sensorineural hearing loss: an immunologic perspective. *J Neuroimmunol*. 2003;138:1-7.
7. Hefeneider SH, McCoy SL, Hausman FA, et al. Autoimmune mouse antibodies recognize multiple antigens proposed in human immune-mediated hearing loss. *Otol Neurotol*. 2004;25:250-256.
8. Kastanioudakis I, Ziavra N, Voulgari PV, et al. Ear involvement in systemic lupus erythematosus patients: a comparative study. *J Laryngol Otol*. 2002;116:103-107.
9. Takatsu M, Higaki M, Kinoshita H, et al. Ear involvement in patients with rheumatoid arthritis. *Otol Neurotol*. 2005;26:755-761.
10. Maciaszczyk K, Waszczykowska E, Pajor A, et al. Hearing organ disorders in patients with systemic sclerosis. *Rheumatol Int*. 2010: May 12. doi: 10.1007/s00296-010-1503-5.
11. Tomasi JP, Lona A, Deggouj N, et al. Autoimmune sensorineural hearing loss in young patients: an exploratory study. *Laryngoscope*. 2001;111:2050-2053.

12. Tebo AE, Szankasi P, Hillman TA, et al. Antibody reactivity to heat shock protein 70 and inner ear specific proteins in patients with idiopathic sensorineural hearing loss. *Clin Exp Immunol.* 2006;146:427-432.

13. Mathews J, Rao S, Kumar BN. Autoimmune sensorineural hearing loss: is it still a clinical diagnosis? *J Laryngol Otol.* 2003;117:212-214.

14. Chau JK, Lin JR, Atashband S, et al. Systematic review of the evidence for the etiology of adult sudden sensorineural hearing loss. *Laryngoscope.* 2010;120(5):1011-1021.

15. Lin HC, Chao PZ, Lee HC. Sudden sensorineural hearing loss increases the risk of stroke: a 5-year follow-up study. *Stroke.* 2008;39(10):2744-2748.

16. Asherson RA, Cervera R. Microvascular and microangiopathic antiphospholipid-associated syndromes: semantic or antisemantic? *Autoimmun Rev.* 2008;7(3):164-167.

17. Wiles NM, Hunt BJ, Callanan V, et al. Sudden sensorineural hearing loss and antiphospholipid syndrome. *Haematologica.* 2006;91(Suppl 12):ECR46.

18. Toubi E, Ben-David J, Kessel A, et al. Autoimmune aberration in sudden sensorineural hearing loss: association with anti-cardiolipin antibodies. *Lupus.* 1997;6:540-542.

19. Heller U, Becker EW, Zenner HP, et al. Incidence and clinical relevance of antibodies to phospholipids, serotonin and ganglioside in patients with sudden deafness and progressive inner ear hearing loss. *HNO.* 1998;46(6):583-586.

20. Toubi E, Ben-David J, Kessel A, et al. Immune-mediated disorders associated with idiopathic sudden sensorineural hearing loss. *Ann Otol Rhinol Laryngol.* 2004;113:445-449.

21. Mouadeb DA, Ruckenstein MJ. Antiphospholipid inner ear syndrome. *Laryngoscope.* 2005; 115(5):879-883.

22. Kang KT, Young YH. Sudden sensorineural hearing loss in a patient with primary antiphospholipid syndrome. *J Laryngol Otol.* 2008;122(2):204-206.

23. Wang JG, Xie QB, Yang NP, et al. Primary antiphospholipid antibody syndrome: a case with bilateral sudden sensorineural hearing loss. *Rheumatol Int.* 2009;29(4):467-468.

24. Compadretti GC, Brandolini C, Tasca I. Sudden SNHL in lupus erythematosus associated with antiphospholipid syndrome. *Ann Otol Rhinol Laryngol.* 2005;114(3):214-218.

25. Hajas A, Szodoray P, Barath S, et al. Sensorineural hearing loss in patients with mixed connective tissue disease: immunological markers and cytokine levels. *J Rheumatol.* 2009;36(9): 1930-1936.

26. Srouji IA, Andrews P, Edwards C, et al. Patterns of presentation and diagnosis of patients with Wegener's granulomatosis: ENT aspects. *J Laryngol Otol.* 2007;121:653-658.

27. Rasmussen N. Management of the ear, nose, and throat manifestations of Wegener granulomatosis: an otorhinolaryngologist's perspective. *Curr Opin Rheumatol.* 2001;13:3-11.

28. Seo P, Min YI, Holbrook JT, et al. Damage caused by Wegener's granulomatosis and its treatment: prospective data from WG etanercept trial. *Arthritis Rheum.* 2005;52(7):2168-2178.

29. Takagi D, Nakamaru Y, Maguchi S, et al. Otologic manifestations of Wegener's granulomatosis. *Laryngoscope.* 2002;112:1684-1690.

30. Lidar M, Carmel E, Kronenberg Y, et al. Hearing loss as the presenting feature of systemic vasculitis. *Ann NY Acad Sci.* 2007;1107:136-141.

31. Martinez DPM, Sivasothy P. Vasculitis of the upper and lower airway. *Best Pract Res Clin Rheumatol.* 2009;23(3):403-417.

32. Stewart C, Cohen D, Bhattacharyya I, et al. Oral manifestations of Wegener's granulomatosis: a report of three cases and a literature review. *J Am Dent Assoc.* 2007;138(3):338-348.

33. Gottschlich S, Ambrosch P, Kramkowski D, et al. Head and neck manifestations of Wegener's granulomatosis. *Rhinology.* 2006;44:227-233.

34. Blaivas AJ, Strauss W, Yudd M. Subglottic stenosis as a complication of Wegener's granulomatosis. *Prim Care Respir J.* 2008;17(2):114-116.

35. Solans-Laque R, Bosch-Gil J, Canela M, et al. Clinical features and therapeutic management of subglottic stenosis in patients with Wegener's granulomatosis. *Lupus.* 2008;17:832-836.

36. Wiik A. Rational use of ANCA in the diagnosis of vasculitis. *Rheumatology (Oxford)*. 2002; 41:481-483.

37. Lohrmann C, Uhl M, Warnatz K, et al. Sinonasal computed tomography in patients with Wegener's granulomatosis. *J Comput Assist Tomogr*. 2006;30:122-125.

38. Jayne D. How to induce remission in primary systemic vasculitis. *Best Pract Res Clin Rheumatol*. 2005;19:293-305.

39. De Groot K, Rasmussen N, Bacon PA, et al. Randomized trial of cyclophosphamide versus methotrexate for induction of remission in early systemic antineutrophil cytoplasmic antibody-associated vasculitis. *Arthritis Rheum*. 2005;52:2461-2469.

40. Nouraei SA, Obholzer R, Ind PW, et al. Results of endoscopic surgery and intralesional steroid therapy for airway compromise due to tracheobronchial Wegener's granulomatosis. *Thorax*. 2008;63:49-52.

41. Bacciu A, Bacciu S, Mercante G, et al. Ear, nose and throat manifestations of Churg-Strauss syndrome. *Acta Otolaryngol*. 2006;126:503-509.

42. Solans R, Bosch JA, Pe'rez-Bocanegra C, et al. Churg-Strauss syndrome: outcome and long term follow-up of 32 patients. *J Rheumatol*. 2001;40(7):763-771.

43. Ovadia S, Dror I, Zubkov T, et al. Churg-Strauss syndrome: a rare presentation with otological and pericardial manifestations: case report and review of literature. *Clin Rheumatol*. 2009;28(Suppl 1):S35-S38.

44. Ishiyama A, Canalis RF. Otological manifestations of Churg-Strauss syndrome. *Laryngoscope*. 2001;111(9):1619-1624.

45. Papadimitraki ED, Kyrmizakis DE, Kritikos I, et al. Ear-nose-throat manifestations of autoimmune rheumatic diseases. *Clin Exp Rheumatol*. 2004;22:485-494.

46. Lahmer T, Treiber M, von Werder A, et al. Relapsing polychondritis: an autoimmune disease with many faces. *Autoimmun Rev*. 2010;9(8):540-546.

47. Zeuner M, Straub RH, Rauh G, et al. Relapsing polychondritis: clinical and immunogenetic analysis of 62 patients. *J Rheumatol*. 1997;24:96-101.

48. McAdam LP, O'Hanlan MA, Bluestone R, et al. Relapsing polychondritis: prospective study of 23 patients and a review of the literature. *Medicine (Baltimore)*. 1976;55:193-215.

49. Michet CJ, McKenna CH Jr, Luthra HS, et al. Relapsing polychondritis. Survival and predictive role of early disease manifestations. *Ann Intern Med*. 1986;104(1):74-78.

50. Sarodia BD, Dasgupta A, Mehta AC. Management of airway manifestations of relapsing polychondritis: case reports and review of literature. *Chest*. 1999;116:1669-1675.

51. Gergely P Jr, Poor G. Relapsing polychondritis. *Best Pract Res Clin Rheumatol*. 2004;18: 723-738.

52. Adliff M, Ngato D, Keshavjee S, et al. Treatment of diffuse tracheomalacia secondary to relapsing polychondritis with continuous positive airway pressure. *Chest*. 1997;112:1701-1704.

53. Behar JV, Choi YW, Hartman TA, et al. Relapsing polychondritis affecting the lower respiratory tract. *AJR Am J Roentgenol*. 2002;178:173-177.

54. Carrion M, Giron JA, Ventura J, et al. Airway complications in relapsing polychondritis. *J Rheumatol*. 1993;20:1628-1629.

55. Cody DT, Sones DA. Relapsing polychondritis: audiovestibular manifestations. *Laryngoscope*. 1971;81(8):1208-1222.

56. Kumakiri K, Sakamoto T, Karahashi T, et al. A case of relapsing polychondritis preceded by inner ear involvement. *Auris Nasus Larynx*. 2005;32(1):71-76.

57. Tsuda T, Nakajima A, Baba S, et al. A case of relapsing polychondritis with bilateral sensorineural hearing loss and perforation of the nasal septum at the onset. *Mod Rheumatol*. 2007;17(2):148-152.

58. Bachor E, Blevins NH, Karmody C. Otologic manifestations of relapsing polychondritis. Review of literature and report of nine cases. *Auris Nasus Larynx*. 2006;33(2):135-141.

59. Morgan RF, Baumgartner CJ. Meniere's disease complicated by recurrent interstitial keratitis: excellent result following cervical ganglionectomy. *West J Surg.* 1934;42:628-631.
60. Cogan DS. Syndrome of nonsyphilitic interstitial keratitis and vestibuloauditory symptoms. *Arch Ophthalmol.* 1945;33:144-149.
61. Cody DTR, Williams HL. Cogan's syndrome. *Laryngoscope.* 1960;70:477.
62. Haynes BF, Kaiser-Kupfer MI, Mason P, et al. Cogan syndrome: studies in thirteen patients, long-term follow-up, and a review of the literature. *Medicine.* 1980;59:426-441.
63. Gluth MB, Baratz KH, Matteson EL, et al. Cogan syndrome: a retrospective review of 60 patients throughout a half century. *Mayo Clin Proc.* 2006;81(4):483-488.
64. Arnold W, Gebbers JO. Serum antibodies against corneal and internal ear tissues in Cogan's syndrome. *Laryngol Rhinol Otol.* 1984;63:428-432.
65. Arnold W, Pfaltz R, Altermatt HJ. Evidence of serum antibodies against inner ear tissues in the blood of patients with certain sensorneural hearing disorders. *Acta Otolaryngol.* 1985;99:437-444.
66. Wolff D, Bernhardt WG, Tsutsumi S, et al. The pathology of Cogan's syndrome causing profound deafness. *Ann Otol Rhinol Laryngol.* 1965;74:507-520.
67. McDonald TJ, Vollertsen RS, Younger BR. Cogan's syndrome: audiovestibular involvement and prognosis in 18 patients. *Laryngoscope.* 1985;95:650-654.
68. Majoor MHJM, Albers FWJ, Casselman JW. Clinical relevance of magnetic resonance imaging and computed tomography in Cogan's syndrome. *Acta Otolaryngol.* 1993;113:625-631.
69. Vollertsen RS, Mcdonald TJ, Younge BR, et al. Cogan's syndrome: 18 cases and a review of the literature. *Mayo Clin Proc.* 1986;61:344-361.

Ophthalmological Emergencies in Rheumatic and Autoimmune Diseases

18

Edward Pringle and Miles Stanford

Abstract Sight-threatening autoimmune conditions affect different parts of the visual pathway. This chapter considers ophthalmic emergencies classified anatomically with a discussion of the underlying autoimmune diseases and treatment options. Ophthalmic complications of immunomodulatory treatments are discussed. Finally, the impact of newer immunomodulatory treatments is reviewed.

Keywords Keratitis • Optic neuropathy • Orbital inflammatory disease • Retinal vasculopathy • Scleritis • Uveitis

18.1
Introduction

Almost any disease process, be it a degeneration, infection, inflammation, tumor, or toxic agent, can affect the visual system. While the range of presenting symptoms may not be diverse, namely, pain, red eye, loss of vision, or double vision, it is the subtleties of the history of the presenting complaint and examination that often lead to a useful differential diagnosis. It is important for the ophthalmologist to be aware that the eye may be the presenting organ in life-threatening vasculitis. Conversely, the internist should be aware that an inflammatory process may cause a potentially blinding disease. In this chapter, we review the ophthalmic emergencies that occur in rheumatic and autoimmune diseases. We do this first by the anatomical structure affected, then by reviewing effects of drugs and immunosuppression.

E. Pringle (✉)
Department of Clinical Ophthalmology, Medical Eye Unit, St. Thomas' Hospital,
160 Gloucester Place, NW1 6DT London, UK
e-mail: edwardpringle@doctors.org.uk

M.A. Khamashta and M. Ramos-Casals (eds.), *Autoimmune Diseases*,
DOI: 10.1007/978-0-85729-358-9_18, © Springer-Verlag London Limited 2011

18.2
Anterior Segment

The anterior segment of the eye involves all structures of the globe anterior to the lens. This includes the anterior sclera, cornea, conjunctiva, and anterior uveal tract (the ciliary body and iris). The blood supply to the anterior segment arises from anterior and long posterior ciliary arteries, which are branches of the ophthalmic artery, which itself is a branch of the internal carotid artery. The anterior and long posterior ciliary arteries anastomose to create the major arterial circle of the iris, which supplies the iris, ciliary body, and the anterior conjunctiva and episclera. The superficial and deep episcleral plexuses which are involved in episcleritis and scleritis, respectively, are branches of this arterial circle.

18.2.1
Anterior Scleritis

18.2.1.1
Epidemiology

Scleritis is an uncommon disease with an estimated prevalence between 3 and 10 per 10,000 of the general population. In the rheumatoid arthritis population, the prevalence increases to approximately 1%. Rheumatoid-associated scleritis accounts for 10–33% of all scleritis.

18.2.1.2
Symptoms and Signs

Anterior scleritis causes a red eye (Fig. 18.1). The hallmark is intense pain (Table 18.1). It may disrupt sleep and is often described as dull or aching pain centered in the orbit or eye. The pain may be modulated by concurrent use of immunosuppressive agents. The inflamed

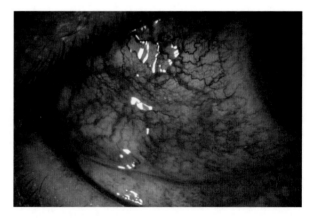

Fig. 18.1 Diffuse anterior scleritis

Table 18.1 Key warning symptoms with in patients with acute red eye

Symptom	Significance
Light sensitivity/photophobia	Any corneal pathology
	Uveitis
Severe pain (may prevent sleeping)	Scleritis
	Acute angle closure glaucoma
Loss of vision	Acute angle closure glaucoma
	Corneal melting
	Longstanding anterior uveitis
	Posterior uveitis

and dilated scleral vessels are more easily visualized at the slit lamp where they are found deep to the overlying conjunctiva and episclera. Instillation of a dilute topical solution of phenylephrine does not blanch the inflamed scleral vessels in scleritis, unlike episcleritis. The inflammation may cause scleral necrosis which may expose the underlying uveal tract and lead to sight-threatening globe perforations. Figure 18.2 shows scleral thinning, which occurs once the active phase of scleritis has settled.

18.2.1.3
Associated Systemic Diseases

Systemic autoimmune diseases are present in up to 50% of patients and include: rheumatoid arthritis, systemic vasculitis (particularly Wegener granulomatosis), systemic lupus erythematosus, inflammatory bowel disease, and relapsing polychondritis. Rheumatoid patients with scleritis tend to have more aggressive systemic disease than those without scleritis. In the rheumatoid patient, when necrotizing anterior scleritis occurs, it correlates with a rheumatoid vasculitis and increased cardiovascular mortality.

Wegener granulomatosis is the most commonly encountered of the systemic vasculitides. Scleritis is an uncommon manifestation of systemic lupus erythematosis, but may be

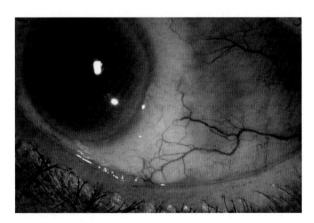

Fig. 18.2 Scleral thinning following an episode of anterior scleritis with necrosis

associated with flares in systemic disease requiring aggressive medical therapy. Although uveitis is the most common ocular manifestation of inflammatory bowel disease, in large series of patients with scleritis, the prevalence of inflammatory bowel disease was 5%. Scleritis is the commonest ocular manifestation of relapsing polychondritis, which is characterized by recurrent potentially destructive inflammation of type II collagen present in the sclera, ears, nose, joints, cardiovascular system, and trachea (which may cause airway collapse).

18.2.1.4
Treatment

Non-necrotizing scleritis may be controlled with nonsteroidal anti-inflammatory drugs. Those who do not respond may need additional immunosuppression to prevent globe perforation from scleral necrosis: It is vital to have an infectious agent excluded (viral, bacterial, fungal, or parasitic) before commencing immunosuppressive therapy. Patients with any evidence of scleral necrosis need immediate high-dose systemic immunosuppression.[1] Corticosteroids can be given as a local orbital floor injection, orally or intravenously depending on the extent and severity of disease. A variety of steroid sparing agents including azathioprine, methotrexate, cyclosporin, mycophenolate, cyclophosphamide, and rituximab have been reported to be effective in case series.

18.2.2
Peripheral Ulcerative Keratitis

18.2.2.1
Symptoms and Signs

Peripheral ulcerative keratitis is a condition whereby the peripheral cornea melts away under the influence of collagenase derived from polymorphonuclear leucocytes secondary to immune complex deposition in inflamed limbal vessels as part of scleritis. It presents with pain, light sensitivity (photophobia), a red eye and may cause loss of vision (Table 18.2). The melting of the corneal stroma causes corneal distortion and reduces vision. This may progress to globe perforation.[2] The slit lamp demonstrates the peripheral crescentic thinning of the cornea, the overlying epithelium maybe intact, and the adjacent sclera maybe injected (Fig. 18.3).

18.2.2.2
Associated Systemic Diseases

Rheumatoid arthritis, systemic lupus erythematosus, Wegener granulomatosis, relapsing polychondritis, polyarteritis nodosa, microscopic polyangiitis, and Churg-Strauss syndrome have all been associated with peripheral ulcerative keratitis.[3,4] As with scleritis, rheumatoid arthritis is the most common association. Case series of rheumatoid patients with peripheral ulcerative keratitis demonstrate higher mortality rates.

Table 18.2 Causes of loss of vision in autoimmune disease

Reason	Diagnostic clues	Example
Refractive change	Vision improves looking through a pinhole, or with glasses This is usually a gradual process (weeks to months), but patients may become suddenly aware of the change when the better eye becomes occluded	Corneal melt associated with vasculitis
Cataracts	Poor red reflex on fundoscopy Usually a gradual process	Posterior subcapsular lens opacities with steroid use
Vitreous hemorrhage	Loss of vision over minutes to hours No red reflex on fundoscopy	Many months following an ischemic retinal vein occlusion
Exudative retinal detachment	Gradual onset loss of vision Severe pain with posterior scleritis Fundoscopy demonstrates the retinal elevations	Posterior scleritis
Retinal vein occlusion	Sudden onset Typical striking fundoscopic appearance with multiple retinal hemorrhages	Macular branch retinal vein occlusion in Behçets disease
Retinal artery occlusion	Sudden onset Superior or inferior field defect in the affected eye Fundoscopic appearances are subtle Foveal 'Cherry red spot' may be seen	Retinal artery occlusion in giant cell arteritis
Retinal microangiopathy	Maybe asymptomatic Maybe vague blurring of vision in either eye Fundoscopy reveals cotton wool spots in the optic disk	Lupus retinopathy
Optic neuritis	Pain on eye movements followed by monocular visual loss Red desaturation (reduced color vision) Relative afferent papillary defect	Multiple sclerosis
Acute ischemic optic neuropathy	Sudden onset of loss of vision Very poor visual acuity Relative afferent papillary defect	Giant cell arteritis
Compressive optic neuropathy from orbital disease	Gradual onset of loss of vision Ocular motility may be disturbed causing double vision Proptosis Relative afferent papillary defect	Thyroid eye disease

18.2.2.3
Treatment

Peripheral ulcerative keratitis when associated with systemic vasculitis may indicate life-threatening disease. Treatment is designed to control pain, prevent globe perforation, and identify any other organ involvement. Local topical treatment is often inadequate, and treatment usually requires potent systemic immunosuppression. In the setting of rheumatoid

Fig. 18.3 Peripheral ulcerative keratitis. The corneal thinning is seen as the slit beam of light passes through the cornea. The yellow stain is due to pooling of fluorescein dye applied during the examination

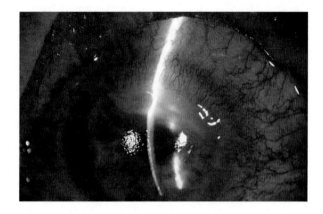

arthritis, high-dose prednisolone with ciclosporin, methotrexate, or azathioprine has been tried, reserving pulsed cyclophosphamide for therapeutic failures.[5] Perforation may need a tectonic corneal graft to maintain the integrity of the globe.[6]

18.2.3
HLA B27 Spondyloarthropathy–Associated Uveitis

18.2.3.1
Symptoms and Signs

Anterior uveitis presents with red eye and photophobia. When untreated, the pain can become severe and vision can been reduced. A hypopyon (a white fluid level of inflammatory cells and debris) may form in the anterior chamber.[7] As the disease evolves, macular edema can occur and reduce central vision. All patients presenting with an anterior uveitis need a detailed examination of the posterior segment to exclude other inflammatory, infective, ischemic, or neoplastic processes which may also cause an anterior uveitis.

18.2.3.2
Associated Systemic Diseases

The lifetime risk of developing anterior uveitis in a patient who is HLA B*27 positive is 1%; this rises to 40% in a patient with associated spondyloarthropathy. Anterior uveitis affects 30% of patients with ankylosing spondylitis,[8] 5% of patients with ulcerative colitis and is well reported in psoriatic patients and those with reactive arthritis.[9,10]

18.2.3.3
Treatment

Patients usually respond well to a tapering course of topical corticosteroids which need to be started early in the disease process to prevent complications. In severe attacks, hourly drops of a strong topical steroid such as dexamethasone 0.1% may not be adequate.

Subconjunctival steroids will often gain control; it is rare that systemic corticosteroids,[11] orbital floor steroids, or intravitreal steroids are required.

18.2.4
Juvenile Idiopathic Arthritis

18.2.4.1
Epidemiology

Juvenile idiopathic arthritis (JIA) is the commonest childhood autoimmune disease affecting 1 in 1,000 children. The frequency of associated uveitis varies with subtype, but is most severe in young girls with pauciarticular disease with antinuclear antibodies.[12]

18.2.4.2
Symptoms and Signs

Early disease is asymptomatic, with symptoms such as visual loss from cataract, glaucoma, or band keratopathy (calcium deposition in the cornea) appearing late in the disease. This has given rise to a variety of screening protocols for different groups. Ocular complications maybe prevented by early detection.[13]

18.2.4.3
Treatment

In sight-threatening disease, methotrexate is often used as the first-line disease-modifying agent. Biologicals targeting tumor necrosis factor alpha-α (TNF-α, such as etanercept, infliximab, and adalimumab), and cytotoxic T-lymphocyte–associated antigen 4 (CTLA-4, such as abatacept) have been approved for use by the Food and Drug Administration in the USA. Anakinra (targets IL-1), rituximab (targets CD20), and tocilizumab (targets IL-6) have also been tried.[14]

18.3
Posterior Segment

The posterior segment of the eye involves the vitreous cavity, retina and retinal vasculature, posterior uveal tract (the choroid), and sclera. The central retinal artery can be considered as an end artery of the ophthalmic artery; at the optic disk, it splits into four branches supplying four quadrants of the inner two-thirds of the retina. The outer third of the retina is supplied by the highly vascularized choroid. The choroid is supplied by the numerous short ciliary arteries and recurrent branches of the long ciliary arteries. The choroid vessels fill hexagonal lobules. If vasculitis affects the short ciliary arteries, this can give rise to watershed filling defects seen with fluorescein angiography. Although this sign is not always present, it is highly specific for a systemic vasculitis.

18.3.1
Posterior Scleritis

18.3.1.1
Symptoms and Signs

Posterior scleritis may present with a white, painful eye. As with anterior scleritis, the hallmark is intense pain especially on eye movement. Loss of vision can occur due to exudative retinal detachment (Fig. 18.4),[15] retinal or choroidal folds, peripheral choroidal detachments (causing secondary angle closure glaucoma), subretinal mass lesion (Fig. 18.5), and optic nerve involvement. These signs may be identified by detailed anterior and posterior segment examination by an ophthalmologist, although 15% of patients may have no abnormal physical signs. In the absence of other physical signs, the diagnosis rests on the history and imaging. B-mode ocular ultrasonography enables visualization of the thickened sclera and fluid within the Tenon capsule. It is quick, sensitive, and noninvasive.

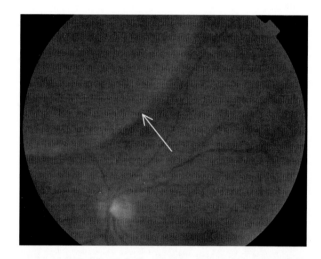

Fig. 18.4 Exudative retinal detachment (*white arrow*)

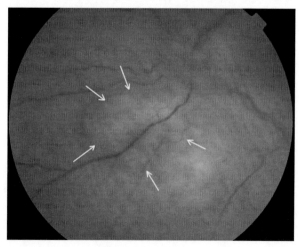

Fig. 18.5 Posterior scleritis presenting with a subretinal mass (*outlined by arrows*)

18.3.1.2
Associated Systemic Diseases

The spectrum of associated diseases is similar to that of anterior scleritis: rheumatoid arthritis, systemic vasculitis (particularly Wegener granulomatosis[16]), systemic lupus erythematosis, inflammatory bowel disease, and relapsing polychondritis.[17]

18.3.1.3
Treatment

As with anterior scleritis, if there is no visual threat, the disease and pain may be treated with nonsteroidal anti-inflammatory drugs. Immunosuppressive agents are often required for unresponsive or sight-threatening diseases, and the same agents are used for anterior scleritis. It is important to have considered and excluded other infective or neoplastic disease processes prior to starting immunosuppression.

18.3.2
Retinal Vascular Occlusions

Retinal vascular occlusions can affect the arterial or venous system. Retinal artery occlusion in the elderly is commonly caused by embolic phenomenon, warranting the same investigation and treatment as a cerebrovascular accident. Importantly, however, it may also be caused by vasculitis, particularly giant cell arteritis, which rapidly progresses to blind both eyes.

When retinal vascular occlusions occur in association with systemic vasculitis, it is not certain whether the mechanism is due to the inflammatory process causing occlusion by infiltration of the vessel wall, immune complex deposition,[18] or other thrombotic consequences of the systemic disease.[19,20] With the exception of giant cell arteritis, systemic vasculitis–associated retinal vascular occlusions generally occur in a younger age group. It is of note that these occlusions are rarely associated with intraocular inflammation, apart from the venous occlusions seen in Behçets disease.

18.3.3
Retinal Artery Occlusion in Inflammatory Disease

18.3.3.1
Symptoms and Signs

Sudden onset monocular blurred vision. Identifying the precise onset of the monocular disturbance may be difficult. The affected retinal arterioles are attenuated, and corresponding retinal sectors are edematous and look slightly pale in comparison to normal. When a central retinal artery is occluded, the entire retina appears pale except the fovea which retains its blood supply from the underlying choroid. This gives rise to the foveal "cherry red spot" seen in central retinal artery occlusions. The slow movement of individual blood cells in the returning retinal venules can be seen.

18.3.3.2
Associated Inflammatory Diseases

All the systemic vasculitides have been associated with retinal arterial disease.[21] It is important to consider giant cell arteritis, systemic lupus erythematosis, antiphospholipid syndrome, scleroderma, and relapsing polychondritis as well as the medium vessel ANCA-positive vasculitides.

18.3.3.3
Treatment

The primary treatment is directed at the underlying inflammatory disease. Giant cell arteritis can rapidly progress to blind both eyes; a high index of suspicion and early treatment with high-dose corticosteroids can save sight in this condition.

18.3.4
Retinal Vein Occlusion in Inflammatory Disease

18.3.4.1
Symptoms and Signs

Sudden onset blurred vision in the affected eye (Table 18.2). Patients are not always aware of a monocular disturbance in vision, and precisely identifying the onset of a vein occlusion is not always possible. If there is associated inflammation of the vitreous gel, known as a vitritis, then the inflammatory cells can be perceived by the patient; this is not true of cells in the anterior chamber. The cells of vitritis are described as floating dots, flies, or cobwebs in the visual space called "floaters." "Floaters" are seen when the vitreous gel contains inflammatory cells (vitritis), red blood cells (vitreous hemorrhage), or if the vitreous body detaches from the retina (posterior vitreous detachment) (Table 18.3).

Multiple retinal hemorrhages are seen when vein occlusions occur (Fig. 18.6). These hemorrhages are in the territory of the draining venule. They may occupy a small sector (branch vein occlusion), the inferior or superior half or the retina (hemi-vein occlusion) or all four retinal quadrants (central retinal vein occlusion).

The retinal veins may also be surrounded by a cuff of inflammatory cells, known as periphlebitis (Fig. 18.7). Retinal infiltrates may also be seen in Behçets disease (Fig. 18.8).

18.3.4.2
Associated Inflammatory Diseases

Behçets disease may present with a retinal vein occlusion and other evidence of intraocular inflammation. Antiphospholipid syndrome can cause retinal vein occlusion without any intraocular inflammation. Sarcoidosis, inflammatory bowel disease, and seronegative arthropathies have all been associated with retinal vein occlusions.

Table 18.3 Causes of visual floaters

Floater type	Cause	Example
Posterior vitreous detachment	Age-related vitreous degeneration	Normal age-related event
Red blood cell in the vitreous	New vessel formation (which bleed) following an ischemic retinal vascular process	Proliferative diabetic retinopathy Ischemic central retinal vein occlusion
White blood cells in the vitreous	Vitritis related to a uveitis	Posterior uveitis
Retinal pigment epithelial cells in the vitreous	Retinal tear or retinal detachment from traction on the retina	Myopic patients retinal detachments. This is usually unrelated to any inflammatory process

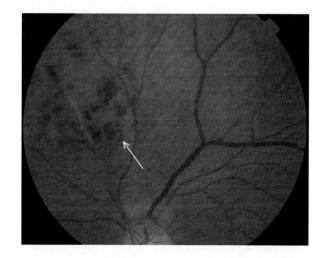

Fig. 18.6 A branch retinal vein occlusion in a patient with Behçets disease. Retinal hemorrhages (*arrowed*) surround the occluded vein

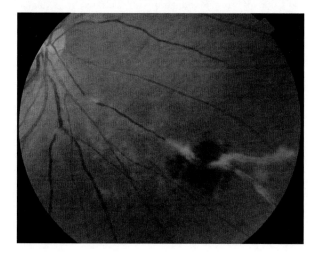

Fig. 18.7 An area of periphlebitis involving a vein inferotemporal to the optic disk

Fig. 18.8 A retinal infiltrate
(*arrowed*) in a patient with
Behçets disease

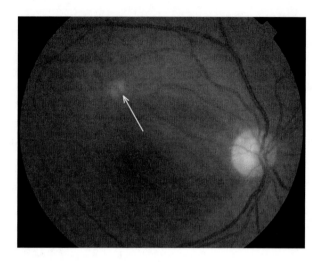

18.3.4.3
Treatment and Complications

The primary treatment is of the underlying inflammatory disease and the associated throm-botic tendencies. Patients with retinal vein occlusions can develop a neovascular response that may require specific ophthalmic treatment. Iris neovascularization can cause blinding and painful glaucoma. Retinal neovascularization can cause bleeding into the vitreous (vit-reous hemorrhage) which may initially be perceived by the patient as floaters, but soon fills the entire vitreous causing loss of vision. Retinal neovascularization may progress and cause tractional retinal detachments with loss of vision. The neovascular response occurs because of retinal ischemia and may been treated with retinal laser photocoagulation,[22] or the instillation of triamcinolone or anti-vascular endothelial growth factor (VEGF) which can be injected into the vitreous cavity. Macular edema may occur following vein occlusion and causes blurring and distortion of central vision. Macular laser, corticosteroids (orally, peribulbar or intravitreal), and intravitreal anti-VEGF agents have been used to treat this.

18.3.5
Ocular Ischemic Syndrome

Occlusion of the ophthalmic artery or all its branches may result in an ocular ischemic syndrome affecting the anterior and posterior segments.

18.3.5.1
Symptoms and Signs

Loss of vision occurs from retinal artery under perfusion or retinal ganglion cell death from raised intraocular pressure (glaucoma). Pain can be caused by corneal epithelial blistering (bullae) secondary to glaucoma. The profound ocular ischemia causes an aggressive intraocular neovascular response leading to new vessel growth on the iris, known as rubeosis. Iris rubeosis may be visualized with slit lamp microscope; if new vessels occlude the trabecular meshwork, the intraocular pressure will rise causing "rubeotic glaucoma."

18.3.5.2
Associated Inflammatory Diseases

Large vessel systemic vasculitis such as giant cell arteritis and Takayasu's arteritis.

18.3.5.3
Treatment

The underlying vasculitis should be controlled. Ocular manifestations are difficult to manage. Retinal laser photocoagulation and intravitreal anti-VEGF agents have been tried to reduce the intraocular neovascular response. When intraocular pressure becomes uncontrolled, topical medical therapies are often futile, surgical drainage procedures have a high failure rate, and occasionally, destruction of the ciliary body, which produces aqueous, may be required and in desperate cases, the eye may need to be enucleated.

18.3.6
Retinal Microangiopathy

18.3.6.1
Symptoms and Signs

Retinal microangiopathy rarely produces symptoms, but is an important sign since it often indicates a major flare of systemic vasculitis usually with renal and cerebral involvement. The hallmark of a retinal microangiopathy is the appearance of multiple cotton wool spots which may be seen at the posterior pole near to the optic disk (Fig. 18.9). They represent disruption of axonal transport in the retinal ganglion cells and mark the borders of an area of inner retinal ischemia.[23]

18.3.6.2
Associated Systemic Diseases

All the systemic vasculitides can present with cotton wool spots. They are commonly seen in systemic lupus, and in this situation, they may herald the onset of a life-threatening renal

Fig. 18.9 Cotton wool spots
around the optic disk

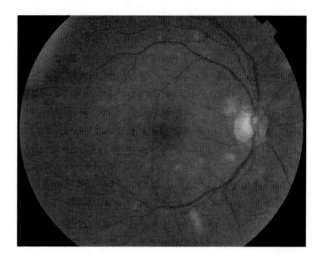

vasculitis. It is important for the ophthalmologist to check the renal function and blood pressure and to urgently involve the internist or rheumatologist.

18.3.6.3
Treatment

The underlying vasculitis should be controlled. The cotton wool spots themselves do not warrant any specific ocular treatment and usually resolve within 6 weeks.

18.3.7
Choroidal Infarction

18.3.7.1
Symptoms and Signs

Blurred vision in one or both eyes. The fundus examination in the early stages may demonstrate pale areas deep to the retina. Over time these evolve into pigmented and hypopigmented scars. Choroidal ischemia can be identified by fluorescein and indocyanine green angiography (Fig. 18.10).

18.3.7.2
Associated Systemic Diseases

All the systemic vasculitides can produce choroidal infarction.[24]

Fig. 18.10 Choroidal infarction in vasculitis. In this fundus fluorescein angiogram, a watershed is seen (*arrowed*) between nonperfused and perfused choroid

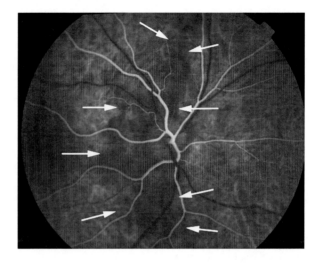

18.4
Optic Nerve

The optic nerve is the continuation of the retinal ganglion cells passing from the optic disk to the optic chiasm. The optic nerve head is supplied by the central retinal artery, the circle of Zinn (formed by the choroid and short posterior ciliary arteries), and small vessels of the pial plexus of the surrounding meninges.

18.4.1
Optic Neuritis in Systemic Vasculitis

18.4.1.1
Symptoms and Signs

Optic neuritis causes pain on eye movement. This may precede visual loss by a few days. The loss of vision is usually monocular (only one nerve affected) and typically affects the central visual field. Blurring of vision may progress over days. Color vision is impaired during optic neuritis, and patients may be aware of "red desaturation" in the affected eye. The pupil responses may be abnormal: A relative afferent pupil defect (RAPD) may be present. Fundoscopy may be entirely normal, or the optic disk may be swollen and hemorrhagic.

Optic neuritis associated with central nervous system demyelination, such as in multiple sclerosis, usually follows a benign course with resolution of pain in the first few weeks and improvement in visual acuity within 5 weeks without treatment. This is not the case in optic neuritis in association with systemic vasculitis where pain or visual loss may be unusually severe or prolonged and requires early treatment.

18.4.1.2
Associated Systemic Diseases

Optic neuritis has been described in association with a variety of systemic vasculitides including rheumatoid arthritis and Wegener granulomatosis.

18.4.1.3
Treatment

These patients require urgent high-dose corticosteroids and/or second-line immunosuppressive agents. Prolonged treatment is often required to prevent visual relapse.

18.4.2
Acute Ischemic Optic Neuropathy

18.4.2.1
Symptoms and Signs

Sudden and profound loss of vision involving the entire visual field (rather than an altitudinal hemifield defect seen in non-arteritic disease) is characteristic of a systemic vasculitis. Systemic vasculitis may affect multiple different vascular territories simultaneously, for example, multiple short posterior ciliary arteries and the central retinal artery. The presence of scalp tenderness, headaches, jaw claudication, or proximal myalgias is suggestive of giant cell arteritis.[25] The optic disk may be pale, swollen, and with associated hemorrhage.[26] (Fig. 18.11). Color vision is reduced and a RAPD present.

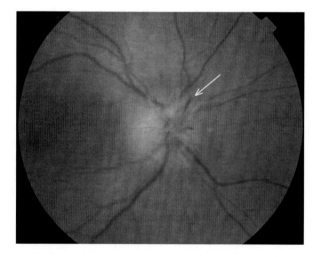

Fig. 18.11 Acute ischemic optic neuropathy. The optic disk is swollen, and nerve fiber layer hemorrhages are present (*arrowed*)

18.4.2.2
Associated Systemic Diseases

Systemic vasculitis, particularly giant cell arteritis.

18.4.2.3
Treatment

This is directed at the underlying vasculitis. Prompt treatment may prevent progression to bilateral blindness.

18.5
Orbit

18.5.1
Orbital Inflammatory Disease

18.5.1.1
Symptoms and Signs

Proptosis occurs when the globe is displaced by mass effect within the orbit. The displacement may be axial (when the mass is behind the globe within the muscle cone of the globe), or non-axial (when the mass is "extra-conal") (Fig. 18.12). Eye movements may be

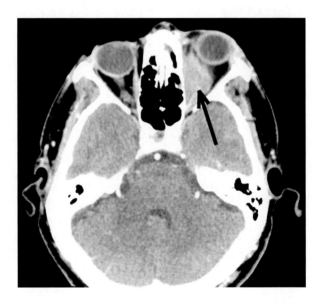

Fig. 18.12 A CT scan of Wegener granulomatous is presenting with an orbital mass (*arrowed*)

restricted causing double vision. Eye movements can be either painful (e.g., orbital myositis) or painless (e.g., thyroid eye disease). If the optic nerve becomes compressed, then loss of vision occurs, field defects may be documented, color vision reduced, and a RAPD present. Visual loss can occur if the cornea is not protected by normal lid closure due to proptosis. This is known as exposure keratopathy, the patient may be light sensitive with reduced vision, and the eye will be red and proptosed. If there is evidence of visual loss, it is important to seek an urgent ophthalmological opinion.

18.5.1.2
Associated Systemic Diseases

Thyroid eye disease, Wegener granulomatosis,[27] lymphoma,[28] sarcoidosis,[29] and idiopathic orbital inflammatory syndrome.[30] Idiopathic orbital inflammatory syndrome can be further classified depending on the predominant structure involved, for example, orbital myositis[31] and superior orbital fissure syndrome.

18.5.1.3
Treatment

Control of the underlying disease process. If vision is compromised by an optic neuropathy or exposure keratopathy, then immunosuppression, orbital radiotherapy, or surgical orbital decompression maybe warranted.[32] The treatment regime depends on urgency and etiology

18.6
The Ocular Effects Drugs Used in Rheumatic and Autoimmune Diseases

Medications used to treat inflammatory disease may have a direct toxic effect on the ocular structures. Furthermore, the effect of immunosuppression may increase the risk of opportunistic infections.

18.6.1
Hydroxychloroquine and Retinopathy

Hydroxychloroquine has been associated with a bull's eye maculopathy, although this is rare. One meta-analysis with over 1,800 patients using hydroxychloroquine identified only one case of visual loss due to retinopathy.[33] It presents with impaired central vision. Monocular field testing can demonstrate small scotomas in the central visual field. In the late stages, a depigmented ring can be seen on fundoscopy around the fovea. These changes are irreversible. Patients can monitor for signs of retinopathy by using an Amsler grid which is a grid held at 30 cm; if distortion or missing patches are seen, then an ophthalmic review is recommended.[34] In the rare instance where a hydroxychloroquine retinopathy is identified, treatment should be withdrawn.

18.6.2
Corticosteroids, Cataracts, and Glaucoma

Corticosteroids are associated with cataract formation which can reduce vision. Typically, it is the posterior aspect of the lens that opacifies beneath the lens capsule known as a posterior subcapsular cataract.[35] If visual impairment affects the quality of life, cataract surgery is indicated.

Topical eye preparations containing corticosteroids have been associated with raised intraocular pressure in approximately 5% of users.[36] Over long periods of time, high intraocular pressure may cause a slow progressive optic neuropathy characterized by enlargement of the optic disk cup (cupping) and visual field loss known as glaucoma. The increased intraocular pressure occurs because of increased resistance through the trabecular meshwork to the drainage of aqueous humor. Intraocular pressure rises are less common with oral corticosteroids because aqueous humor production is also reduced.

18.6.3
Infectious Uveitis in the Immunosuppressed Patient

The development of intraocular inflammation or uveitis, in an immunosuppressed patient, raises the possibility of an infectious uveitis.

18.6.3.1
Signs and Symptoms

Patients may present with unilateral or bilateral features including red eye, pain, light sensitivity, floaters, and blurred vision. The immunosuppression may mask the symptoms and signs. There may be evidence of sepsis with night sweats and weight loss; there may be an obvious portal of entry or stigmata of an infective source such as endocarditis. Frequently, however, there are no other systemic features of infection.

Ophthalmic examination may reveal an anterior uveitis, vitritis, retinitis, or choroiditis. Certain infections cause particular patterns of infectious uveitis. Cytomegalovirus[37] may cause a very mild anterior uveitis and slowly progressive retinitis characterized by white retinal necrosis with hemorrhage (Fig. 18.13). *Mycobacterium tuberculosis*[38] can cause a choroiditis with choroidal granulomas; these are discrete lesions seen deep to the retina and have a creamy yellow color (Fig. 18.14).

18.6.3.2
Treatment

First, the organism needs to be identified. In the case of viral retinitis, this requires a vitreous biopsy in which the viral genome can be identified by amplification using the polymerase chain reaction (PCR). Other organisms may be identified indirectly by growth from blood cultures or aspirates from infective emboli. Fungi and other organisms may occasionally only be isolated by diagnostic vitreous or chorioretinal biopsy. Once the infectious agent has been identified, appropriate anti-infective agents can be used.[39] For

Fig. 18.13 CMV retinitis in an immunosuppressed patient. White areas of retinal necrosis (*black arrow*) are seen with areas of retinal hemorrhage (*white arrow*)

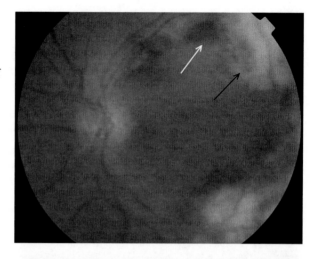

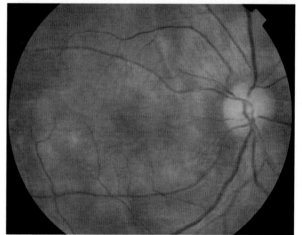

Fig. 18.14 Multiple tuberculous choroidal granulomas. These poorly defined creamy yellow lesions are in the choroid, deep to the retina

infectious uveitis, this may be delivered orally, intravenously or intravitreally. The embolizing source of the infection will require separate treatment.

18.7
New Therapies

18.7.1
Etanercept in Uveitis

Etanercept has anecdotally been reported as a cause of uveitis in patients with spondyloarthropathies. The temporal association has been identified in a number of case reports;[40] however, case-controlled observational studies on the incidence of uveitis in patients using etanercept report conflicting results.[41,42]

18.7.2
Rituximab and Scleritis

Rituximab has been shown to gain control of scleritis refractory to multiple other agents. Case reports have described remission in idiopathic, rheumatoid, and Wegener granulomatosis–associated scleritis.[43,44]

18.7.3
Infliximab and Juvenile Idiopathic Arthritis

A randomized controlled trial comparing infliximab with methotrexate to placebo with methotrexate for 14 weeks (until both arms were given methotrexate with infliximab at different doses) recruited 122 children with polyarticular JIA previously refractory to methotrexate. It demonstrated a higher response rate in the infliximab group at 14 weeks; however, the difference was not statistically significant.[45]

18.7.4
Interferon Alpha 2a and Behçet Disease

A case series of 32 patients with severe refractory uveitis reported treatment with subcutaneous interferon α2a three times a week. Twenty eight patients responded to the treatment, and during follow-up, relapse rate reduced; however, on discontinuing therapy, the relapse rate increased.[46]

18.8
Conclusions

Awareness of the painful or blinding complications of autoimmune diseases enables timely liaison between the internist and ophthalmologist. Prompt treatment reduces morbidity from visual loss, and mortality from systemic consequences of uncontrolled disease. While newer biological agents are improving the ability to control disease, systemic immuno-modulation can itself precipitate unwanted ocular effects.

References

1. Albini TA, Rao NA, Smith RE. The diagnosis and management of anterior scleritis. *Int Ophthalmol Clin*. 2005;45(2):191-204.
2. Galor A, Thorne JE. Scleritis and peripheral ulcerative keratitis. *Rheum Dis Clin North Am*. 2007;33(4):835-854.
3. Pakrou N, Selva D, Leibovitch I. Wegener's granulomatosis: ophthalmic manifestations and management (Review). *Semin Arthritis Rheum*. 2006;35(5):284-292.

4. Malik R, Culinane AB, Tole DM, Cook SD. Rheumatoid keratolysis: a series of 40 eyes. *Eur J Ophthalmol*. 2006;16(6):791-797.
5. Liu DT, Chan AY. Use of intravenous cyclophosphamide in the prevention of corneal melt: justified or not? *Rheumatology*. 2006;45(7):920 (author reply 921-922).
6. Casas VE, Kheirkhah A, Blanco G, Tseng SC. Surgical approach for scleral ischemia and melt. *Cornea*. 2008;27(2):196-201.
7. Zaidi AA, Ying GS, Daniel E, et al. Hypopyon in patients with uveitis. *Ophthalmology*. 2010;117(2):366-372.
8. Zeboulon N, Dougados M, Gossec L. Prevalence and characteristics of uveitis in the spondyloarthropathies: a systematic literature review. *Ann Rheum Dis*. 2008;67(7):955-959.
9. Chang JH, McCluskey PJ, Wakefield D. Acute anterior uveitis and HLA-B27. *Surv Ophthalmol*. 2005;50(4):364-388.
10. Chang JH, Raju R, Henderson TR, McCluskey PJ. Incidence and pattern of acute anterior uveitis in Central Australia. *Br J Ophthalmol*. 2010;94(2):154-156.
11. Ali A, Samson CM. Seronegative spondyloarthropathies and the eye (Review). *Curr Opin Ophthalmol*. 2007;18(6):476-480.
12. Woreta F, Thorne JE, Jabs DA, Kedhar SR, Dunn JP. Risk factors for ocular complications and poor visual acuity at presentation among patients with uveitis associated with juvenile idiopathic arthritis. *Am J Ophthalmol*. 2007;143(4):647-655.
13. Benezra D, Cohen E, Behar-Cohen F. Uveitis and juvenile idiopathic arthritis: a cohort study. *Clin Ophthalmol*. 2007;1(4):513-518.
14. Hayward K, Wallace CA. Recent developments in anti-rheumatic drugs in pediatrics: treatment of juvenile idiopathic arthritis. *Arthritis Res Ther*. 2009;11(1):216.
15. Dodds EM, Irarrázaval LA, Scarfone A, Gáspari E. Bilateral posterior scleritis. *Ocul Immunol Inflamm*. 1997;5(4):267-269.
16. Pecorella I, La Cava M, Mannino G, Pinca M, Pezzi PP. Diffuse granulomatous necrotizing scleritis. *Acta Ophthalmol Scand*. 2006;84(2):263-265.
17. Kim RY, Loewenstein JI. Systemic diseases manifesting as exudative retinal detachment. *Int Ophthalmol Clin*. 1998;38(1):177-195.
18. Nag TC, Wadhwa S. Vascular changes of the retina and choroid in systemic lupus erythematosus: pathology and pathogenesis. *Curr Neurovasc Res*. 2006;3(2):159-168.
19. Coroi M, Bontas E, Defranceschi M, Bartos D, Dorobantu M. Ocular manifestations of antiphospholipid (Hughes)' syndrome – minor features? *Oftalmologia*. 2007;51(3):16-22.
20. Au A, O'Day J. Review of severe vaso-occlusive retinopathy in systemic lupus erythematosus and the antiphospholipid syndrome: associations, visual outcomes, complications and treatment. *Clin Experiment Ophthalmol*. 2004;32(1):87-100.
21. Stanford MR, Verity DH. Diagnostic and therapeutic approach to patients with retinal vasculitis. *Int Ophthalmol Clin*. 2000;40(2):69-83.
22. Sivaraj RR, Durrani OM, Denniston AK, Murray PI, Gordon C. Ocular manifestations of systemic lupus erythematosus. *Rheumatology*. 2007;46(12):1757-1762.
23. McLeod D. Why cotton wool spots should not be regarded as retinal nerve fibre layer infarcts. *Br J Ophthalmol*. 2005;89:229-237.
24. Cohen S, Gardner F. Bilateral choroidal ischemia in giant cell arteritis. *Arch Ophthalmol*. 2006;124(6):922.
25. Hayreh SS. Ischemic optic neuropathy. *Prog Retin Eye Res*. 2009;28(1):34-62.
26. Luneau K, Newman NJ, Biousse V. Ischemic optic neuropathies. *Neurologist*. 2008;14(6): 341-354.
27. Vischio JA, McCrary CT. Orbital Wegener's granulomatosis: a case report and review of the literature. *Clin Rheumatol*. 2008;27(10):1333-1336.
28. Demirci H, Shields CL, Karatza EC, Shields JA. Orbital lymphoproliferative tumors: analysis of clinical features and systemic involvement in 160 cases. *Ophthalmology*. 2008;115(9):1626-1631.

29. Mavrikakis I, Rootman J. Diverse clinical presentations of orbital sarcoid. *Am J Ophthalmol.* 2007;144(5):769-775.
30. Lutt JR, Lim LL, Phal PM, Rosenbaum JT. Orbital inflammatory disease. *Semin Arthritis Rheum.* 2008;37(4):207-222.
31. Costa RM, Dumitrascu OM, Gordon LK. Orbital myositis: diagnosis and management. *Curr Allergy Asthma Rep.* 2009;9(4):316-323.
32. Swamy BN, McCluskey P, Nemet A, et al. Idiopathic orbital inflammatory syndrome: clinical features and treatment outcomes. *Br J Ophthalmol.* 2007;91(12):1667-1670.
33. Silman A, Shipley M. Ophthalmological monitoring for hydroxychloroquine toxicity: a scientific review of available data. *Br J Rheumatol.* 1997;36(5):599-601.
34. Tehrani R, Ostrowski RA, Hariman R, Jay WM. Ocular toxicity of hydroxychloroquine. *Semin Ophthalmol.* 2008;23(3):201-209.
35. Wang JJ, Rochtchina E, Tan AG, Cumming RG, Leeder SR, Mitchell P. Use of inhaled and oral corticosteroids and the long-term risk of cataract. *Ophthalmology.* 2009;116(4):652-657.
36. Clark AF, Wordinger RJ. The role of steroids in outflow resistance. *Exp Eye Res.* 2009;88(4): 752-759.
37. Wiegand TW, Young LH. Cytomegalovirus retinitis. *Int Ophthalmol Clin.* 2006;46(2):91-110.
38. Tabbara KF. Tuberculosis. *Curr Opin Ophthalmol.* 2007;18(6):493-501 (Review).
39. Cordero-Coma M, Anzaar F, Yilmaz T, Foster CS. Herpetic retinitis. *Herpes.* 2007;14(1):4-10.
40. Taban M, Dupps WJ, Mandell B, Perez VL. Etanercept (enbrel)-associated inflammatory eye disease: case report and review of the literature. *Ocul Immunol Inflamm.* 2006;14(3):145-150.
41. Lim LL, Fraunfelder FW, Rosenbaum JT. Do tumor necrosis factor inhibitors cause uveitis? A registry-based study. *Arthritis Rheum.* 2007;56(10):3248-3252.
42. Sieper J, Koenig A, Baumgartner S, et al. Analysis of uveitis rates across all etanercept ankylosing spondylitis clinical trials. *Ann Rheum Dis.* 2010;69(1):226-229 (Epub).
43. Kurz PA, Suhler EB, Choi D, Rosenbaum JT. Rituximab for treatment of ocular inflammatory disease: a series of four cases. *Br J Ophthalmol.* 2009;93(4):546-548.
44. Onal S, Kazokoglu H, Koc A, Yavuz S. Rituximab for remission induction in a patient with relapsing necrotizing scleritis associated with limited Wegener's granulomatosis. *Ocul Immunol Inflamm.* 2008;16(5):230-232.
45. Ruperto N, Lovell DJ, Cuttica R, et al. A randomized, placebo-controlled trial of infliximab plus methotrexate for the treatment of polyarticular-course juvenile rheumatoid arthritis. *Arthritis Rheum.* 2007;56(9):3096-3106.
46. Gueudry J, Wechsler B, Terrada C, et al. Long-term efficacy and safety of low-dose interferon alpha2a therapy in severe uveitis associated with Behçet disease. *Am J Ophthalmol.* 2008; 146(6):837-844 (e1).

Emergencies for the Vascular Surgeon

19

Ashish S. Patel and Matthew Waltham

Abstract Systemic autoimmune diseases can result in a variety of vascular abnormalities, usually due to either vessel wall inflammation or clotting abnormalities. Acute vascular emergencies secondary to these abnormalities commonly occur due to thrombosis with subsequent ischemia or infarction, aneurysm formation, or hemorrhage. A range of vessels can be affected depending on the type and severity of the autoimmune disease, and patients can present with a range of symptoms to vascular surgeons in the emergency setting. Medical management of the underlying systemic disease is the preferred choice of treatment in autoimmune vascular emergencies, but life-/limb-threatening ischemia or hemorrhage of the cerebrovascular/brachiocephalic, upper limb, renal, gastrointestinal, or lower limb vessels often requires emergency vascular surgery. Traditional open vascular surgery is high-risk, especially in this group of patients, and is rapidly being replaced by less invasive endovascular procedures, including percutaneous transluminal balloon angioplasty/stenting, mechanical thrombectomy, and thrombolysis. Emergency endovascular repair of ruptured aneurysms/dissections is now also performed routinely in specialist vascular centers. A multidisciplinary team approach is essential in the treatment of patients with complex and acute autoimmune diseases and should involve specialist physicians, hematologists, and interventional radiologists as well as vascular and endovascular surgeons.

Keywords Aortic aneurysm • Aortic dissection • Deep venous thrombosis. • Endovascular surgery • Intra-arterial digital subtraction angiography • Mesenteric angina • Percutaneous transluminal balloon angioplasty • Thrombolysis • Upper/lower limb ischemia

A.S. Patel (✉)
Academic Department of Surgery, Cardiovascular Division,
King's College London, St Thomas' Hospital, First Floor, North Wing,
Westminster Bridge Road, London SE1 7EH, UK
e-mail: ashish.s.patel@kcl.ac.uk

M.A. Khamashta and M. Ramos-Casals (eds.), *Autoimmune Diseases*,
DOI: 10.1007/978-0-85729-358-9_19, © Springer-Verlag London Limited 2011

19.1
Introduction

Acute vascular emergencies associated with autoimmune diseases usually result as a consequence of vessel wall inflammation. They include thrombosis with subsequent ischemia or infarction, aneurysm formation, and hemorrhage. A range of target vessels can be affected, and patients present with a range of symptoms to vascular surgeons in the emergency setting. In this chapter, we outline the common presenting features of some of these conditions and describe the vascular surgical interventions available.

19.2
Acute Ischemia of the Lower Limb

Acute limb ischemia is defined by the *Trans-Atlantic Inter-Society Consensus* (TASC) as a sudden decrease or worsening in limb perfusion causing a potential threat to extremity viability.[1] The two major causes are acute thrombosis and embolus. The development of symptoms in acute lower limb ischemia depends on the anatomical localization and extent of the lesion. Sudden occlusion of an artery is commonly due to embolic disease but, in the patient with vasculitis, can result as a consequence of acute thrombosis. Acute arterial thrombosis of the lower limb is a diagnosis that can be made accurately based on clinical symptoms and signs. When appropriate, it should be complemented with supplementary investigations and, in the emergency setting of lower limb ischemia due to vasculitis, it is essential to decide whether treatment should be initiated urgently or whether it is safe to delay treatment in order to obtain further anatomical information with a diagnostic investigation.

19.2.1
Presenting Symptoms and Signs

The symptoms of an acutely ischemic limb can be dramatic and include intense pain, pallor, paresthesia, paralysis, pulselessness and poikilothermia. In less severe cases (usually as a result of thrombosis of a short segment of vessel with adequate collateral blood flow), the patient may have moderate pain and pallor with little deficit of motor or sensory nervous function. Intense pain can then develop, followed by paresthesia and numbness progressing to a loss of sensation. Light touch and proprioception are often lost first, whereas decreased temperature sense and two-point discrimination are late signs. Finally, deep pain and pressure senses are lost. An inability to dorsiflex and plantar flex the toes or ankle signifies rigidity of the crural muscles (*rigor mortis*). The ankle-brachial pressure index (ABPI), which is a ratio of the ankle and brachial blood pressures, may be misleading in patients with vasculitis as the arteries may be incompressible giving a falsely high pressure at the ankle.

19.2.2
Investigations

If the leg is viable and further investigations are indicated, ultrasound duplex scanning can be performed to assess the patency of the larger vessels. Duplex scanning is, however, operator dependent and accurate, reliable information on the run-off distal, crural and pedal vessels can be difficult to obtain. Contrast-enhanced multi-slice computed-tomography (CT) scanning, especially after three-dimensional reconstruction, can provide adequate imaging of the large vessels and the distal run-off but can also be hampered by the presence of highly calcified vessels. Magnetic resonance angiography (MRA), if available in the emergency setting, avoids this problem and does not expose the patient to toxic contrast agents or radiation.[2] Techniques into imaging the perfusion of the ischemic muscle with magnetic resonance scans are also under development but further work is needed. Intra-arterial digital subtraction angiography (IADSA) with use of contrast, therefore, remains the standard for imaging as this provides detailed and selective imaging of affected vessels and allows for endovascular procedures to be performed, such as stenting, thrombolysis, or suction/aspiration of thrombus.

19.2.3
Treatment of Lower Limb Thrombosis

Providing that the limb is viable, catheter-directed intra-arterial thrombolysis (with access often gained via the contralateral femoral artery) over a period of hours is the preferred mode of treatment for acute thromboses.[3] Successful thrombolysis alleviates symptoms, lyses the thrombus, provides anatomical information on the run-off vessels and may prevent the need for further surgery, or limit the extent of major surgery required subsequently.[4] Recombinant tissue-type plasminogen activator (rt-PA), rather than urokinase or streptokinase, is currently the preferred thrombolytic agent because of its rapid onset of action and reduced allergic side-effect profile. Thrombolysis is associated with a risk of hemorrhagic complications, such as stroke, and is contraindicated in patients who have had a recent hemorrhagic stroke, recent surgery, or a bleeding diathesis and in patients who are pregnant. Other endovascular procedures can also be performed during thrombolysis, including suction embolectomy/thrombectomy, transluminal balloon angioplasty, and/or stenting of the affected vessel or vessels (see Fig. 19.1). Thrombolysis can also be performed on previous bypass (vein or prosthetic) grafts (see Fig. 19.2).

For thromboses which are not suitable for endovascular procedures (more often these are the larger vessels such as the common femoral artery), local thrombo-endarterectomy with or without vein patching can be performed via the femoral or popliteal arteries. New rotary-type mechanical thrombectomy endovascular devices and stent-grafts are, however, being developed for use on these larger vessels, and in specialist vascular units, percutaneous thrombectomy is rapidly becoming the first-line treatment for acute thromboses. Embolectomy procedures are also performed via the groin and can be carried out under local or general anesthesia depending on the patient's general condition. A Fogarty balloon embolectomy catheter is used to remove the embolus as well as any thrombus which

Fig. 19.1 IADSA of a 46-year-old lady with anti-phospholipid syndrome showing stenosis of the distal popliteal artery (**a**, *black arrow*). Note the previous stent within the proximal section of the popliteal artery (**a** and **b**, *white arrows*). The patient was treated with intraluminal balloon angioplasty of the affected segment (**b**, *black arrow*) followed by insertion of a stent (**c**, *arrow*). Post-intervention angiogram shows improved blood flow through the popliteal artery to the distal crural vessels

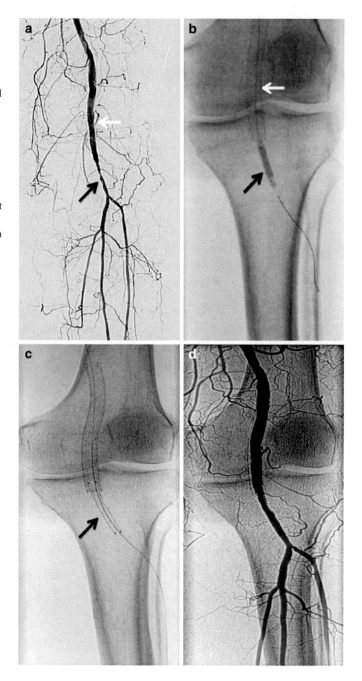

may have extended either proximally and/or distally. Following adequate revascularization, patients may require prophylactic fasciotomies of the lower limb as there is a high risk of the development of compartment syndrome after revascularization of the acutely ischemic limb.

Fig. 19.2 A case of a patient with severe anti-phospholipid syndrome and previous multiple stents (which subsequently occluded) within the right superficial femoral artery for lower limb ischemia. The patient underwent an emergency femoral-popliteal bypass procedure but was re-admitted a few months later with acute ischemia of the same leg. The angiogram (**a**) shows the previous occluded stents, but no flow within the bypass graft. This thrombosis was treated with an intra-arterial infusion of rt-TPA (**b**) shows the angiogram after an initial rt-PA bolus. 24 h later (**c**), a check angiogram confirmed successful lysis of the thrombus and restoration of flow within the graft

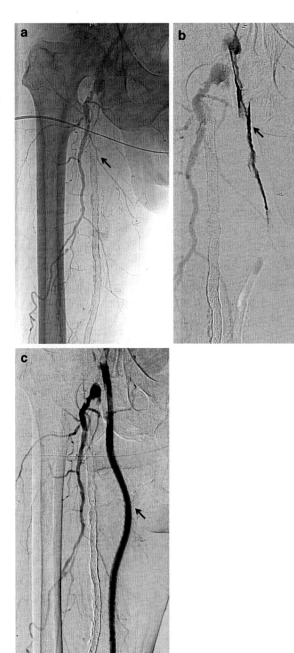

19.2.4
Thromboangitis Obliterans (Buerger's Disease)

Buerger's disease is characterized by occlusive disease of small- and medium-sized arteries, thrombophlebitis of the superficial or deep vein(s), and Raynaud's syndrome.

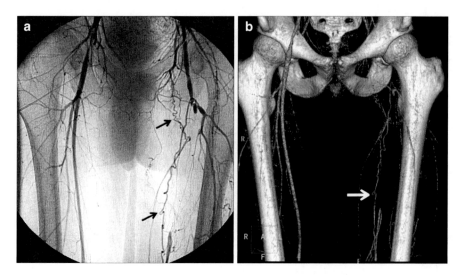

Fig. 19.3 A 24-year-old man with Buerger's disease and ischemia of the left leg resulting in severe claudication. An IADSA shows occlusion of the left superficial femoral artery with an extensive collateral network forking a corkscrew appearance (**a**, *arrows*). This can clearly be seen on the reconstructed images (**b**, *arrow*)

Patients usually present with the usual symptoms and signs of arterial occlusive disease, ranging from progressive intermittent claudication (pain when walking which is resolved by rest) to short-distance claudication, rest pain and/or tissue loss (skin ulceration/gangrene of the digits). It usually occurs in young (usually under the age of 30), male patients. Angiography classically reveals a smooth outline of the artery proximal to the occlusion in comparison to the irregular appearance of atheromatous lesions. Tapering and abrupt occlusion are seen with extensive collateral networks around the occlusion which form a corkscrew appearance (see Fig. 19.3).

Open arterial reconstructive surgery can be problematic and of little value in this group of patients since the disease is often distal and multifocal. Transluminal angioplasty of the anterior tibial or tibioperoneal trunk vessels can be used to improve distal blood flow but is limited for patients with rest pain and tissue loss.

19.3
Mesenteric Ischemia

Acute mesenteric ischemic, although a rare manifestation of the vasculitides, is a life-threatening vascular emergency.[5] Mesenteric vascular disease may be arterial or venous. The diagnosis can be difficult to make as there is no single clinical feature which can be conclusive. Accurate and early diagnosis, therefore, usually depends on a high index of clinical suspicion.

19.3.1
History and Examination

The superior mesenteric artery (SMA) is the most common site of thromboembolic or vasculitic occlusion. In acute occlusions, the patient complains of sudden and constant, severe epigastric or periumbilical pain. This can be associated with vomiting and bloody diarrhea. The symptoms of acute mesenteric ischemia are often out of proportion to the clinical signs, which are often either lacking or nonspecific. The patient is usually writhing around, unless they have generalized peritonitis. The abdomen may be clinically distended without any signs of peritonism. The bowel sounds can be absent or normal and a bruit may be heard. Clinical features of peritonism (local or generalized guarding with rebound tenderness) are an indication of severe and advanced intestinal ischemia and infarction. Acute-on-chronic mesenteric ischemia is usually due to thrombosis of the SMA. The patient will usually have a history of "mesenteric angina" which manifests as postprandial epigastric or periumbilical pain, typically starting 20–30 min after eating, lasting up to 60–90 min. As a result of this, they may also have a history of food fear and subsequent weight loss.

19.3.2
Investigations

Blood tests in acute mesenteric ischemia may reveal a raised lactate level and a leukocytosis. Arterial blood gases may also reveal a marked metabolic acidemia. Ischemic damage to the mucosa of the gut may result in loss of the mucosal barrier, and patients may have systemic signs of sepsis and multiorgan failure due to translocation of gut bacteria, endotoxins, and cytokines. Plain radiographs of the abdomen may reveal nonspecific bowel dilatation, gas in the bowel wall, or air in the portal venous system as a late finding. The presence of gas bubbles in the mesenteric veins is rare but pathognomic. An erect chest radiograph may reveal a pneumoperitoneum. However, plain radiographs are generally not helpful and non-contrast- and contrast-enhanced CT is more helpful in revealing SMA or superior mesenteric vein thrombosis, portal venous gas and/or ischemia of the bowel wall and other organs (such as liver and splenic infarcts). Other nonspecific findings include distended, thickened bowel and air-fluid levels. The new generation of multi-slice CT scanners can now provide much more accurate assessment of the small bowel and mesenteric vessels and can make a diagnosis of mesenteric ischemia with 93% and 96% sensitivity and specificity, respectively.[6] Mesenteric angiography, where lateral views of the visceral aorta and its branches are taken, is the gold standard for confirmation of the diagnosis. Selective angiography of mesenteric arteries can also diagnose peripheral splanchnic disease. Mesenteric angiography can be used to show intestinal arterial vasospasm as well as confirm the extent of the disease.

19.3.3
Surgical Treatment

If there is evidence of peritonitism, the patient should, after initial resuscitation, have an emergency laparotomy without mesenteric angiography. Otherwise, mesenteric angiography provides a diagnosis and the option to proceed to treatment in selected cases of subacute mesenteric ischemia.[7] Percutaneous transluminal angioplasty with stenting is a valuable treatment option in selected patients where open bowel surgery is not necessary. Patients who present early without any clinical or radiographic features of bowel necrosis or peritonitis may also be treated with a trial of thrombolytic therapy for acute thrombotic disease. If emergency laparotomy is required, the degree and extent of bowel viability is assessed – ischemic bowel is dull gray with no peristalsis. Infarcted bowel is purple/black and friable, and there are often multiple areas of perforations. In cases of extensive and unreconstructable bowel ischemia, there may be insufficient residual bowel to sustain life, and so, no further surgical treatment is performed and the patient is treated palliatively. If sufficient bowel remains, revascularization may be performed prior to bowel resection. Ischemic bowel is resected with the aim of preserving as much bowel as possible to minimize the risk of creating a short gut syndrome. If arterial reconstruction is planned, this is usually performed before any bowel resection is considered because precarious segments of intestine may recover, allowing resection of clearly ischemic bowel only. For short, lesions, localized thrombo-embolectomy, with or without endarterectomy and vein patching, may be the procedure of choice. SMA reconstruction can be performed using a bypass graft from the aorta to the distal, patent SMA or by implanting the healthy part of the SMA onto the aorta.[8] Generally, prosthetic grafts are avoided, especially if there is bowel perforation, and either direct SMA implantation or reversed saphenous vein is used.

If there is a high risk of the patient developing abdominal compartment syndrome after revascularization for acute mesenteric ischemia, the abdomen may be left often via a laparostomy while the patient is managed in the intensive care unit. A second-look laparotomy is generally performed 24–48 h after initial surgery where the bowel is re-inspected to assess the viability of the marginally perfused areas as well as any anastomosis.

19.4
Takayasu's Arteritis

Takayasu's disease is a nonspecific inflammatory process of the aorta, the pulmonary arteries, and their major branches. This can result in stenosis or aneurysm formation. Patients with aortitis, usually young women, most commonly present as a result of symptoms from the thoracic aorta or subclavian arteries but can also present as a result of embolic disease to other vessels. Emergencies for vascular surgeons, therefore, include upper/lower limb ischemia, mesenteric/renal ischemia, neurological or ocular symptoms, and ruptured aortic aneurysms.

19.4.1
Signs and Symptoms

Patients with upper limb pathology present with claudication and will describe symptoms of pain, numbness, and fatigue resulting from repetitive arm movements and sustained arm elevation. Arterial pulses in the affected arm may be diminished, and a bruit may be audible over the subclavian artery. A reduced blood pressure in the affected arm is common.

Symptoms from carotid artery disease include headaches, transient visual disturbances (such as amaurosis fugax), transient ischemic attacks, or stroke. Symptoms from vertebral artery disease or a subclavian artery with a dominant vertebral artery include posterior circulation neurological symptoms, including dizziness or syncope. These symptoms can be reproduced clinically when the ipsilateral arm is exercised and retrograde flow through the vertebral artery to supply the subclavian artery distal to the stenosis results in compromised posterior cerebral blood flow – this is called subclavian steal syndrome.

Patients with acute renal artery stenosis can present with variable symptoms, including flank pain, nausea, vomiting and micro- or macroscopic haematuria. Uncontrolled hypertension may also be a presenting feature,

19.4.2
Diagnosis

IADSA is essential in patients with Takayasu's arteritis, and all the brachiocephalic vessels should be imaged. This may reveal a critical stenosis (as well as pre- and post-stenotic dilatation of the affected vessel), obstruction and/or aneurysm formation. CT angiography is currently the noninvasive investigation of choice and also allows imaging of other organs such as the kidneys. Magnetic resonance angiography of the aorta and large arteries avoids the risk of arterial puncture and exposure to iodinated contrast or radiation and is usually the investigation of choice in young women.

19.4.3
Treatment

Although steroids may relieve the early symptoms, they do not treat established occlusive lesions. The principles of arterial reconstructive surgery for either thrombotic or embolic disease are similar to those for atherosclerotic occlusive disease. Emergency reconstructive surgery is indicated for patients with cerebral ischemia, severe hypertension as a result of coarctation or renal artery stenosis, limb-threatening ischemia, and symptomatic aneurysms.

- Carotid artery surgery is usually performed for symptomatic cases with a stenosis greater than 70%. Common techniques include resection with vein grafting, aortocarotid or carotid-sublclavian bypass rather than subclavian-carotid bypass grafting.
- For patients with acute renal artery stenosis, treatment options include percutaneous transluminal angioplasty with or without renal artery stent placement or open aortorenal bypass surgery. For patients with symptomatic subclavian artery stenosis, extraanatomical bypass surgery such as a carotid-subclavian bypass procedure can be performed. The anastomoses are generally made at disease-free sites to minimize future risk of aneurysm formation and occlusion. Percutaneous transluminal angioplasty and

stenting may be offered as an alternative treatment, but there is a risk of long-term restenosis/occlusion.

- The presence of either a symptomatic fusiform aneurysm or any saccular aneurysm is an indication for urgent vascular surgery. The traditional surgical procedure of choice is open resection and repair with a prosthetic graft, but this may be superseded by endovascular stent grafting techniques in the very near future.
- For aortic regurgitation, valvular surgery with aortic root replacement may be necessary.

19.5
Periarteritis Nodosa (Polyarteritis)

Periarteritis nodosa (PAN) is an inflammatory disease of small- and medium-sized arteries. In addition to the cerebrovascular, renal, and gastrointestinal syndromes associated with this condition, inflammatory destruction of the media of affected vessels can also result in formation of microaneurysms in these organs. Spontaneous rupture of these aneurysms in young men with PAN is not uncommon, and patients may present with severe flank/abdominal pain or massive gastrointestinal bleeding. Emergency CT angiography or IADSA should be performed to locate the source of the bleeding, and percutaneous transcatheter selective embolisation of bleeding microaneurysms can be potentially life-saving in this group of patients.

19.5.1
Summary

The evolution of endovascular and imaging techniques over the last few decades has equipped vascular surgeons with an array of treatment modalities for thrombotic and embolic vasculitic diseases. Nevertheless, vascular surgical intervention should be reserved for patients with life- or limb-threatening symptoms and medical management remains the mainstay of treatment in the majority of patients.

19.6
Inflammatory Aortic Aneurysms

Approximately 5–10% of abdominal aortic aneurysms (AAA) are inflammatory. They most commonly affect the infrarenal portion of the abdominal aorta. In contrast to atherosclerotic aneurysms, inflammatory aneurysms are associated with marked thickening of the aneurysm wall, fibrosis of the adjacent retroperitoneum, and adherence of surrounding structures to the anterior aneurysm wall.[9] Inflammatory aneurysms have been associated with several autoimmune conditions, including Wegener's granulomatosis, Henoch–Schonlein purpura, polyarteritis nodosa, and autoimmune thyroid disease.

19.6.1
Signs and Symptoms

In contrast to atherosclerotic aneurysms, the majority (80%) of patients with inflammatory aneurysms are symptomatic at time of presentation. Localized symptoms include abdominal and back pain and systemic symptoms such as fever, malaise, and weight loss may also be present. Surgical treatment should be expedited in patients presenting with inflammatory aneurysms if the diameter of the aorta is greater than 5.5 cm. In certain cases, smaller aneurysms may also be treated as the presence of symptoms may indicate impending rupture. Anterior rupture of an AAA results in free bleeding into the peritoneum, and few patients reach hospital alive. Posterior rupture often results in a retroperitoneal hematoma, and this group of patients may present with severe abdominal pain and clinical features of shock. Other symptoms include lower limb ischemia secondary to hypovolemia or distal embolisation and high-output cardiac failure in patients with aortocaval fistulae. Aortocaval fistulae and aortoduodenal fistulae (which present as massive catastrophic rectal bleeding) are more common in patients with inflammatory aneurysms.

19.6.2
Investigations

Blood tests in patients with inflammatory aneurysms may reveal features of systemic inflammation with raised C-reactive protein (CRP) and/or erythrocyte sedimentation rate (ESR) levels. Contrast-enhanced CT scans will reveal the aneurysm with a thickened aortic wall and surrounding periaortic inflammation and fibrosis.

19.6.3
Treatment

Open surgical repair of inflammatory aneurysms was first attempted in the 1970s.[10] Surgical repair is particularly challenging as a result of heavy adhesions between the aneurysm and the duodenum, inferior vena cava and ureters. Studies have shown that inflammatory aneurysms can be treated equally as effectively with endovascular stent grafting.[11] With this technique, the aorta is accessed via the common femoral arteries, which are exposed surgically and the endovascular stent graft is deployed under radiological guidance within the aorta to exclude the aneurysm from the circulation. The majority of specialist vascular centers now offer emergency endovascular aneurysm repair (EVAR) for ruptured aneurysms/dissections (Fig. 19.4).

Fig. 19.4 A 56-year-old patient admitted with sudden onset chest and back pain. A CT angiogram (**a**) showed intramural hematoma within the descending thoracic aorta which required emergency endovascular surgery. An IADSA (**b**) taken during the procedure confirmed the lesion (*arrow*). An endovascular stent graft (**c**) was successfully deployed into the thoracic aorta to seal the "primary tear"

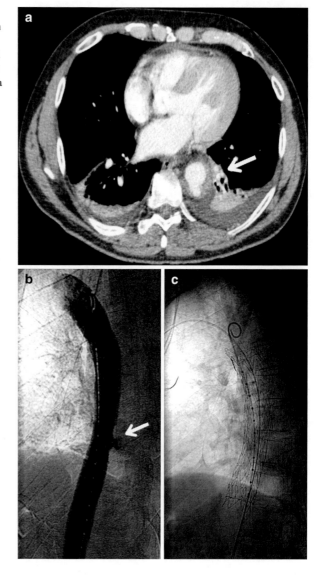

19.7
Venous Thrombosis

Patients with autoimmune diseases, particularly anti-phospholipid syndrome and systemic lupus erythematous, are at increased risk of venous thrombosis as a result of hypercoagulability. Deep venous thrombosis (DVT) is a serious and potentially life-threatening condition that can lead to sudden death as a result of pulmonary embolism. The long-term sequelae of venous thrombosis can include the development of a post-thrombotic limb in

23–60% of patients, resulting in significant morbidity.[12] The most common location of a DVT is the lower leg in the distribution of the popliteal and crural veins. However, in patients with autoimmune diseases, other less common sites of venous thromboses also include the more proximal iliofemoral, iliocaval, or axillary veins. There is a higher risk of pulmonary embolism with more proximal thromboses.

19.7.1
Symptoms and Signs

The patient will usually present with pain and swelling of the affected limb. The clinical features may include calf tenderness, edema, visible dilated superficial veins and rubor. These may be associated with a low-grade pyrexia. In cases of a more proximal (e.g., iliofemoral) thrombosis which extends into the inferior vena cava, the patient may have severe groin pain, dilated superficial veins visible over the anterior abdominal wall and marked swelling of the entire limb. As a result of increased compartmental pressure, impaired tissue perfusion may result in *phlegmasia cerulea dolens*. This can be mistaken for acute arterial ischemia. Patients with subclavian-axillary vein thromboses present with similar symptoms of upper limb swelling, pain, venous engorgement and mild cyanosis.

19.7.2
Investigations

The investigation of choice for a definitive diagnosis is venous duplex ultrasonography. Other imaging modalities include contrast-enhanced venous-phase CT angiography or venography in cases where interventional treatment is planned (see below).

19.7.3
Treatment

The majority of DVTs are treated with low-molecular-weight heparin followed by oral anticoagulation, limb elevation and compression. However, in selected cases (e.g., a fresh thrombus in a young patient presenting with phlegmasia), more aggressive surgical options should be considered. These include open thrombectomy or percutaneous catheter-directed thrombectomy with or without thrombolysis (Fig. 19.5). Open surgical thrombectomy usually requires general anesthesia. After exposure of the femoral vein, a venous Fogarty catheter is introduced into the iliac vein and the thrombus is removed. Endovascular options, which can be performed under local anesthesia, include catheter-directed thrombolysis or percutaneous mechanical thrombectomy (which also reduces the dose of thrombolytic drug required to lyse the clot). If an iliac vein stenosis is uncovered on completion venography, a self-expanding stent can be also be deployed. For most patients suitable for intervention, percutaneous techniques are usually first choice[13], whereas open surgical thrombectomy is usually considered in those where thrombolysis is contraindicated.

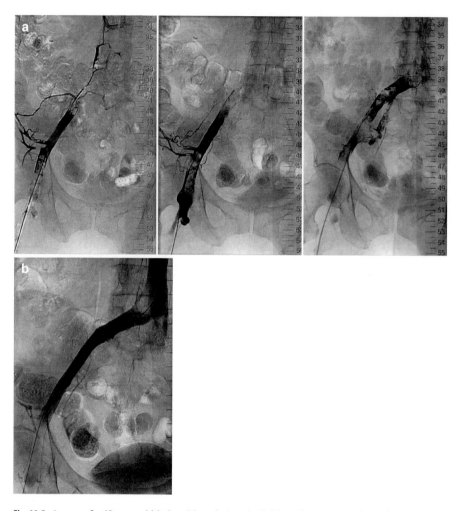

Fig. 19.5 A case of a 68-year-old lady with anti-phospholipid syndrome presenting with an acutely cold, swollen right leg with marked edema. A diagnosis of phlegmasia cerulea dolens secondary to a massive iliofemoral DVT was made and emergency venography was subsequently performed. This confirmed a DVT, with extensive thrombus within the right common and external iliac veins extending into the inferior vena cava (**a**). The patient underwent percutaneous mechanical thrombectomy followed by catheter-directed thrombolysis for 24 h. A check angiogram confirmed lysis of the thrombus (**b**) and her symptoms subsequently resolved

In subclavian-axillary vein thrombosis, catheter-directed thrombolysis can be an effective first-line treatment in selected cases and, if successful, can prevent the disabling post-phlebitic consequences of subclavian-axillary vein thromboses that can be treated with oral anticoagulation only.

19.7.4
Superficial Thrombophlebitis

Superficial thrombosis or thrombophlebitis is an inflammatory reaction as a result of thrombosis of a superficial vein and may present as an emergency to the vascular surgeon. It is associated with autoimmune conditions including anti-phospholipid syndrome, SLE, polyarteritis nodosa, and Buerger's disease. The patient presents with tenderness and redness along the course of a superficial vein. Intermittent bleeding may occur if the inflammation extends through the vein wall. Venous duplex ultrasonography can confirm the diagnosis and should be repeated to ensure that the disease is not migrating into the deep venous system as this can have severe consequences as a result of pulmonary embolus. Leg elevation and compression, low-molecular-weight heparins, and non-steroidal anti-inflammatory drugs are the most effective current therapeutic options for superficial thrombrophlebitis.[14] For severe cases not responding to these treatments, emergency surgical ligation of the affected vein under general anesthesia may be required.

19.8
Conclusion

Systemic autoimmune diseases can cause a variety of vascular abnormalities, usually as a result of either vessel wall inflammation or clotting abnormalities. Acute emergencies secondary to these abnormalities are commonly due to thrombosis, aneurysm formation, or hemorrhage. There are a plethora of emergency presentations depending on the vessel(s) affected as well as the severity of the underlying disease. Medical management of the systemic disease is the preferred treatment in this group of patients and can prevent the need for emergency surgery. However, when life or limb is threatened, emergency vascular surgery is often necessary. Arterial and venous occlusive or hemorrhagic lesions can be treated by vascular surgeons with traditional open surgery along with aggressive control of the underlying systemic disease by specialist physicians. More recently, with improved imaging modalities and modern endovascular techniques, major open vascular reconstructive surgery can be avoided with the goal of reducing trauma and morbidity and improving outcomes in this high-risk group of patients.

References

1. Norgren L, Hiatt WR, Dormandy JA, Nehler MR, Harris KA, Fowkes FG. Inter-society consensus for the management of peripheral arterial disease (TASC II). *J Vasc Surg.* 2007;45 (Suppl S):S5-S67.
2. Chan D, Anderson ME, Dolmatch BL. Imaging evaluation of lower extremity infrainguinal disease: role of the noninvasive vascular laboratory, computed tomography angiography, and magnetic resonance angiography. *Tech Vasc Interv Radiol.* 2010;13(1):11-22.

3. Comerota AJ, Gravett MH. Do randomized trials of thrombolysis versus open revasculariza-tion still apply to current management: what has changed? *Semin Vasc Surg.* 2009;22(1): 41-46.
4. Rutherford RB. Clinical staging of acute limb ischaemia as the basis for choice of revascular-ization method: when and how to intervene. *Semin Vasc Surg.* 2009;22(1):5-9.
5. Rits Y, Oderich GS, Bower TC, et al. Interventions for mesenteric vasculitis. *J Vasc Surg.* 2010;51(2):392-400.
6. Menke J. Diagnostic accuracy of multidetector CT in acute mesenteric ischaemia: systematic review and meta-analysis. *Radiology.* 2010;256(1):93-101.
7. Resch TA, Acosta S, Sonesson B. Endovascular techniques in acute arterial mesenteric ischae-mia. *Semin Vasc Surg.* 2010;23(1):29-35.
8. Wyers MC. Acute mesenteric ischaemia: diagnostic approach and surgical treatment. *Semin Vasc Surg.* 2010;23(1):9-20.
9. Rasmussen TE, Hallett JW Jr. Inflammatory aortic aneurysms. A clinical review with new perspectives in pathogenesis. *Ann Surg.* 1997;225(2):155-164.
10. Walker DI, Bloor K, Williams G, Gillie I. Inflammatory aneurysms of the abdominal aorta. *Br J Surg.* 1972;59(8):609-614.
11. Tang T, Boyle JR, Dixon AK, Varty K. Inflammatory abdominal aortic aneurysms. *Eur J Vasc Endovasc Surg.* 2005;29(4):353-362.
12. Ashrani AA, Heit JA. Incidence and cost burden of post-thrombotic syndrome. *J Thromb Thrombolysis.* 2009;28(4):465-476.
13. Comerota AJ. Randomized trial evidence supporting a strategy of thrombus removal for acute DVT. *Semin Vasc Surg.* 2010;23(3):192-198.
14. Di NM, Wichers IM, Middeldorp S. Treatment for superficial thrombophlebitis of the leg. *Cochrane Database Syst Rev.* 2007;(2):CD004982.

Suggested Reading

Branchereau A, Jacobs M. *Vascular emergencies.* 1st ed. Oxford: Blackwell; 2003.
Waltham M, Burnand KG. Surgical treatments. In: Asherson R, Cervera R, eds. *Vascular manifes-tations of systemic autoimmune diseases.* 1st ed. Boca Raton: CRC Press; 2001:529.

Complicated Pregnancies in Patients with Autoimmune Systemic Diseases

20

Guillermo Ruiz-Irastorza and Munther A. Khamashta

Abstract Systemic autoimmune diseases (SAD) are complex conditions with the potential for severe multiorgan involvement. Many patients are young women, thus potentially subject to one or more pregnancies during the course of their disease. An integrated multidisciplinary approach is essential in order to assure a correct diagnosis and management of pregnancy complications in this group of women.

Keywords Antiphospholipid syndrome • Miscarriage • Preeclampsia • Pregnancy • Systemic lupus erythematosus • Systemic sclerosis

Systemic autoimmune diseases (SAD) are complex conditions with the potential for severe multiorgan involvement. Many patients are young women, thus potentially subject to one or more pregnancies during the course of their disease. The old classical dogma stating that pregnancy was usually contraindicated in women with SAD is fortunately obsolete, for most of these patients can complete successful pregnancies. However, the chance for serious complications is not negligible (Table 20.1).

Systemic lupus erythematosus (SLE) may flare,[1] residual renal impairment may worsen[2] and there is a risk of suffering hypertension or preeclampsia, thrombosis, miscarriage, and growth restriction and prematurity.[3] Recent data from a national study in the US confirm these fears.[4] It identified 13,555 deliveries between 2000 and 2003, in women with a diagnosis of SLE at discharge. Women with a diagnosis of lupus were more likely to suffer from pregestational diabetes mellitus, hypertension, pulmonary hypertension (PH), renal failure, and thrombophilia. The chance of suffering pregnancy complications was two- to fourfold higher: preeclampsia happened in 22.5% of women with lupus vs. 7.6% in the general population, preterm labor in 20.8% vs. 8.1%, and intrauterine growth restriction in 5.6% vs. 1.5%, respectively. Moreover, medical complications such as stroke, pulmonary

G. Ruiz-Irastorza (✉)
Autoimmune Disease Research Unit, Department of Internal Medicine,
Hospital de Cruces, University of the Basque Country,
Pza Cruces s/n, Barakaldo, Bizkaia 48903, Spain
e-mail: r.irastorza@euskaltel.net

M.A. Khamashta and M. Ramos-Casals (eds.), *Autoimmune Diseases*,
DOI: 10.1007/978-0-85729-358-9_20, © Springer-Verlag London Limited 2011

Table 20.1 Potential pregnancy complications of systemic autoimmune diseases

Systemic lupus erythematosus	Lupus flare
	Worsening organ damage
	Hypertension
	Preeclampsia
	Miscarriage
	Fetal loss
	Prematurity
Antiphospholipid syndrome	Thrombosis
	Preeclampsia
	Miscarriage
	Fetal loss
	Intrauterine growth restriction
	Prematurity
Systemic sclerosis	Worsening gastroesophageal reflux
	Scleroderma renal crisis
	Heart failure in women with pulmonary hypertension
	Respiratory insufficiency in women with interstitial lung disease

embolus, deep vein thrombosis, major infections, bleeding, and thrombocytopenia were two to eight times more frequent among women with SLE.

Seventy six percent of the 63 women from the LUMINA cohort who became pregnant during the follow-up presented complications.[5] Moreover, these authors reported a significant, albeit modest, increase in irreversible damage postpartum, which was especially determined by disease activity and the presence of damage before conception. However, treatment-related variables were not entered in the model. In other studies, corticosteroid use, as well as disease activity, has been associated with prematurity and general adverse pregnancy outcome.[6,7]

Antiphospholipid syndrome (APS) has been associated with a wide range of potential pregnancy complications, including miscarriage, fetal death, intrauterine growth restriction, prematurity, and preeclampsia.[8] A recent large population-based study showed that women with positive antiphospholipid antibodies (aPL) had an increased risk of preeclampsia/eclampsia (OR 2.93) and placental insufficiency (OR 4.58). The risk increased further in those aPL-positive women with a concomitant diagnosis of SLE.[9]

Compared with SLE and APS, systemic sclerosis has a lower incidence and a higher mean age of onset, around the early 40s.[10] Nonetheless, women with systemic sclerosis, particularly those with early-onset disease, may face the possibility of pregnancy. Common manifestations, such as Raynaud's and gastroesophageal reflux, may be affected by pregnancy (improving or worsening, respectively) without a critical influence on its course. This is not the case of major organ involvement, particularly renal and cardiopulmonary. Scleroderma renal crisis is a dreadful complication of systemic sclerosis with a grim prognosis. Maternal cardiorespiratory overload is the rule in normal pregnancy, especially in the last trimester and delivery, and, in women with significant arterial pulmonary hypertension or restrictive lung disease, may lead to life-threatening situations.[11] Moreover, in a recent population-based survey of around 14,000,000 obstetric hospitalizations, the 695 women with systemic sclerosis had an increased risk of having suffered hypertensive disorders (OR 3.95) and intrauterine growth restriction (OR 3.67).[12] However, preeclampsia has not been a significant problem in most cohorts of pregnant women with scleroderma.[10]

20.1
High-Risk Pregnancy Situations

20.1.1
Lupus Flare

Whether pregnancy increases lupus activity has been a question of debate for years. Now, it is generally agreed that SLE is more likely to flare in unselected women.[1,13] However, women with lupus in longstanding remission are much more likely to complete uneventful pregnancies from a lupus point of view.[14,15] Data from the Hopkins Lupus Cohort showed an increased chance for developing lupus nephritis;[16] however, flares during pregnancy are not usually severe.[1]

One of the recently identified factors that increases the risk for lupus flares during pregnancy is hydroxychloroquine discontinuation. In a small randomized controlled trial, Levy et al. showed that women taking hydroxychloroquine during pregnancy had lower activity scores and lower doses of prednisone at delivery.[17] Clowse et al. obtained similar results in a prospective cohort study, in which women not taking hydroxychloroquine, and, specially, those who had withdrawn it, had more flares, higher activity scores, and needed higher doses of prednisone.[18]

Lupus flares are also a problem for the baby. The impact of lupus activity on pregnancy outcome has been recently addressed.[19] Women with high lupus activity during pregnancy had a higher chance of miscarriage, prematurity, and perinatal death. In addition, increasing doses of prednisone used to treat flares may contribute to complications, and many other drugs are contraindicated during this period (see below), making treatment much more problematic.

Clinical and immunological features of lupus activity may be difficult to recognize during pregnancy. Fatigue and mild arthralgia are common among normal pregnant women. Edema normally appears during the last phases of pregnancy and, if symmetrical and without accompanying hypertension or proteinuria, is not a warning sign. Mild anemia and thrombocytopenia are also common in pregnant women. Lupus activity scales specific for pregnancy have been established;[20,21] however, experienced clinical judgment is the best way to evaluate lupus activity during pregnancy in daily practice.

20.1.2
Lupus Nephritis

Lupus nephritis is a clinical challenge, especially during pregnancy. The risk of suffering a renal flare seems variable, particularly related to SLE status at the time of conception and the history of previous renal involvement. Therefore, patients with recent active nephritis are at the highest risk, while those in longstanding remission with no past kidney disease are at the lowest.[2]

A second important point is the recognition of renal activity during pregnancy. Urinary protein excretion normally rises during pregnancy in women with residual proteinuria, thus not always reflecting active disease.[2] Complement levels normally increase during pregnancy, thus limiting their utility as markers of active lupus. Proteinuria, hypertension, and decline in renal function can also be seen in preeclampsia. In fact, the differential diagnosis between these two conditions is difficult, as both conditions can coexist. Women with renal disease are at a higher risk for hypertensive complications during pregnancy.[22] Rising uric acid levels point to preeclampsia while the presence of hematuria and/or cellular casts, extrarenal activity, rising anti-DNA antibody levels, and falling complement levels (even within normal limits for non-pregnant patients) point to lupus nephritis.[22] Supporting therapy and labor induction in severe cases is commonly indicated.

Management of active lupus nephritis is also conflicting during pregnancy. Most immunosuppressive drugs, with the exception of azathioprine and cyclosporin, are contraindicated during pregnancy,[23] making it difficult to treat proliferative forms. Antiproteinuric drugs such as angiotensin-converting enzyme inhibitors and angiotensin receptor antagonists can neither be employed during the full course of pregnancy due to the risk of renal failure and oligoamnios, as well as reported congenital malformations in babies born to women receiving angiotensin-converting enzyme inhibitors during the first trimester of pregnancy.[2,24] Thus, pulse steroids followed by a combination of prednisone (aiming for a rapid reduction to maintenance doses <7.5 mg/day), hydroxychloroquine, and azathioprine are the usual therapy.[3] Intravenous immunoglobulins can be safely used in pregnant women[23] and are thus an option in active cases in order to buy time before labor induction can be performed.

The last issue is the impact of renal disease on pregnancy outcome. A recent study from the Toronto Lupus Cohort compared the course of 81 women with lupus renal involvement, suffered within 6 months preconception and delivery, and 112 without.[25] They found a significant increase in the frequency of hypertension and a lower mean weight at birth in the group of patients with renal disease. On the other hand, complications such as preeclampsia or perinatal death were infrequent in both groups. A live baby was the result of almost 60% of pregnancies overall, without significant differences between women with or without nephritis.

However, other studies have shown a higher impact of renal disease on pregnancy outcome. A small retrospective study from Saudi Arabia found a significantly higher frequency of pregnancy complications among those women with active lupus nephritis, as compared with those in remission (fetal loss 52% vs. 30%, complicated premature deliveries, 36% vs. 16%, respectively).[26] An observational study by Imbasciati et al., including 113 pregnancies in 81 women with lupus renal disease, identified hypocomplementemia and the combined variable proteinuria >1 gr/day or glomerular filtration rate below ml/min/1.73 m[2] as independent predictors of adverse fetal or maternal outcomes.[27] Of note, treatment with low-dose aspirin was associated with an improvement of pregnancy outcome in this series. A recent review by Germain and Nelson-Piercy identified women with baseline serum creatinine levels higher than 2.5–2.8 mg/dl (220–250 μmol/l) as those most likely to suffer postpartum renal function decline as well as complications during pregnancy.[28] A recently published systematic review and meta-analysis found that lupus women with past nephritis or active nephritis were more likely to suffer hypertension and prematurity.[29] In addition, those with a history of nephritis also had a higher risk for preeclampsia.[29]

In view of these data, lupus renal disease does not generally preclude pregnancy. However, women with either active disease or established severe renal impairment and/or proteinuria should be monitored with vigilance, in view of the increased risk of both maternal and fetal complications. Low-dose aspirin is useful in these patients, including its effect in preventing preeclampsia in high-risk pregnancies (see below).

20.1.3
Preeclampsia

Apart from renal disease, a recent systematic review has identified several predictors of preeclampsia, such as a previous history of preeclampsia (odds ratio 7.19) and the presence of APS (odds ratio 9.72).[30] Preeclampsia has no effective therapy other than delivery. Thus, prevention is the main goal. A recent meta-analysis has shown a statistically significant reduction in the frequency of pregnancy complications among women at high risk for preeclampsia who took low-dose aspirin.[31] Recurrent preeclampsia, preterm delivery before 34 weeks, perinatal death, small babies at birth, and any serious adverse outcome were all significantly reduced by around 10%. Extrapolating these data, treatment with low-dose aspirin during pregnancy would be indicated in women with SAD with aPL, history of preeclampsia, hypertension, and/or renal disease.

20.1.4
Antiphospholipid Syndrome

The presence of aPL is one of the most important predictors of adverse pregnancy outcome, both in women with and without SLE. A recent survey of 141,286 women delivering in Florida in 2001 found positivity for aPL in 88 of them.[9] This subgroup was more likely to have preeclampsia/eclampsia, placental insufficiency, and a longer duration of admission. Similar data were obtained in a Japanese study, in which women with positive aPL were at a higher risk for hypertension, preeclampsia, fetal death, growth restriction, and prematurity.[32] Combined positivity for both anticardiolipin antibodies (aCL) and lupus anticoagulant (LA) multiplied the risk. Triple aPL positivity (LA plus aCL plus anti-β2-glycoprotein I) was also associated with prematurity and lower birth weight in a Italian study,[33] as was the history of maternal thrombosis. In keeping with these data, a recent study from London also showed a worse obstetric profile in women with previous thrombosis.[34] Thus, aPL positivity is a risk marker for pregnancy complications, this risk being modulated by both immunological (the more number of positive aPL, the worst) and clinical profiles (women with previous thrombosis are at the highest risk).

Severe preeclampsia complicated by HELLP syndrome (hemolysis, elevated liver enzymes, low platelets) may occasionally develop in pregnant women with APS. A recent

Table 20.2 Suggested regimens for the treatment of antiphospholipid syndrome in pregnancy

Antiphospholipid syndrome without prior thrombosis
(a) Recurrent early (pre-embryonic or embryonic) miscarriage
    Low-dose aspirin ALONE OR PLUS:
    LMWH: usual prophylactic doses (e.g., enoxaparin 40 mg/day sc. or dalteparin 5,000 U/day, sc.)
(b) Fetal death (>10 weeks gestation) or prior early delivery (<34 weeks gestation) due to
    severe preeclampsia or placental insufficiency
    Low-dose aspirin PLUS:
    LMWH: usual prophylactic doses (e.g., enoxaparin 40 mg/day sc. or dalteparin 5,000 U/
    day, sc.)

Antiphospholipid syndrome with thrombosis
    Low-dose aspirin PLUS:
    LMWH: usual therapeutic dose (e.g., enoxaparin 1 mg/kg sc. or dalteparin 100 U/kg, sc.
    every 12 h or enoxaparin 1.5 mg/kg/day sc. or dalteparin 200 U/kg/day sc.)

LMWH low-molecular-weight heparin

retrospective series of 16 cases (14 during pregnancy, 2 postpartum) showed a high rate of fetal death: The baby died in 6 out of 14 episodes of HELLP starting in the second or third trimesters.[35] Therapy with low-dose aspirin and low-molecular-weight heparin substantially decreased the risk of HELLP in subsequent pregnancies. However, HELLP recurred in one woman fully treated. Thus, close monitoring should be performed in all cases.

Low-dose aspirin should be taken by all women with aPL in order to decrease the risk of miscarriage[36] and preeclampsia.[31,36] Preconceptional treatment has improved results in some series.[37] Since warfarin is contraindicated during organogenesis and complicated to use afterward, due to an increased risk of fetal bleeding,[23] full antithrombotic-dose heparin, preferably low molecular weight, is given to women with previous thrombosis. For women without thrombosis, treatment should be individualized (Table 20.2). There is general agreement in treating those with fetal (late) deaths with aspirin plus low-dose heparin, although most data for this subgroup come from observational studies.[36,38] On the other hand, according to some clinical trials, some women suffering early miscarriages only may do well with low-dose aspirin alone,[36] although current guidelines recommend the universal combination of aspirin and heparin.[38] In all cases, women should be informed of the different treatment possibilities and the final option be assumed by the patient, the physician, and the obstetrician. Adequate postpartum thromboprophylaxis with low-dose, low-molecular-weight heparin is important in all women with aPL, although the duration is a matter of debate. Four to six weeks is the usual recommendation;[38] however, a recent British consensus document advocates shorter courses.[39]

20.1.5
Neonatal Lupus and Congenital Heart Block

Neonatal lupus (NNL) syndromes is a rare complication affecting children born to mothers with lupus, Sjögren's syndrome, and, even, asymptomatic women, whose most serious form of presentation is congenital heart block (CHB). This syndrome is closely related to the presence of maternal anti-Ro and anti-La antibodies. These antibodies gain access to the fetal circulation during the active transport of IgG across the placenta that happens between the 16th and 30th weeks of gestation. The prevalence of CHB among newborns of anti-Ro-positive women with known connective tissue diseases is around 2%.[40] However, this risk increases to 18% in younger siblings of an infant with CHB.[41] The actual prevalence may be even higher, since incomplete forms of CHB have been described, including first-degree heart block that can progress during childhood.[41] Most children affected with CHB would need a permanent pacemaker, and around 20% may die in the perinatal period.[41]

Serial fetal echocardiograms must be performed between 18 and 28 weeks of pregnancy to all women with anti-Ro and/or anti-La antibodies. If a case of incomplete heart block, myocarditis, ascites, or hydrops is identified, therapy with fluorinated steroids – dexamethasone or betamethasone, which crosses the placental barrier – is recommended since there is a chance for reversibility (total or partial).[41] Recently, two clinical trials have failed to reduce the expected rate of recurrent CHB (20%) in women treated with IVIG during pregnancy.[42,43] On the other hand, a recent case-control study has suggested a protective effect of hydroxychloroquine on the development of cardiac manifestations in children with NNL born to mothers with lupus and anti-Ro/anti-La antibodies.[44]

Other clinical manifestations, including photosensitive skin rash (Fig. 20.1), hepatitis, and thrombocytopenia, are also part of the NNL syndromes spectrum. Unlike CHB, these mild forms of NNL disappear as maternal antibodies are cleared from the baby's circulation.[41]

20.1.6
Pulmonary Hypertension

Pulmonary Hypertension (PH) is defined by a resting mean pulmonary artery pressure ≥25 mm/Hg, measured by right heart catheterization.[45] Systemic sclerosis is an important cause of PH, accounting for most cases of pulmonary arterial hypertension (PAH) secondary to connective tissue diseases.[46] In addition, patients with systemic sclerosis, SLE, inflammatory myopathies, Sjögren's syndrome and APS, can develop PH secondary to interstitial lung disease or chronic thromboembolism.[46]

The prognosis of PAH has significantly improved with the development of effective therapies, including prostacyclin analogues, endothelin-receptor antagonists, phosphodiesterase inhibitors, and nitric oxide.[47] Unfortunately, endothelin-receptor antagonists are contraindicated during pregnancy. Thus, therapy in pregnant women should be based on oral sildenafil, intravenous prostacyclin analogues, inhaled iloprost and nitric oxide, as well as LMWH, since long-term anticoagulation is recommended in all patients with idiopathic and connective tissue disease–related PAH and chronic thromboembolic PH.[48]

Pregnancy and labor, however, are very high-risk situations for women with PH. Pregnancy-related mortality has been estimated to be over 30%.[48,49] Thus, experts agree that PH should be considered a major contraindication for pregnancy and effective contraception recommended to affected fertile women.[48] Pregnancy termination should be

Fig. 20.1 Typical neonatal lupus rash (**a**), with spontaneous resolution 3 months later (**b**)

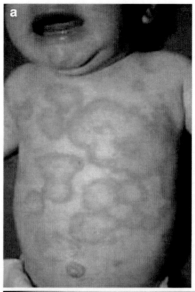

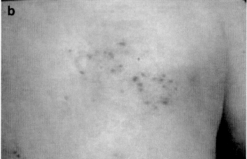

discussed if a woman with PH becomes pregnant. However, if the patient decides to go on with pregnancy, multidisciplinary management in a center with experience in treating patients with PH is warranted. A recent series of nine cases managed in a referral center, receiving targeted therapy with combinations of inhaled iloprost, intravenous epoprostenol, and oral sildenafil plus prophylactic LMWH, reported nine live babies, all delivered between 32 and 37 weeks except for a very premature baby of 26 weeks.[50] One mother died in the postpartum period. Elective Cesarean section under combined epidural/spinal anesthesia is recommended by these authors.[50]

In summary, PH should be considered a very high-risk condition in pregnant women, with high maternal mortality that justifies the contraindication of pregnancy. However, if pregnancy occurs and the fully informed woman refuses termination of pregnancy, these patients must be managed by a combined team including physicians with experience in PH, in a center with fully equipped intensive care and neonatal units. Combined therapy with inhaled iloprost, oral sildenafil, intravenous prostacy-clin analogues, and LMWH with close monitorization of hemodynamic parameters is warranted.[48,50]

20.1.7
Scleroderma Renal Crisis

Scleroderma renal crisis constitutes one of the most feared complications of systemic scle-rosis, with a high rate of associated progression to end-stage renal disease and mortality.[51] Several clinical and immunological factors help identify scleroderma patients at high risk for developing this condition: early (<4 years) diffuse disease, rapid progression of skin thickening, presence of pericardial effusion, positivity for anti-RNA polymerase III anti-bodies, and treatment with high-dose steroids.[51] Early and aggressive treatment with ACE inhibitors is mandatory.

Should scleroderma renal crisis develop in a pregnant woman, it must be considered a medical and obstetric emergency. Differential diagnosis includes severe preeclampsia with HELLP syndrome, with whom scleroderma renal crisis shares many features, like hypertension and microangiopathic anemia but not liver involvement. Despite formal con-traindication in pregnancy, therapy with ACE should be instituted early.[52] Prematurity is almost the rule in this setting, but with adequate management, both mother and child can survive.[10]

Blood pressure should be closely monitored in women with systemic sclerosis and high-risk features for scleroderma renal crisis. Likewise, women with early aggressive disease should be discouraged from getting pregnant until the disease has stabilized.[10] A previous history of scleroderma renal crisis is not a contraindication for pregnancy, provided there is clinical stability and no major organ damage.[51]

20.2
General Management Plan

Adequate pregnancy care of women with connective tissue diseases rests on the three pillars of a coordinated medical-obstetrical care, an agreed and well-defined management protocol and a good neonatal unit. Preconceptional counseling is essential in order to estimate the chance of both fetal and maternal problems and to provide the patient with reliable informa-tion regarding her specific risk for complications and the expected management plan (Tables 20.3 and 20.4). A complete set of autoantibodies should be available before preg-nancy, including aPL, both aCL and LA, anti-Ro and anti-La antibodies, and, in women with systemic sclerosis, anti-RNA polymerase II should be anti-RNA polymerase III anti-bodies, if available. Women with active disease should delay pregnancy until a quiescent phase of the disease, especially those with renal, cardiopulmonary, or neurological involve-ment, thrombosis. Women with early diffuse scleroderma should also postpone pregnancy until the disease has stabilized. Women with a high degree of irreversible damage are more

Table 20.3 Preconceptional visit checklist

Age?
Any previous pregnancy?
Previous pregnancy complications?
Presence of severe irreversible organ damage?
History of renal, heart, or lung disease?
Recent or current lupus activity?
Presence of antiphospholipid antibodies/syndrome?
Recent thrombosis?
Early (<4 years) diffuse systemic sclerosis?
Positivity of anti-Ro/anti-La?
Current treatment: any "forbidden" drugs?
Smoking?

Table 20.4 High-risk features for pregnancy in women with systemic autoimmune diseases

Previous poor obstetric history
Lupus nephritis
Renal failure
Heart failure
Pulmonary hypertension
Interstitial lung disease
Active disease
Early (<4 years) diffuse systemic sclerosis
Systemic sclerosis with pericardial effusion
High degree of irreversible organ damage
High-dose steroid therapy
Presence of antiphospholipid antibodies/syndrome
Presence of anti-Ro/La antibodies
Multiple pregnancy
Age over 40 years

likely to suffer complications and even further damage during and after pregnancy particularly those with chronic renal, lung, or heart disease. Pregnancy may be contraindicated in some situations (Table 20.5).

This is also the time to evaluate the safety of the treatment received by the patient. Most forbidden medications can (and should) be stopped at this point and be substituted by alternative drugs (Table 20.6). Smoking should be also strongly discouraged.

Women considered to be at high risk should be best managed in a combined medical-obstetrical clinic throughout the whole pregnancy. The general schedule includes more frequent visits as pregnancy progresses. Blood pressure should be measured on each visit, but women with hypertension, previous preeclampsia, or past or present renal involvement should also ideally provide additional home measurements. Likewise, regular urine analysis is essential to detect proteinuria, which could be the first sign of impending preeclampsia or renal lupus flare.

Table 20.5 Contraindications to pregnancy in women with systemic autoimmune diseases

Severe pulmonary hypertension (estimated systolic PAP > 50 mmHg or symptomatic)
Severe restrictive lung disease (FVC < 1 l)
Heart failure
Chronic renal failure (Cr ≥ 3 mg/dl)
Previous severe preeclampsia or HELLP despite therapy with aspirin and heparin
Stroke within the previous 6 months
Severe lupus flare within the previous 6 months
Early (<4 years) active diffuse systemic sclerosis

PAP pulmonary arterial pressure, *FVC* forced vital capacity

Table 20.6 Summary of drugs permitted and contraindicated during pregnancy

Permitted	Contraindicated
Immunosuppressive drugs	
Azathioprine[a]	Cyclophosphamide
Cyclosporine	Methotrexate
	Mycophenolate mofetil
Corticosteroids	
Prednisone/prednisolone[a]	Dexamethasone[b]
Methyl-prednisolone	
Antimalarials	
Hydroxychloroquine[a]	
Chloroquine[a]	
Antihypertensive drugs	
Methyl-dopa[a]	ACE inhibitors[a]
Labetalol[a]	Angiotensin receptor antagonists
Nifedipine[a]	Diuretics
Anticoagulant and antiaggregant drugs	
Heparin and LMWH[a]	Warfarin[a]
Aspirin (low dose)[a]	
Other	
Immunoglobulins[a]	NSAIDs (third trimester)
Vitamin D[a]	
Sildenafil	Bosentan

ACE angiotensin-converting enzyme, *LMWH* low-molecular-weight heparins, *NSAIDs* nonsteroidal anti-inflammatory drugs
[a]Drugs allowed during breast feeding
[b]Except for *in utero* treatment of fetal myocarditis, *hydrops fetalis*, or immature babies

Doppler studies of the placental vessels are very useful to estimate placental function and to predict the occurrence of complications such as preeclampsia and fetal distress. Uterine Doppler studies are recommended in women at high risk for preeclampsia (those with aPL, renal disease, hypertension, previous preeclampsia, multiple pregnancy, and age over 40), first done around the 20th week and repeated 4 weeks later if abnormal. Umbilical

Doppler ultrasound after the 24th week may show absent or even reverse diastolic flow, a sign of impending placental insufficiency and fetal distress. The finding of abnormal Doppler studies is considered an adverse prognostic sign that increases the risk of adverse outcomes. On the other hand, the negative predictive value of this test is higher as repeated normal results are associated with very low frequency of obstetric complications.[53,54] Repeated ultrasound examination of baby's heart is needed between the 18th and 28th weeks when the mother is anti-Ro and/or anti-La positive in order to detect congenital heart block.[41]

The postpartum period should be considered high risk for women with SLE and APS, with several possible complications such as, lupus flares and thrombosis. A close surveillance within the first 4 weeks after delivery is thus warranted.

References

1. Ruiz-Irastorza G, Lima F, Alves J, et al. Increased rate of lupus flare during pregnancy and the puerperium: a prospective study of 78 pregnancies. *Br J Rheumatol.* 1996;35:133-138.
2. Day CJ, Lipkin GW, Savage CO. Lupus nephritis and pregnancy in the 21st century. *Nephrol Dial Transplant.* 2009;24:344-347.
3. Ruiz-Irastorza G, Khamashta MA. Lupus and pregnancy: ten questions and some answers. *Lupus.* 2008;17:416-420.
4. Clowse MEB, Jamison M, Myesr E, James AH. A national study of the complications of lupus in pregnancy. *Am J Obstet Gynecol.* 2008;199:127.e1-127.e6.
5. Andrade RM, McGwin G Jr, Alarcon GS, et al. Predictors of post-partum damage accrual in systemic lupus erythematosus: data from LUMINA, a multiethnic US cohort (XXXVIII). *Rheumatology.* 2006;45:1380-1384.
6. Chakravarty EF, Colón I, Langen ES, et al. Factors that predict prematurity and preeclampsia in pregnancies that are complicated by systemic lupus erythematosus. *Am J Obstet Gynecol.* 2005;192:1897-1904.
7. Andrade R, Sanchez ML, Alarcon GS, et al. Adverse pregnancy outcomes in women with systemic lupus erythematosus from a multiethnic US cohort: LUMINA (LVI). *Clin Exp Rheumatol.* 2008;26:268-274.
8. Ruiz-Irastorza G, Khamashta MA. Managing lupus patients during pregnancy. *Best Pract Res Clin Rheumatol.* 2009;23:575-582.
9. Nodler J, Moolamalla SR, Ledger EM, Nuwayhid BS, Mulla ZD. Elevated antiphospholipid antibody titers and adverse pregnancy outcomes: analysis of a population-based hospital dataset. *BMC Pregnancy Childbirth.* 2009;9:11.
10. Steen VD. Pregnancy in scleroderma. *Rheum Dis Clin North Am.* 2007;33:345-358.
11. Ruiz-Irastorza G, Khamashta MA, Hughes GRV. Heart disease, pregnancy and systemic autoimmune diseases. In: Oakley C, Warnes CA, eds. *Heart disease in pregnancy.* 2nd ed. Oxford: Blackwell Publishing; 2007:136-150.
12. Chakravarty EF, Khanna D, Chung L. Pregnancy outcomes in systemic sclerosis, primary pulmonary hypertension, and sickle cell disease. *Obstet Gynecol.* 2008;111:927-934.
13. Petri M, Howard D, Repke J. Frequency of lupus flare in pregnancy. The Hopkins Lupus Pregnancy Center experience. *Arthritis Rheum.* 1991;34:1538-1545.
14. Urowitz MB, Gladman DD, Farewell VT, Stewart J, McDonald J. Lupus and pregnancy studies. *Arthritis Rheum.* 1993;36:1392-1397.

15. Le Thi Huong D, Wechsler B, Vauthier-Brouzes D, et al. Outcome of planned pregnancies in systemic lupus erythematosus: a prospective study on 62 pregnancies. *Br J Rheumatol.* 1997;36:772-777.
16. Petri M. The Hopkins Lupus Pregnancy Center: ten key issues in management. *Rheum Dis Clin North Am.* 2007;33:227-235.
17. Levy R, Vilela V, Cataldo M, et al. Hydroxychloroquine (HCQ) in lupus pregnancy: double-blind and placebo-controlled study. *Lupus.* 2001;10:401-404.
18. Clowse M, Magder L, Witter F, Petri M, Petri M. Hydroxychloroquine in lupus pregnancy. *Arthritis Rheum.* 2006;54:3640-3647.
19. Clowse MEB, Magder LS, Petri M. The impact of increased lupus activity on obstetric outcomes. *Arthritis Rheum.* 2005;52:514-521.
20. Buyon JP, Kalunian KC, Ramsey-Goldman R, et al. Assessing disease activity in SLE patients during pregnancy. *Lupus.* 1999;8:677-684.
21. Ruiz-Irastorza G, Khamashta MA, Gordon C, et al. Measuring systemic lupus erythematosus activity during pregnancy: validation of the Lupus Activity Index in Pregnancy scale. *Arthritis Rheum.* 2004;51:78-82.
22. Mackillop LH, Germain SJ, Nelson-Piercy C. Systemic lupus erythematosus. *Br Med J.* 2007;335:933-936.
23. Ostensen M, Khamashta M, Lockshin M, et al. Anti-inflammatory and immunosuppressive drugs and reproduction. *Arthritis Res Ther.* 2006;8:209-227.
24. Cooper WO, Hernandez-Diaz S, Arbogast PG, et al. Major congenital malformations after first-trimester exposure to ACE inhibitors. *N Engl J Med.* 2006;354:2443-2451.
25. Gladman DD, Tandon A, Ibañez D, Urowitz M. The effect of lupus nephritis on pregnancy outcome and fetal and maternal complications. *J Rheumatol.* 2010;37:754-758.
26. Rahman FZ, Rahman J, Al-Suleiman SA, Rahman MS. Pregnancy outcome in lupus nephropathy. *Arch Gynecol Obstet.* 2005;271:222-226.
27. Imbasciati E, Tincani A, Gregorini G, et al. Pregnancy in women with pre-existing lupus nephritis: predictors of fetal and maternal outcome. *Nephrol Dial Transplant.* 2009;24:519-525.
28. Germain S, Nelson-Piercy C. Lupus nephritis and renal disease in pregnancy. *Lupus.* 2006;15:148-155.
29. Smyth A, Oliveira G, Lahr B, Bailey K, Norby S, Garovic V. A systematic review and meta-analysis of pregnancy outcomes in patients with systemic lupus erythematosus and lupus nephritis. *Clin J Am Soc Nephrol.* 2010;5(11):2060-2068. Epub 2010 May 25.
30. Milne F, Redman C, Walker J, et al. The pre-eclampsia community guideline (PRECOG): how to screen for and detect onset of pre-eclampsia in the community. *Br Med J.* 2005;330:576-580.
31. Askie LM, Duley L, Henderson-Smart DJ, Stewart LA. On behalf of the PARIS Collaborative Group. Antiplatelet agents for prevention of pre-eclampsia: a meta-analysis of individual patient data. *Lancet.* 2007;369:1791-1798.
32. Yamada H, Atsumi T, Kobashi G, et al. Antiphospholipid antibodies increase the risk of pregnancy-induced hypertension and adverse pregnancy outcomes. *J Reprod Immunol.* 2009;79:188-195.
33. Ruffatti A, Calligaro A, Hoxha A, et al. Laboratory and clinical features of pregnant women with antiphospholipid syndrome and neonatal outcome. *Arthritis Care Res.* 2010;62:302-307.
34. Bramham K, Hunt BJ, Germain S, et al. Pregnancy outcome in different clinical phenotypes of antiphospholipid syndrome. *Lupus.* 2010;9:58-64.
35. Le Thi Thuong D, Tieulié N, Costedoat N, et al. The HELLP syndrome in the antiphospholipid syndrome: retrospective study of 16 cases in 15 women. *Ann Rheum Dis.* 2005;64:273-278.
36. Ruiz-Irastorza G, Crowther MA, Branch DW, Khamashta MA. Antiphospholipid syndrome. *Lancet.* 2010;376(9751):1498-1509. Epub 2010 Sep 6.

37. Carmona F, Font J, Cervera R, Muñoz F, Cararach V, Balasch J. Obstetrical outcome of pregnancy in patients with systemic lupus erythematosus. A study of 60 cases. *Eur J Obstet Gynecol Reprod Biol.* 1999;83:137-142.

38. Bates SM, Greer IA, Pabinger I, Sofaer S, Hirsh J. Venous thromboembolism, thrombophilia, antithrombotic therapy, and pregnancy: American College of Chest Physicians Evidence-Based Clinical Practice Guidelines (8th Edition). *Chest.* 2008;133:844S-886S.

39. Royal College of Obstetricians and Gynaecologists. Reducing the risk of thrombosis and embolism during pregnancy and the puerperium. *Green Top Guideline* n 37; November 2009.

40. Brucato A, Frassi M, Franceschini F, et al. Risk of congenital complete heart block in newborns of mothers with anti-Ro/SSA antibodies detected by counterimmunoelectrophoresis: a prospective study of 100 women. *Arthritis Rheum.* 2001;44:1832-1835.

41. Izmirly PM, Rivera TL, Buyon JP. Neonatal lupus syndromes. *Rheum Dis Clin N Am.* 2007;33:267-285.

42. Friedman D, Llanos C, Izmirly PM, et al. Evaluation of fetuses in a study of intravenous immunoglobulin as preventive therapy for congenital heart block: Results of a multicenter, prospective, open-label clinical trial. *Arthritis Rheum.* 2010;62:1138-1146.

43. Pisoni C, Brucato A, Ruffatti A, et al. Failure of intravenous immunoglobulin to prevent congenital heart block: Findings of a multicenter, prospective, observational study. *Arthritis Rheum.* 2010;62:1147-1152.

44. Izmirly PM, Kim MY, Llanos C, et al. Evaluation of the risk of anti-SSA/Ro-SSB/La antibody-associated cardiac manifestations of neonatal lupus in fetuses of mothers with systemic lupus erythematosus exposed to hydroxychloroquine. *Ann Rheum Dis.* 2010;69(10): 1827-1830. Epub 2010 May 6.

45. Badesch DB, Champion HC, Sanchez MA, et al. Diagnosis and assessment of pulmonary arterial hypertension. *J Am Coll Cardiol.* 2009;54:S55-S66.

46. Simonneau G, Robbins IM, Beghetti M, et al. Updated clinical classification of pulmonary hypertension. *J Am Coll Cardiol.* 2009;54:S43-S54.

47. Humbert M, Sitbon O, Simonneau G. Treatment of pulmonary arterial hypertension. *N Engl J Med.* 2004;351:1425-1436.

48. National Pulmonary Hypertension Centres of the UK and Ireland. Consensus statement on the management of pulmonary hypertension in clinical practice in the UK and Ireland. *Heart.* 2008;94:S1-S41.

49. Bonnin M, Mercier FJ, Sitbon O, et al. Severe pulmonary hypertension during pregnancy. Mode of delivery and anesthetic management of 15 consecutive cases. *Anesthesiology.* 2005;102:1133-1137.

50. Kiely DG, Condliffe R, Webster V, et al. Improved survival in pregnancy and pulmonary hypertension using a multiprofessional approach. *Br J Obstet Gynaecol.* 2010;117:565-574.

51. Steen VD. Scleroderma renal crisis. *Rheum Dis Clin North Am.* 2003;29:315-333.

52. Miniati I, Guiducci S, Mecacci F, Mello G, Matucci-Cerinic M. Pregnancy in systemic sclerosis. *Rheumatology (Oxford).* 2008;47(Suppl 3):iii16-iii18.

53. Le Thi Huong D, Wechsler B, Vauthier-Brouzes D, et al. The second trimester Doppler ultrasound examination is the best predictor of late pregnancy outcome in systemic lupus erythematosus and/or the antiphospholipid syndrome. *Rheumatology (Oxford).* 2006;45:332-338.

54. Castellino G, Capucci R, Govoni M, Mollica G, Trotta F. Uterine artery Doppler in predicting pregnancy outcome in women with connective tissue disorders. *Rheumatology (Oxford).* 2006;45:1174-1175.

The Complex Management of Viral-Related Autoimmune Diseases

21

Dimitrios Vassilopoulos and Spilios Manolakopoulos

Abstract Viral-associated autoimmune syndromes are usually encountered during the acute and/or chronic phase of viral infections due to hepatitis B virus (HBV), hepatitis C virus (HCV), or human immunodeficiency virus (HIV). The management of these autoimmune manifestations with antirheumatic drugs could lead in certain situations to exacerbation or worsening of the underlying viral infection with potentially harmful effects to the host. In most cases, therapeutic approaches combining immunosuppressive with antiviral agents are needed for the better management of these difficult-to-treat patients. In this chapter, recent advances in the treatment of viral-associated autoimmune diseases are presented.

Key Words Arthritis • Autoimmune diseases • Hepatitis B virus • Hepatitis C virus • Human immunodeficiency virus • Sjögren's Syndrome • Vasculitis

21.1
Introduction

Viruses have been implicated for a long time in the pathogenesis of various organ-specific (such as thyroiditis, diabetes mellitus type I) or systemic (systemic lupus erythematosus – SLE, Sjögren's syndrome, vasculitides) autoimmune diseases.[1] Their role as triggering factors and/or causative agents of autoimmune diseases has been suggested from animal studies as well as from epidemiological and clinical studies in human autoimmune diseases. Despite the abundance of data implicating viruses in autoimmunity, only in a few clinical settings, their pathogenetic role has been unequivocally proven.

The most common viruses associated with the development of autoimmune manifestations include the hepatitis B virus (HBV), the hepatitis C virus (HCV) and the human immunodeficiency virus (HIV).[2]

D. Vassilopoulos (✉)
Associate Professor of Medicine-Rheumatology, 2nd Department of Medicine,
Athens University School of Medicine, Hippokration General Hospital, Athens, Greece
e-mail: dvassilop@med.uoa.gr

M.A. Khamashta and M. Ramos-Casals (eds.), *Autoimmune Diseases*,
DOI: 10.1007/978-0-85729-358-9_21, © Springer-Verlag London Limited 2011

Autoimmune syndromes can arise either during the acute or chronic phase of a viral infection. The management of viral-related autoimmune diseases is complicated by the need to strike a balance between the beneficial effect of immunosuppressive therapies on the underlying autoimmune disease and their detrimental effect on viral replication in target organs (i.e., liver for chronic hepatitis B, immune system in HIV).[2] In this chapter, the treatment of the most common virus-associated autoimmune syndromes, including clinical situations with organ- or life-threatening complications, is reviewed.

21.2
Hepatitis B Virus Infection

Autoimmune manifestations in HBV-infected patients can occur either during the acute or chronic phase of the infection.[3]

21.2.1
HBV-Related Serum Sickness-Like Syndrome

A proportion of patients with acute hepatitis B (5–15%) can present with an immune complex–mediated serum sickness–like syndrome, manifesting by fever, poly-arthralgias/arthritis of the small joints, or more rarely with a small-vessel vasculitis affecting mainly the skin (presenting with an urticarial, petechial, or purpuric rash).[4,5] Typically, the clinical manifestations are present during the pre-icteric phase of acute hepatitis B, lasting a few weeks and resolving spontaneously with the appearance of jaundice.

Immune complexes containing hepatitis B surface antigen (HBsAg) and antibodies against HBsAg (anti-HBs) which are deposited in synovial tissues and vessel walls are considered to play a pathogenetic role in this inflammatory process.

Nonspecific serological findings during this period can cause diagnostic confusion including the frequent presence of rheumatoid factor (RF) and low complement levels (C3 and C4).[4] A high clinical suspicion should direct the search for an underlying acute HBV infection in such cases based on the findings of elevated aminotransferases (AST/ALT) in the majority of cases. The serological findings are typical of acute hepatitis B with positive HBsAg and high-titer IgM antibodies against the core antigen (IgM anti-HBc). HBV DNA can be positive, although its absence does not exclude the possibility of acute hepatitis B, since in certain cases, a vigorous host immune response can lead to early viral clearance at the expense of severe hepatocellular injury manifested by highly elevated levels of aminotransferases and even hepatic failure.

Typically, the skin and joint manifestations of HBV-associated serum sickness–like syndrome last 2–3 weeks and subside with the appearance of jaundice.[4] Given the transient nature and favorable outcome of this syndrome, no specific immunosuppressive therapy is required. Furthermore, according to the most recent guidelines, there is no need for antiviral treatment in such patients since the majority of adult patients recover spontaneously (>95%).[6,7] Only for patients with fulminant hepatitis B or protracted disease, oral antiviral therapy with oral nucleoside or nucleotide analogues may be indicated. The choice of a specific agent should take into account HBV DNA levels, other comorbidities (i.e., renal dysfunction), and the rapidity of onset of action of the different antiviral agents. The preferred approach should be decided in consultation with an expert in the treatment of HBV infection (hepatologist).

21.2.2
HBV-Related Polyarteritis Nodosa

21.2.2.1
Clinical Manifestations and Laboratory Findings

Polyarteritis nodosa (PAN) is the prototype and best studied virus-associated vasculitic syndrome so far.[8] Initially HBV was considered as the most common etiologic factor for PAN, with studies from France in the 1970s showing a prevalence of HBV infection reaching almost 40% among patients with newly diagnosed PAN. The development of vaccines against HBV and their administration to people at risk may explain the dramatic decrease of the number of new cases in the same patient population (<20%) while studies from other areas of the world have shown a much lower prevalence of HBV infection among PAN patients (<10%).[9]

HBV-associated PAN usually appears during the acute or early chronic phase of HBV infection and is characterized by segmental inflammation of predominantly medium-sized vessels (mainly arteries).[9,10] An immune complex–mediated inflammatory process, similar to the "serum sickness–like" syndrome described in the pre-icteric phase of acute hepatitis B, with deposition of HBsAg, complement, and immunoglobulins in vessel walls, is the presumed pathogenetic mechanism. It is still unclear why in certain cases after acute hepatitis B, a small-vessel vasculitis with predominant skin involvement develops while in other cases, medium size vasculitis predominates.

The clinical manifestations of HBV-associated PAN reflect the multisystemic nature of the disease.[9,10] These include constitutional symptoms like weight loss, fever, arthralgias/myalgias, or symptoms attributed to the specific organ involvement such as peripheral neuropathy (mononeuritis multiplex or peripheral polyneuropathy), gastrointestinal (abdominal ischemia), or renal (hypertension, renal failure) involvement. According to the results from a recent large retrospective study from France, HBV-associated PAN runs a more severe course with more frequent nerve, gastrointestinal, and heart involvement compared to non-HBV-associated PAN whereas skin involvement appears to be less frequent (~35%).[9]

Anemia, mild leukocytosis, thrombocytosis, and elevated acute phase reactants such as erythrocyte sedimentation rate (ESR) and C-reactive protein (CRP) are common nonspecific laboratory findings.[8,9] Serological markers suggestive of acute hepatitis B are present in the majority of patients including HBsAg, HBeAg, high-titer serum HBV DNA, and IgM anti-HBc. It should be noted though that approximately one-third of patients with HBV-associated PAN have normal aminotransferases, emphasizing the need for screening for an underlying HBV infection in cases suspicious for PAN even without obvious abnormalities in liver enzymes.[9]

Definite diagnosis of HBV-associated PAN requires either a positive biopsy from an affected organ (skin, muscle, nerve, GI) revealing the characteristic necrotizing arteritis of medium-sized vessels or an abnormal angiogram showing the distinctive microaneurysms or stenotic lesions of medium-sized vessels (abdominal, renal arteries). In a recent study, approximately 70% of patients with HBV-associated PAN had abnormal abdominal or renal angiograms.[9] Biopsies of muscles and/or nerves provide the best tissues for an accurate diagnosis of PAN, demonstrating the characteristic segmental areas of vascular inflammation and fibrinoid necrosis (sensitivity: 65–83%).[8,9]

21.2.2.2
Treatment

Treatment of patients with HBV-associated PAN is a challenging undertaking for the physicians caring for these patients since the majority of patients require initially immunosuppressive therapy with high-dose corticosteroids.[9,10] In severe cases or in patients with steroid-resistant or relapsing disease, another immunosuppressive agent (cyclophosphamide, azathioprine) is usually added (see Fig. 21.1). Use of these agents though, without appropri-

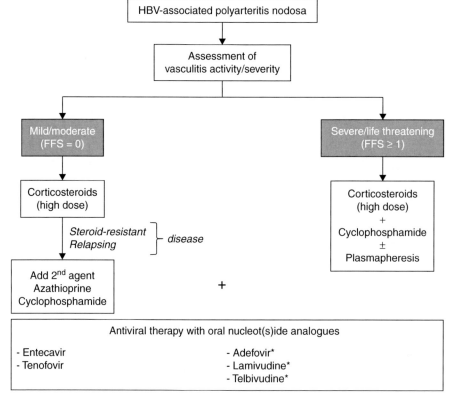

Fig. 21.1 A therapeutic algorithm for patients with hepatitis B virus (*HBV*)–associated polyarteritis nodosa (*PAN*) is presented. Patients are initially categorized as suffering from mild/moderate or severe PAN according to the five factor score (FFS: elevated serum creatinine levels: >140 μmol/l or 1.58 mg/dl, proteinuria: >1 g/day, severe gastrointestinal tract involvement, cardiomyopathy, central nervous system involvement).[11] All patients should receive concomitantly antiviral therapy with one of the above oral nucleoside or nucleotide analogues. (*Note*: *These agents should be used only in inactive HBsAg carriers (see text for definition) scheduled for short courses of immunosuppression (<12 months))

ate antiviral therapy, can lead to fulminant liver failure or even death, due to rebound HBV viremia and enhanced host immune response against virus-infected hepatocytes.

Although case reports and small uncontrolled studies have suggested a favorable response to antiviral treatment alone, the majority of patients require combination therapy with antivirals and immunosuppressives.[9,10] In Fig. 21.1, a therapeutic algorithm is proposed. The initial immunosuppressive regimen should be chosen according to the severity of vasculitis. In patients without adverse prognostic factors, high-dose steroids alone may suffice.[9,10] For steroid-resistant or relapsing disease, azathioprine or cyclophosphamide is the alternative therapeutic option. There are limited data for the efficacy of newer agents such as mycophenolate mofetil as maintenance therapy in this setting. For patients with severe gastrointestinal, renal, cardiac, or central nervous system involvements (Five Factor Score or FFS ≥ 1),[11] the addition of cyclophosphamide is indicated (pos or IV).[9,10] For life-threatening disease, plasmapheresis could be added.[9,10]

Whatever immunosuppressive regimen is selected, the addition of antiviral therapy from the beginning with one of the approved oral nucleoside or nucleotide analogues is imperative.[4,6,7] The selection of the most appropriate antiviral agent should be based on specific viral (HBV DNA levels, state of viral infection, i.e., HBsAg carrier state vs. chronic hepatitis B), host (presence of advanced liver fibrosis/cirrhosis, presence or absence of renal dysfunction), and drug (rapidity of onset of action) characteristics.[4] Therapeutic decisions as well as the issue of performing a baseline liver biopsy should be discussed with a hepatologist.

The duration of antiviral therapy depends on the HBV infection status as well as the predicted duration of immunosuppressive therapy. For patients with chronic hepatitis B or cirrhosis, long-term antiviral therapy regardless of the duration of immunosuppressive therapy is needed while for inactive HBsAg carriers (defined by normal or near-normal ALT levels, undetectable or low serum HBV DNA levels-<2,000 IU/ml, absence of significant liver inflammation or fibrosis in liver biopsy), continuation of antiviral therapy for 6–12 months after cessation of immunosuppressive therapy is indicated, according to the most recent guidelines.[4,6,7] Frequent monitoring of HBV DNA, HBsAg, and liver function is crucial for this group of patients. For patients who achieve viral clearance (HBsAg loss), no further antiviral therapy is required.

According to a recent large retrospective study from France, the overall long-term mortality rate of HBV-associated PAN is high (~34%) with a 10-year survival rate of 54%.[9] In patients with severe disease, deaths usually occur early in the disease course and are primarily related to the vasculitic process itself (70% during the first year after diagnosis). In such cases, the most common cause of death was severe GI involvement.[9] These data emphasize the need for early aggressive immunosuppressive treatment in patients with severe disease and adverse prognostic factors. Despite its severe course, HBV-associated PAN rarely relapses after clinical remission has been achieved (<10%).[9]

21.2.3
Other HBV-Related Rheumatic Diseases

A direct association between chronic HBV infection and autoimmune diseases is rare. Among these manifestations are HBV-associated cryoglobulinemic vasculitis, leukocytoclastic vasculitides, Henoch–Schönlein purpura and membranous nephropathy. In such cases, the treatment approach does not differ significantly from the one described above for HBV-associated PAN.

In most cases, rheumatologists encounter patients with coexisting autoimmune diseases such as SLE, RA, and vasculitides in the context of a known or newly diagnosed chronic HBV infection.[4] The incidence of HBV infection among the rheumatic population of patients does not seem to differ from that of the general population.

Immunosuppression has been shown to induce HBV reactivation at a rate that ranges from 20% to 70%, depending on the immunosuppressive regimen, its dose, and duration of administration as well as the state of the underlying chronic HBV infection (chronic hepatitis B, inactive HBsAg carrier state).[12] Patients with chronic hepatitis B (evidenced by elevated levels of AST/ALT, increased serum HBV DNA levels – >20,000 IU/ml, significant liver inflammation, and/or fibrosis in liver biopsy) are particularly at high risk for HBV reactivation that can lead to exacerbation of liver inflammation and in certain cases to hepatic failure.[4,12]

Although most data regarding HBV reactivation have been gathered over the last two decades from patients with hematologic or neoplastic diseases receiving chemotherapeutic schemes, recent studies have emphasized the potential of antirheumatic drugs to induce such HBV reactivation without appropriate antiviral prophylaxis.[4,13] Among rheumatic therapies those that have been definitely associated with HBV reactivation include high-dose steroids, anti-TNF agents, immunosuppressives such as cyclophosphamide and B-cell-depleting agents (rituximab).[4,13] Rarely, commonly used DMARDs such as methotrexate can also cause HBV reactivation.[4,13]

In a recent review of the literature, 73% of rheumatic patients receiving anti-TNF agents without prophylactic treatment with antivirals displayed viral reactivation.[14] On the contrary, preemptive use of an oral anti-HBV agent can prevent HBV reactivation in most patients (>90%) with chronic HBV infection treated with anti-TNF agents.[15]

International Guidelines and expert opinion recommend that all patients with autoimmune diseases scheduled to receive immunosuppressives should be screened for an underlying HBV infection (HBsAg, anti-HBc, anti-HBs).[4,6,7,13] Patients with chronic HBV infection (HBsAg+) should receive antiviral treatment prior to or at the time of the initiation of immunosuppressive therapy. Interferon-alpha (IFN-a) is contraindicated in these patients due to its frequent side effects (cytopenias) and the potential to exacerbate the underlying rheumatic disease.

Thus, therapy should be initiated with one of the approved oral nucleoside or nucleotide analogues (lamivudine, adefovir, entecavir, telbivudine, tenofovir).[6,7] These antivirals have simplified the treatment of chronic hepatitis B due to their safety profile and ease of administration. Despite their effectiveness in reducing HBV viral load, during chronic administration, drug-induced resistant viral strains may emerge. The rate of drug-induced viral resistance during chronic treatment differs significantly among the different agents as shown in Table 21.1.[6,7] The decision about the most appropriate antiviral agent should be individualized in consultation with a hepatologist and in accordance to recently published treatment guidelines (as presented for patients with HBV-associated PAN above, Fig. 21.1).[6,7] The duration of antiviral therapy depends on the status of the chronic HBV infection and the duration of the planned immunosuppressive therapy. Since most of these patients require long-term or even life-long immunosuppressive therapy, antiviral agents

Table 21.1 Rates of drug-induced viral resistance in patients with chronic hepatitis B during prolonged treatment with oral antivirals

Antiviral agent	Rate of viral resistance (years of follow-up)
Lamivudine	65% (5 years)
Adefovir	29% (5 years)
Telbivudine	22% (2 years)
Entecavir	1.2% (6 years)
Tenofovir	0% (3 years)

Source: Data from references European Association for the Study of the Liver[7], Heathcote et al.[37], Marcellin et al.[38], and Tenney et al.[39]
The rates of viral resistance during chronic treatment for chronic hepatitis B (HBeAg + or −) are shown for the different oral antiviral agents

with low risk for drug-induced viral resistance should be chosen (entecavir, tenofovir), especially for patients with underlying chronic hepatitis B. Special attention should be given in patients receiving rituximab, since there have been reports from the Oncology literature for HBV reactivation even in patients with resolved or occult HBV infection (HBsAg-, anti-HBc+, anti-HBs±).[16] So far, there has not been a consensus regarding antiviral prophylaxis in these cases;[6,7] thus, frequent measurement of HBsAg (every 3–6 months) and/or HBV DNA is recommended in order to diagnose early viral reactivation and initiate antiviral therapy.

21.3
Hepatitis C Virus Infection

Chronic HCV infection, caused by a parenterally transmitted hepatotropic RNA virus (HCV), remains a worldwide public health problem with more than 170 million people affected.[16] People at risk include injection drug uses, those who had been transfused with blood or blood-derived products prior to 1992 and those with multiple sex partners.[17] The majority of adult patients (55–85%) exposed to HCV develop chronic infection. Depending on a number of factors such as advanced age, alcohol abuse, presence of liver steatosis, and coinfections (HIV), around 20% of patients develop end-stage liver disease and 10% hepatocellular carcinoma during the course of their chronic infection.[17] The vast majority of infected patients are asymptomatic; thus, screening for HCV infection with anti-HCV antibodies (confirmed by an HCV RNA assay for those found positive) is recommended for all rheumatic patients, especially those scheduled for antirheumatic treatment.

Since the discovery of HCV in the early 1990s, a number of autoimmune phenomena (clinical and laboratory) have been attributed to the virus.[17] The capacity of HCV not only to infect hepatocytes but also to bind and activate B lymphocytes is the presumed pathogenetic mechanism behind these autoimmune manifestations. The best studied

HCV-associated autoimmune diseases include inflammatory arthritis, cryoglobulinemic vasculitis, and sialadenitis (Sjögren's like).

21.3.1
HCV-Associated Arthritis

21.3.1.1
Clinical and Laboratory Findings

Articular symptoms (arthralgias or inflammatory arthritis) are not uncommon in the HCV population (2–30%); these can be due to a coexistent – unrelated to HCV – arthropathy (SLE, RA, fibromylagia, etc.), mixed cryoglobulinemia (MC), HCV-associated inflammatory arthritis, and more rarely due to the antiviral therapy itself (IFN-a).[18]

In less than 5% of patients with chronic HCV infection, an inflammatory arthritis directly related to HCV has been reported.[19] Most patients present with a symmetric polyarthritis of the small joints (MCPs, PIPs, ankles) while in 20%, a mono- or oligo-arthritic pattern is seen.

A coexisting inflammatory (RA, SLE, Sjögren's syndrome, myositis, etc.) or noninflammatory (fibromyalgia) rheumatic disorder is probably the most common form of arthritis in this population. Since chronic HCV infection (without articular manifestations) can share clinical and laboratory findings with these disorders such as sicca symptoms, fatigue, positive rheumatoid factor (RF, 40–65%), cytopenias, anti-nuclear antibodies (ANA, 10%), or low C4 levels, a careful approach is needed for making the correct diagnosis. The presence of certain laboratory (anti-CCP for RA, anti-dsDNA for SLE, anti-Ro/La for Sjogren's syndrome) or radiological (erosive articular changes in RA) findings are helpful for the differential diagnosis.[18]

21.3.1.2
Treatment

There are limited data on the treatment of HCV-associated arthritis; analgesics, low-dose corticosteroids (<10 mg/day), and rarely DMARDs or anti-TNF agents have been used[19] without significant side effects.

For patients with a coexisting inflammatory arthritis (RA, spondyloarthritis, SLE, etc.), before starting antirheumatic therapy, a thorough assessment of the severity of chronic HCV infection (mild hepatitis, fibrosis, advanced fibrosis-cirrhosis) is imperative and should be performed in consultation with a hepatologist.[4,20] Laboratory (prothrombin time, INR, albumin), imaging (ultrasound of the upper abdomen, transient elastography), and invasive (liver biopsy) techniques are usually required for an accurate assessment. Based on these findings, a decision regarding the most appropriate and less hepatotoxic antirheumatic therapy can be made.

For patients with advanced fibrosis or with clinical evidence of decompensated cirrhosis (ascites, encephalopathy, coagulopathy), immunosuppressive medications should be used with extreme caution.[21] Potentially hepatotoxic DMARDs such as methorexate and leflunomide should be avoided while anti-TNF or B-cell-depleting agents (rituximab) can be used only in case of severe or life-threatening disease complications.

In patients with less advanced disease and stable liver function, these medications can be used with close monitoring of liver function. Biologic agents such as anti-TNF[22] and B-cell-depleting (rituximab)[23,24] agents have been used for a short period of time (up to 2 years) in rheumatic patients with chronic HCV infection without any significant effect on HCV RNA levels or, more importantly, liver function.

21.3.2
HCV-Associated Cryoglobulinemic Vasculitis

21.3.2.1
Clinical and Laboratory Findings

Although cryoglobulins are detected in approximately half of the patients with chronic HCV infection, less than 5% of these patients develop the full blown syndrome of mixed cryoglobulinemia manifested by arthralgias/myalgias, purpura, peripheral neuropathy, membranoproliferative glomerulonephritis, etc.[25] HCV-associated MC can run either an indolent course characterized by bouts of recurrent purpura in the lower extremities or, more rarely, an aggressive course with severe peripheral polyneuropathy and/or glomerulonephritis leading to renal failure. In the latter scenario, immediate therapeutic action is needed in order to avoid organ damage and prolong survival.

21.3.2.2
Treatment

The goals of therapy in HCV-associated MC are dual: to suppress the inflammatory process and to eradicate the virus.[25] Antiviral therapy–induced HCV clearance almost universally leads to sustained clinical remission of MC. The current standard of care for patients with chronic hepatitis C is the administration of pegylated IFN-a (2a or 2b, subcutaneously once a week) in combination with ribavirin (800–1,200 mg/day pos) for 6–12 months (depending on viral genotype and on treatment response to antiviral therapy).[17] Sustained viral clearance is achieved in approximately half of the patients with this regimen. The response to antiviral therapy in patients with HCV-associated MC does not seem to differ from patients with chronic hepatitis C without MC.[25]

There are several caveats though in administering antiviral therapy in patients with HCV-associated MC. It is well established that IFN-a can induce vasculitic exacerbation (especially in patients with severe vasculitic manifestations) while at the same time, it can cause bone marrow suppression (cytopenias).[25] Ribavirin and IFN-a should be used with extreme caution and in reduced doses in patients with renal dysfunction (creatinine clearance <60 ml/min/1.73 m^2).[17] while IFN-a-based regimens cannot be used in patients with decompensated cirrhosis.[17] Thus, in such cases, immunosuppressive therapy alone is the only available therapeutic option.

In general, for patients with mildly or moderately active vasculitis, antiviral therapy can be administered alone (with or without the addition of low-dose corticosteroids, <10 mg/day) for 6–12 months while for patients with severe or life-threatening vasculitis (severe glomerulonephritis, peripheral neuropathy, digital ulcers or necrosis, gastrointestinal involvement), antiviral therapy should be delayed until vascular inflammation has subsided with the appropriate immunosuppressive therapy (Fig. 21.2).

Most data regarding immunosuppressive therapy in the setting of HCV-associated MC are available for corticosteroids, cyclophosphamide, plasmapheresis, and lately on rituximab.[24–26] Older series in patients with "essential" mixed cryoglobulinemia from Italy[27] have clearly shown that high-dose corticosteroids in combination with cyclophosphamide did not have an adverse effect on liver function in this patient population when given for an extended period of time. More recently, a number of promising data have been accumulated showing that rituximab, used either as monotherapy or in combination with antiviral therapy, is a safe and efficacious option for HCV-associated MC.[23,24,28] The combination of antiviral therapy

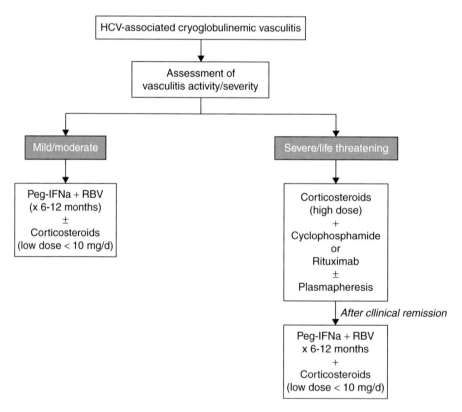

Fig. 21.2 The therapeutic approach for patients with hepatitis C virus (*HCV*)-associated cryoglobulinemic vasculitis is depicted. Peg-IFN-a: Pegylated interferon-a (-2a or -2b), RBV: ribavirin (800–1,200 mg/day, according to weight and viral genotype). The doses of Peg-IFN-a and RBV should be adjusted in patients with renal dysfunction (creatinine clearance <60 ml/min/1.73 m^2)[17]

(pegylated IFN-a and ribavirin) and rituximab led to complete clinical remission in 55–73% of cases with much lower relapse rates (~20%) compared to combination antiviral therapy alone (36–60%).[23,24] It is also reassuring that rituximab alone has been used in patients with advanced liver disease (cirrhosis), without inducing liver decompensation.[26]

Despite these encouraging results, there are certain issues regarding rituximab therapy in patients with HCV-associated MC that need to be explored further. First, there are no long-term data (>5 years) regarding its safety (effect on liver function, infection rate). Secondly, special caution is needed in patients with high baseline cryocrit (≥1 g/l) levels and low C4 values, since serious serum sickness–like reactions and exacerbation of vasculitis have been reported due to the formation of immune complexes between rituximab and cryoglobulins (IgM$_\kappa$).[29] Whether plasmapheresis should be performed first followed by rituximab infusions in such severe cases remains to be proven. Third, there is currently no consensus regarding the correct timing of initiation of combination antiviral therapy and rituximab in patients with severe HCV-associated MC.[23,24] Probably, the best course of action is to delay antiviral therapy until clinical remission has been achieved by the immunosuppressive therapy (corticosteroids, rituximab).

21.4
Human Immunodeficiency Virus Infection

Autoimmune manifestations in patients with HIV infection have declined significantly in frequency and severity with the introduction of highly active antiretroviral therapy (HAART) in the late 1990s.[30] Despite these optimistic advancements, in certain patients with severe autoimmune manifestations, the issue of administering immunosuppressive therapies frequently arises.[3] Such cases include patients with severe HIV-associated inflammatory arthropathy, HIV-associated myositis, patients with coexisting autoimmune diseases such as SLE, RA, vasculitis, etc. In the past, there were reports of patients who developed infectious complications with the administration of immunosuppressives including DMARDs (methotrexate) and anti-TNF agents.[31] These were mainly seen in HIV patients with advanced disease and uncontrolled viral replication. More recent data have indicated that in carefully selected HIV patients with inflammatory arthropathies the use of DMARDs or anti-TNF agents was not associated with serious adverse events.[32–36] Thus, in general, in patients with severe autoimmune manifestations who receive appropriate antiretroviral therapy and maintain CD4 counts >200/μl with low or undetectable HIV RNA levels, immunosuppressive therapy can be administered under close monitoring.

References

1. Calabrese LH. Emerging viral infections and arthritis: the role of the rheumatologist. *Nat Clin Pract Rheumatol.* 2008;4:2-3.
2. Vassilopoulos D, Calabrese LH. Virally associated arthritis 2008: clinical, epidemiologic, and pathophysiologic considerations. *Arthritis Res Ther.* 2008;10:215.

3. Calabrese LH, Zein N, Vassilopoulos D. Safety of antitumour necrosis factor (anti-TNF) therapy in patients with chronic viral infections: hepatitis C, hepatitis B, and HIV infection. *Ann Rheum Dis*. 2004;63(Suppl 2):ii18-ii24.
4. Vassilopoulos D, Manolakopoulos S. Rheumatic manifestations of hepatitis. *Curr Opin Rheumatol*. 2010;22:91-96.
5. Dienstag JL. Hepatitis B virus infection. *N Engl J Med*. 2008;359:1486-1500.
6. Lok ASF, McMahon BJ. AASLD Practice Guidelines. Chronic hepatitis B: Update 2009. Accessed at www.aasld.org on September 1 2010.
7. European Association for The Study of the Liver. EASL Clinical Practice Guidelines: management of chronic hepatitis B. *J Hepatol*. 2009;50:227-242.
8. Guillevin L, Mahr A, Callard P, et al. Hepatitis B virus-associated polyarteritis nodosa: clinical characteristics, outcome, and impact of treatment in 115 patients. *Medicine (Baltimore)*. 2005;84:313-322.
9. Pagnoux C, Seror R, Henegar C, et al. Clinical features and outcomes in 348 patients with polyarteritis nodosa: a systematic retrospective study of patients diagnosed between 1963 and 2005 and entered into the French Vasculitis Study Group Database. *Arthritis Rheum*. 2010; 62:616-626.
10. Stone JH. Polyarteritis nodosa. *JAMA*. 2002;288:1632-1639.
11. Guillevin L, Lhote F, Gayraud M, et al. Prognostic factors in polyarteritis nodosa and Churg-Strauss syndrome. A prospective study in 342 patients. *Medicine (Baltimore)*. 1996;75:17-28.
12. Hoofnagle JH. Reactivation of hepatitis B. *Hepatology*. 2009;49:S156-S165.
13. Calabrese LH, Zein NN, Vassilopoulos D. Hepatitis B virus (HBV) reactivation with immunosuppressive therapy in rheumatic diseases: assessment and preventive strategies. *Ann Rheum Dis*. 2006;65:983-989.
14. Zingarelli S, Frassi M, Bazzani C, et al. Use of tumor necrosis factor-alpha-blocking agents in hepatitis B virus-positive patients: reports of 3 cases and review of the literature. *J Rheumatol*. 2009;36:1188-1194.
15. Vassilopoulos D, Apostolopoulou A, Hadziyannis E, et al. Long-term safety of anti-TNF treatment in patients with rheumatic diseases and chronic or resolved hepatitis B virus infection. *Ann Rheum Dis*. 2010;69:1352-1355.
16. Yeo W, Chan TC, Leung NW, et al. Hepatitis B virus reactivation in lymphoma patients with prior resolved hepatitis B undergoing anticancer therapy with or without rituximab. *J Clin Oncol*. 2009;27:605-611.
17. Ghany MG, Strader DB, Thomas DL, et al. Diagnosis, management, and treatment of hepatitis C: an update. *Hepatology*. 2009;49:1335-1374.
18. Vassilopoulos D, Calabrese LH. Rheumatic manifestations of hepatitis C infection. *Curr Rheumatol Rep*. 2003;5:200-204.
19. Rosner I, Rozenbaum M, Toubi E, et al. The case for hepatitis C arthritis. *Semin Arthritis Rheum*. 2004;33:375-387.
20. Vassilopoulos D, Calabrese LH. Risks of immunosuppressive therapies including biologic agents in patients with rheumatic diseases and co-existing chronic viral infections. *Curr Opin Rheumatol*. 2007;19:619-625.
21. Saag KG, Teng GG, Patkar NM, et al. American College of Rheumatology 2008 recommendations for the use of nonbiologic and biologic disease-modifying antirheumatic drugs in rheumatoid arthritis. *Arthritis Rheum*. 2008;59:762-784.
22. Ferri C, Ferraccioli G, Ferrari D, et al. Safety of anti-tumor necrosis factor-alpha therapy in patients with rheumatoid arthritis and chronic hepatitis C virus infection. *J Rheumatol*. 2008;35:1944-1949.
23. Dammacco F, Tucci FA, Lauletta G, et al. Pegylated interferon-alpha, ribavirin, and rituximab combined therapy of hepatitis C virus-related mixed cryoglobulinemia: a long-term study. *Blood*. 2010;116:343-353.

24. Saadoun D, Resche RM, Sene D, et al. Rituximab plus Peg-interferon-alpha/ribavirin compared with Peg-interferon-alpha/ribavirin in hepatitis C-related mixed cryoglobulinemia. *Blood*. 2010;116:326-334.
25. Vassilopoulos D, Calabrese LH. Hepatitis C virus infection and vasculitis. Implications of antiviral and immunosuppressive therapies. *Arthritis Rheum*. 2002;46:585-597.
26. Petrarca A, Rigacci L, Caini P, et al. Safety and efficacy of rituximab in patients with hepatitis C virus-related mixed cryoglobulinemia and severe liver disease. *Blood*. 2010;116:335-342.
27. D'Amico G, Colasanti G, Ferrario F, et al. Renal involvement in essential mixed cryoglobulinemia. *Kidney Int*. 1989;35:1004-1014.
28. Cacoub P, Delluc A, Saadoun D, et al. Anti-CD20 monoclonal antibody (rituximab) treatment for cryoglobulinemic vasculitis: where do we stand? *Ann Rheum Dis*. 2008;67:283-287.
29. Sene D, Ghillani-Dalbin P, Amoura Z, et al. Rituximab may form a complex with IgMkappa mixed cryoglobulin and induce severe systemic reactions in patients with hepatitis C virus-induced vasculitis. *Arthritis Rheum*. 2009;60:3848-3855.
30. Walker UA, Tyndall A, Daikeler T. Rheumatic conditions in human immunodeficiency virus infection. *Rheumatology (Oxford)*. 2008;47:952-959.
31. Aboulafia DM, Bundow D, Wilske K, et al. Etanercept for the treatment of human immunodeficiency virus-associated psoriatic arthritis. *Mayo Clin Proc*. 2000;75:1093-1098.
32. Cepeda EJ, Williams FM, Ishimori ML, et al. The use of anti-tumour necrosis factor therapy in HIV-positive individuals with rheumatic disease. *Ann Rheum Dis*. 2008;67:710-712.
33. Linardaki G, Katsarou O, Ioannidou P, et al. Effective etanercept treatment for psoriatic arthritis complicating concomitant human immunodeficiency virus and hepatitis C virus infection. *J Rheumatol*. 2007;34:1353-1355.
34. Sellam J, Bouvard B, Masson C, et al. Use of infliximab to treat psoriatic arthritis in HIV-positive patients. *Joint Bone Spine*. 2007;74:197-200.
35. Bartke U, Venten I, Kreuter A, et al. Human immunodeficiency virus-associated psoriasis and psoriatic arthritis treated with infliximab. *Br J Dermatol*. 2004;150:784-786.
36. Gaylis N. Infliximab in the treatment of an HIV positive patient with Reiter's syndrome. *J Rheumatol*. 2003;30:407-411.
37. Heathcote EJ, Gane EJ, de Man RA, et al. Three years of tenofovir disoproxil (TDF) treatment in HBeAg – positive patients (HBeAg+) with chronic hepatitis B (study 103). *Hepatology*. 2009;50(Suppl 4):533A-534A.
38. Marcellin P, Buti M, Krastev Z, et al. Three years of tenofovir disoproxil fumarate (TDF) treatment in HBeAg – negative patients with chronic hepatitis B (study 102). *Hepatology*. 2009;50(Suppl 4):532A-533A.
39. Tenney DJ, Pokornowski KA, Rose RE, et al. Entecavir maintains a high genetic barrier to HBV resistance through 6 years in naive patients. *J Hepatol*. 2009;50(Suppl 1):S10.

The Role of Intravenous Immunoglobulins in the Management of Acute Complex Autoimmune Conditions

22

Rotem Kedar, Yehuda Shoenfeld, and Howard Amital

Abstract Intravenous immunoglobulin (IVIG) was used in the past to treat immune deficiency states. Recently, it is more employed over the counter for treatment of autoimmune diseases. Only a few randomized controlled studies were performed in autoimmune diseases (AITP, polymyositis), but it seems that in many refractory cases, case reports and small series indicate a successful avenue. Moreover, by and large, the therapy although quite expensive is associated with low risks and especially if delivered properly (i.e., slow infusion, not more than 28 g/day, etc.) Recently, novel aspects of IVIG led to the generation of a new kind of IVIG, called specific IVIG, still not in clinical use but very promising.

Keywords Autoantibodies • Autoimmunity • AITP • IVIG • SLE • Systemic sclerosis

Intravenous immunoglobulin (IVIG), an immunomodulatory agent, is used to treat various autoimmune diseases, including autoimmune thrombocytopenia (AITP), Kawasaki disease, systemic lupus erythematosus, multiple sclerosis, myasthenia gravis, antiphospholipid syndrome, and others. In some cases, such as AITP and Kawasaki disease, its use is well established and commonly used, while in others, our knowledge is based mainly on case reports and uncontrolled trials. Thus, IVIG is used as salvage treatment, once all other approved options have been exhausted and failed.

22.1
Mechanisms of Action

The various mechanisms through which IVIG affects autoimmune diseases are not fully recognized and understood, but several mechanisms have been suggested[1]:

H. Amital (✉)
Department of Medicine 'B', Chaim Sheba Medical Centre,
Tel-Hashomer 52621, Israel
e-mail: hamital@netvision.net.il

M.A. Khamashta and M. Ramos-Casals (eds.), *Autoimmune Diseases*,
DOI: 10.1007/978-0-85729-358-9_22, © Springer-Verlag London Limited 2011

1. The most extensively studied mechanism was described in AITP, where the therapeutic effect was attributed to interference with Fc receptor (FcR)–mediated platelet clearance by phagocytic cells. Administration of IVIG results in a decreased clearance of anti-D-coated autologous erythrocytes in vivo,[2] and peripheral blood monocytes of IVIG-treated patients with AITP exhibit a decreased ability to form rosettes with IgG-coated erythro-cyte.[3] The binding of the injected immunoglobulins to macrophage FcR hinders the clearance of antibody-coated cells in the reticuloendothelial system. Furthermore, IVIG binding to inhibitory FcγRIIb on macrophages leads to the deactivation of phagocytosis.[4] The Fc portion of IgG interacts with FcR. Free monomeric IgG will compete with antibody–antigen complexes for activation of the FcR (such as FcγRI and FcγRIII), albeit with lower avidity.[2]

2. IVIG also abrogates the ability of aggregated IgG to lead to complement activation – The Fc portion of IgG competes for complement components, and although IVIG can activate complement,[5] it also appears to scavenge C3a and C5a, thus conferring an anti-inflammatory effect.[6]

3. The $F(ab)_2$-binding site region of IgG represents a "species repertoire" within IVIG that has a range of mechanistic effects. In IVIG replacement therapy for primary antibody deficiencies, it is the repertoire against pathogens that is of critical importance, while with IVIG for autoimmune disease, a range of effects has been demonstrated. Intact IgG, but not Fc fragments, suppresses in vitro T-cell responses to mitogens and anti-gens.[7] IVIG manipulates the idiotypic network via the binding of idiotypic (Id) and antiidiotypic antibodies.[8] In normal serum, autoreactive IgG may be constantly blocked by Id/anti-Id interactions with IgM.[9] IVIG saturates the regulating mechanism of auto-reactive IgG and participates in the formation of autoimmune complexes, which may participate in the therapeutic effects of IVIG, particularly in diseases where immune complexes play an important role.[10]

4. Other postulated mechanisms of IVIG action have been suggested, including enhancement of suppressor activity, complement regulation, modulation of T and B lympho-cyte activities, induction of apoptosis in lymphocytes and monocytes, and neutralization of pathogenic antibodies,[11] as well as shortening the half-life of naturally occurring IgG.[12]

IVIG treatment is generally a safe treatment, but it is not free of side effects. Most adverse events are mild, and include headache, fever, nausea, diarrhea, blood pressure changes, and tachycardia. However, some severe side effects, including renal failure and thromboembolic events, as well as IgA deficiency–related anaphylactic reactions may occur. Risk factors include advanced age, previous thromboembolic diseases, previous renal failure, immobilization, diabetes mellitus, hypertension, and dyslipidemia.[13] These risk factors should be taken into consideration when deciding whether to treat patients, and in any case, the administration must be slow, and proper hydration must be maintained. In the coming chapter, we discuss the clinical aspects of IVIG therapy in acute pure and infection-related autoimmune conditions.

22.2
IVIG Treatment in Cardiac Emergencies

22.2.1
Dilated Cardiomyopathy/Inflammatory Cardiomyopathy

Dilated cardiomyopathy (DCM) – myocardial dilatation and dysfunction – is the most common cause of heart failure in young patients. The majority of cases are sporadic, and a viral (adenovirus and Coxackievirus) or immune pathogenesis is suspected.[14] Despite this, inflammation is rarely seen in biopsies, and immunosuppressive therapy is basically not effective in treating DCM. However, uncontrolled series suggest that IVIG treatment might affect the recovery of patients with recent-onset dilated cardiomyopathy[15,16] and peripartum cardiomyopathy.[17]

Supported by these encouraging data, a small (62 patients) prospective randomized placebo-controlled double-blind trial [the IMAC (Intervention in Myocarditis and Acute Cardiomyopathy)[18] trial] was designed to test the effect of intravenous immunoglobulin treatment on the left ventricle ejection fraction in adults with recent onset of idiopathic dilated cardiomyopathy or myocarditis. The treated patients received 2 g/kg IVIG (divided to two doses). However, this trial failed to prove any advantage for the treatment since no significant difference in left ventricular ejection fraction and functional capacity between the two groups was recorded. It is worth mentioning though that the rate of spontaneous recovery in the untreated group of this study was greater than previously reported in the literature. Furthermore, the authors suggest that a prolonged treatment, rather than a single dose, might be more beneficial; this suggestion is based on a report of patients with congestive heart failure (other ischemic or DCM) that were treated with a 26-week course of IVIG, with a significant improvement of left ventricular function and a decrease in inflammatory mediators levels.[19]

22.2.2
Myocarditis

Myocarditis is an inflammatory process with myocardial involvement, usually following a flu-like illness. The clinical presentation varies, and can range from subclinical to fulminant heart failure. Viral infections are the leading cause of myocarditis, but the cardiac injury most probably arises from immunologic reaction and not from viral toxicity (e.g., antibodies against self-antigen). Although an autoimmune mechanism has been postulated in the pathogenesis of myocarditis, treatment with immunosuppressive agents has not been shown to provide any benefit. However, there is evidence suggesting that IVIG may have a therapeutical role. Eleftheriou et al.[20] presented two cases of acute and potentially lethal myocarditis in adults that were treated with IVIG (in addition to standard of care, including wide-range antibiotics, β-blocker, and ACE-inhibitor). IVIG treatment was given at an early stage, with rapid stabilization and improvement (much faster than known for conventional treatment only). Kato et al.[21] present a case of a 45-year-old man with fulminant myocarditis that required ventricular-assisted devices to maintain hemodynamic stability. He was treated with high-dose IVIG with rapid (12–24 h) improvement in left ventricular ejection fraction. Concomitantly, a significant decrease in inflammatory cytokines levels was noted. Somewhat stronger evidence is brought by Haque et al.[22] This group conducted a small study, comparing supportive care with and without adding IVIG for severe cases of acute myocarditis in children (12–13 children in each group). In this study, the IVIG group had a significantly higher survival rate compared to the other group. However, the recovery of the left ventricular function did not significantly differ between the two groups.

In all three cases, IVIG treatment was initiated at early stages. Other reports, in which IVIG treatment was initiated during later phases, resulted with a less favorable outcome. Some cases of myocarditis are associated with systemic autoimmune diseases. Case reports showing benefit of IVIG use for treating myocarditis associated with lupus,[23] dermatomyositis/polymyositis, Kawasaki syndrome,[23] and adult-onset Still's disease[24] have been reported.

22.2.3
Pericarditis

Chronic idiopathic pericarditis (CIP) complicates one-fourth of patients with acute idiopathic pericarditis. It is a chronic disease characterized by recurrence of chest pain, fever, dyspnea, biochemical markers of systemic inflammation, and typical ECG changes in the presence or absence of pericardial effusion. It is considered an immune-mediated inflammatory disease of the pericardium, and usually treated with NSAIDs, corticosteroids, and colchicine, but some patients are unresponsive to treatment. Peterlana et al.[25] describe four patients suffering from CIP, who were unresponsive to standard care. They were treated with high-dose IVIG – three patients had complete remission and were able to stop steroid treatment completely. The fourth had a partial response and needed low-dose steroid treatment to prevent flares. Similar results were obtained by Tona et al.[26]

Some cases of pericarditis are related to systemic autoimmune diseases. IVIG treatment was reported to be beneficial in cases of lupus-related pericarditis[27] and systemic juvenile idiopathic arthritis–related pericarditis.[28]

22.3
IVIG Treatment in Neurological Emergencies

22.3.1
Guillain–Barré Syndrome (GBS)

GBS[29-31] is a common cause of neuromuscular paralysis occurring 1.2–2.3 per 100,000 worldwide. It affects both children and adults. The incidence increases with age, and men are 1.5 times more likely to be affected than women. It is a postinfectious disorder that usually occurs in otherwise healthy people, and is not typically associated with other autoimmune or systemic disorder. Clinically, GBS is characterized by a rapidly progressive bilateral and relatively symmetric weakness of the limbs, with or without involvement of respiratory muscles or cranial nerve–innervated muscles. Patients have decreased or absent tendon reflexes. Pain frequently occurs (and even precedes weakness) and may cause severe complaints. Sensory and autonomic symptoms can also occur. CSF examination typically shows an increased protein level with a normal white cell count. Electromyography (EMG) can be helpful in confirming the diagnosis, as well as in subclassifying GBS into subgroups such as acute motor axonal neuropathy (AMAN) and acute inflammatory demyelinating polyneuropathy (AIDP). By definition, maximal weakness is reached within 4 weeks; thereafter, patients enter a plateau phase that ranges from days to several months. This phase is followed by a much slower recovery phase. The severity of the symptoms varies between mild (patients still able to walk) and severe (bedridden, need artificial ventilation).

GBS is caused by an infection-induced aberrant immune response that damages peripheral nerves. The most frequently identified preceding infection is by *Campylobacter jejuni*. Other associated infectious agents include cytomegalovirus, Epstein–Barr virus, *Mycoplasma pneumoniae*, and *Haemophilus influenza*. GBS has also been reported to occur shortly after vaccines, operations, and stressful events, but the causality and pathophysiology in these cases is still debated. Autoantibodies to various peripheral nerve gangliosides were reported in about half the patients. It is presumed that a lipo-oligosaccharide expressed on *Campylobacter jejuni* mimics the carbohydrate of gangliosides and induces autoantibodies production by means of molecular mimicry. Myelin destruction is believed to be mediated through a number of effector mechanisms: Activated macrophages are believed to invade myelin or release injurious molecules, circulating antibodies may cause myelin damage by activating the complement system and assembling the membrane attack complex or binding to Fc receptors of activated macrophages that invade the myelinated nerve fibers.

Treatment of GBS patients include supporting treatment (monitoring of pulmonary functions and autonomous functions, mechanical ventilation if needed, pain control, preventing and treating infections and deep vein thrombosis, prevention of decubitus ulcers and contractures), as well as immunomodulatory treatment (intravenous immunoglobulin and plasmapheresis). Plasmapheresis was suggested as an effective treatment for GBS during the 1980s (the North American PE study[32] and the French Cooperative Group on Plasma exchange in GBS[33,34]). When using plasmapheresis, the usual regimen is five times during 2 weeks, with a total exchange of about five plasma volumes. It is most effective when started early (during the first 2 weeks), but is still beneficial during the first 4 weeks. In 1992, the first randomized control trial comparing the use of IVIG and plasma exchange was published.[35] One hundred and fifty patients who had GBS for less than 2 weeks were treated with either five plasma exchanges (each of 200–250 ml/kg of body weight) or five doses of a preparation of intravenous immune globulin (0.4 g/kg/day). At 4 weeks, more patients in the IVIG group had improved by at least one grade on a seven-point scale of motor function (34% in the plasma exchange group, 53% in the IVIG group, $p = 0.024$). The rate of improvement was also faster, and patients in this group had less complication and less need for artificial ventilation. The authors concluded that treatment with intravenous immune globulin is at least as effective as plasma exchange and may be superior. Since then, several other trials were conducted. Most studies used the 0–6 disability scale

(0 – healthy, 1 – minor symptoms, capable of manual work, 2 – able to walk without support but incapable of manual work, 3 – able to walk with support, 4 – confined to bed or chair, 5 – requiring assisted ventilation, 6 – dead) or similar. Improvement is considered a change in one point 4 weeks after randomization. A short summary of some of the relevant trials is given in Table 22.1.

Table 22.1 Major studies dealing with IVIG administration in acute neurological conditions

Study	Design and number of patients	Treatment modalities	Outcome
Pilot trial of immunoglobulin versus plasma exchange in patients with Guillain–Barré syndrome. Brill et al.[36]	Randomized control trial. 50 patients, unable to perform manual work	IVIG 0.5 g/kg/day for 4 days or 5 PE amounting to 200–250 ml/kg over 7–10 days	There was no significant difference in the clinical results. More complications in the plasma exchange group.
Randomized trial of plasma exchange, intravenous immuno-globulin, and combined treatment in Guillain–Barré syndrome. PSGBS group[37]	Randomized control trial. 383 patients, within 14 days of onset of symptoms, unable to walk independently	IVIG 0.4 g/kg/day for 5 days or 5–6 PE amounting to 250 ml/kg over 8–13 days, or PE followed by IVIG (same regimens)	No significant difference between the three groups.
A preliminary randomized study comparing intrave-nous immunoglobulin, plasma exchange, and immune absorption in patients with Guillain–Barré syndrome. Diener et al.[38]	Randomized control trial. 74 patients.	IVIG 0.4 g/kg/day for 5 days or 5 PE amounting to 200–250 ml/kg within 14 days, or immune absorption on five occasions within 14 days.	No significant difference between the groups.
Intravenous immune globulins in patients with Guillain–Barré syndrome and contraindications to plasma exchange: 3 days versus 6 days. Raphael et al.[39]	Randomized control trial. 39 patients.	IVIG 0.4 g/kg/day for 3 days or for 6 days.	The trial was terminated prema-turely, but the results showed a trend in favor of the higher dose.
Intravenous immuno-globulin treatment in children with Guillain–Barré syndrome. Gürses et al.[40]	Randomized control trial. 18 patients (children).	IVIG 1 g/kg/day for 2 days or supportive treatment alone.	A larger proportion of the treated group recovered full strength after 4 weeks; the median time to recover unaided walking was shorter in the treated group.

The Cochrane collaboration reviewed the aforementioned studies, as well as several others.[41] In meta-analysis, there was no significant difference between plasma exchange and intravenous immunoglobulin (as previously mentioned, plasma exchange was proven superior to no treatment in previous trials). In each of the trials reviewed, there were more adverse events in the plasma exchange group compared to the IVIG group (mete-analysis was not done since the definition to adverse events plasma exchange was different in each trial). Moreover, the relative risk for treatment discontinuation was 0.14 less in the IVIG group (this is not surprising since giving IVIG is a logistically and medically easier than plasma exchange). It is worth mentioning that combining both treatments did not improve the results.[37]

According to the evidence-based guidelines on the use of intravenous immune globulins in neurologic conditions,[42] IVIG is recommended as a treatment option for GBS within 2 weeks of symptoms onset for patients with grade 3 severity symptoms or greater, and for patients with less than grade 3 severity symptoms whose symptoms are progressing. It can also be considered for patients who responded to IVIG but had relapse, and for variants of GBS. Similarly, the American Academy of neurology guidlines[43] concluded that plasmapheresis and IVIG are equally efficacious. Plasmapheresis is recommended for non-ambulatory patients presenting within 4 weeks and ambulatory patients presenting within 2 weeks (5–6 1.0–1.5 volume exchanges over 7–10 days). IVIG (0.4 g/kg q 24 h for 5 days) is recommended for patients who required aid to walk presenting within 2 (possibly up to 4) weeks. Corticosteroids are not recommended.

22.3.2
Encephalitis

22.3.2.1
Infectious and Postinfectious Encephalitis

Acute infectious (viral) encephalitis is a complex neurological syndrome, characterized by encephalopathy, focal deficits, seizures, and fever, with significant morbidity and mortality. Postinfectious encephalitis[44,45] is clinically similar, but it develops several days to weeks after an infection (viral of bacterial) or a vaccine. In this case, no pathogen can be isolated from CSF cultures, and pathology examinations reveal inflammation and demyelination. The most common form of postinfectious encephalitis is ADEM – acute disseminated encephalomyelitis, but other, rarer form such as acute hemorrhagic leukoencephalitis and Bickerstaff's brainstem encephalitis also occur. IVIG is administrated in these cases with two aims: first, to increase viral clearance due to antibody-dependent neutralization, and second, postinfectious encephalitis is an immune-mediated mechanism, and like other immune- and inflammation-mediated diseases, might respond to intravenous immunoglobulin treatment. The data regarding the use of IVIG for treating infectious and postinfectious encephalitis is scarce and comprises mainly of case reports.

West Nile virus is an emerging cause for encephalitis. There is no specific treatment for it, and patients are treated with supportive care. In 2003, Ben-Nathan et al. used a murine model of West Nile encephalitis and demonstrated that IVIG preparation containing anti-West Nile virus antibodies (i.e., pooled from populations in which West Nile virus infection rates are high) can be used both to treat West Nile fever[46] if given shortly after exposure. This result is supported by data obtained from other animal models;[47,48] based on this information, Makhoul et al.[49] used IVIG to treat eight adult patients suffering from West Nile encephalitis during the outbreak in Israel in 2007, with good results. The timing of treatment administration is also important. According to animal models, the virus invades the brain as early as day 3 after infection, and according to animal models, the window for successful administration of antibodies closes 4–6 days after infections.[50] In this series, of the eight patients, the six who received the IVIG early (before day 6) improved rapidly, while the two who only started treatment at day 6 and 19 died. There was comparison to untreated patients.

Acute measles encephalitis is an immune-mediated disorder that complicates 1:1,000 cases of acute measles and is associated with high rates of mortality. Nakajima et al.[51] describe two patients with acute measles encephalitis–induced coma. Both were treated with high-dose IVIG and steroids with a rapid response and recovered from their coma within 24 h. Van Dam et al.[52] describe a case of a 19-year-old soldier, who suffered from severe postvaccinia encephalitis and was treated with wide-range antibiotic, corticosteroids, and high-dose IVIG. The patient gradually improved and was discharged from the hospital by day 37 and was back to full active service after 3 months.

Japanese encephalitis is the most common cause of viral encephalitis in Asia. It has a high mortality rate (25–30%), and neuropsychiatric sequelae occur in 50% of the patients. Cases of successfully treating Japanese encephalitis[53] and Mycoplasma pneumonia encephalitis using high-dose IVIG have also been described.[54]

The "Evidence-based guidelines on the use of IVIG for neurologic conditions"[42] recommends IVIG as a treatment option for ADEM when corticosteroid treatment fails or is contraindicated.

22.3.2.2
Lupus Encephalitis

There are a few reports on the use of IVIG in CNS lupus. Sherer et al.[55] report of a 28-year-old patient with systemic lupus erythematosus who developed within a few hours motor and sensory aphasia, rotator nystagmus with deviation of the eyes, and severe nuchal rigidity. An extensive series of imaging and laboratory tests were interpreted as normal, except for an elevated opening pressure at lumbar puncture, cerebrospinal fluid inflammatory findings, and asymmetrical cortical perfusion on single-photon emission computed tomography. The patient received one course of high-dose intravenous immunoglobulin (IVIG) and within 5 days her condition returned to that of 3 months before admission. Other patients, with lupus psychosis, also responded to IVIG treatment.[56,57]

22.3.2.3
Rasmussen's Encephalitis

Rasmussen's encephalitis is a rare syndrome, affecting mostly children. It is characterized by focal seizures, progressive neurological deterioration, hemispheric atrophy, and inflammatory histopathology.[58] Conventional antiepileptic treatment has only a limited control over the seizures, and currently, the only treatment that effectively halts the progression of the disease is surgical exclusion of the affected hemisphere. Trying to avoid this radical procedure, several medical treatments have been tried, including corticosteroids, plasma exchange, and IVIG. The experience of IVIG treatment is based on case reports with mixed results.[59-64] The "Evidence-based guidelines on the use of IVIG for neurologic conditions"[42] suggests IVIG as a short-term temporizing measure for patients with Rasmussen's encephalitis, but states that the treatment is not recommended for long therapy, since surgical therapy is still the standard of care.

22.3.2.4
Autoimmune Subacute Encephalitis and Paraneoplastic Brainstem Encephalitis

Subacute encephalopathies are neurological diseases causing insidious impairment of consciousness over weeks or months. Hashimoto's encephalitis is associated with elevated levels of antithyroperoxidase, antithyroglobulin, and anti-NH_2-terminal of enolase, or antithyrotropin antibodies. It responds well to treatment with steroids and plasmapheresis and has good prognosis. Voltage-gated potassium channel antibody (VGKCab)–associated encephalitis is a paraneoplastic or nonparaneoplastic disorder characterized by amnesia, delirium, and seizures with good response to intravenous immune globulin, plasma exchange, and steroids.[65] Mittal et al.[66] present two cases of mixed syndrome who were treated with high-dose steroids and either plasmapheresis or IVIG with a slow improvement.

In paraneoplastic neurological syndromes, the most frequently found antineuronal antibodies are anti-Hu, anti-Yo, and anti-CRMP5. Fumal et al.[67] describe a case of paraneoplastic brainstem encephalitis with the rare anti-Ri antibodies that was treated with high-dose IVIG with clinical improvement.

22.4
IVIG Treatment in Nephrologic Emergencies: Lupus Nephritis

Systemic lupus erythematosus (SLE) is a multisystemic autoimmune disease with great diversity of clinical manifestations, ranging from mild clinical finding with typical abnormal laboratory tests to a life-threatening condition.[68] Lupus nephritis is one of the most serious manifestations of systemic lupus erythematosus (SLE). It is histologically evident in most patients with SLE, even those without clinical manifestations of renal disease. When symptoms occur, they are generally related to hypertension, proteinuria, and renal failure. The pathophysiology of lupus nephritis is autoimmune, e.g., autoantibodies directed against nuclear elements form immune complexes. These immune complexes form deposits in the kidneys, activate the complement cascade, and initiate an immune response that damages the kidney. Lupus nephritis is usually treated with corticosteroids and immunosuppressive agents, namely cyclophosphamide, azathioprine, or mycophenolate mofetil. Unfortunately, not all patients respond to this treatment; since most of the patients are young women, exposure to continuous chemotherapy might cause premature ovarian failure, and increases the odds of developing acute myeloid leukemia and hemorrhagic cystitis. In addition, prolonged treatment with immunosuppressive agents is related to increased susceptibility to infections. Hence, new therapeutic options are constantly sought.

IVIG is successfully used to treat a broad spectrum of lupus manifestations, including thrombocytopenia, leucopenia, autoimmune hemolytic anemia, pleural effusion, pericarditis, cerebritis, and others.[68] Several studies analyzed the benefits of IVIG in lupus nephritis, most only include a small number of patients. The largest study, conducted by Monova et al.,[69] involved 116 patients, 58 of which suffered from lupus glomerulonephritis. The patients were treated with 85 mg/kg/24 h three times every other day. The course could be repeated after 1–3 months, according to the clinical response. Out of the 58 lupus nephritis patients, 12 had complete response (unchanged or improved renal functions, disappearance of edema, normalization of hemoglobin, serum protein and albumin values, proteinuria <0.5 g/24 h) and 27 had partial response. The results were better for WHO classes II and III, compared with classes IV and V. In patients with thrombocytopenia and leucopenia, leukocyte and platelet counts returned to normal limits. When mechanism of action is concerned, the authors reported a significant decrease in anti-DNA antibodies and ANA titer.

The results of several other, smaller studies and case reports are summarized in the Table 22.2.

In most of the cases described above, IVIG treatment improved proteinuria and renal function. Some studies demonstrated serologic changes: increase in C3 and C4 levels and decrease in anti-dsDNA antibodies and antinuclear antibodies. One study also demonstrated a reduction in immune deposits viewed on biopsy.[70]

However, since renal failure is an infrequent complication of IVIG, using IVIG to treat renal disease is a double-edged sword. The occurrence of renal failure after IVIG treatment is not disease specific, and is most probably the consequence of sucrose nephropathy. Sucrose is a stabilizer within the IVIG preparation that can cause osmotic nephrosis (biopsy shows vacuolization of proximal tubules and swelling and narrowing of the tubular lamina). IVIG-induced renal failure usually occurs in less than 7 days postadministration. More than 80% of the cases are reversible and are resolved within 2–60 days. However, 28–40% may have severe symptoms requiring dialysis. Age, volume depletion, and preexisting renal insufficiency lower the threshold for renal toxicity following IVIG treatment. Orbach et al.[75] reviewed 78 cases reported in the literature and 120 cases reported to the FDA between 6/1985 and 11/1988 of renal failure following IVIG treatment. Thus far, it seems that the benefits of the treatment exceed the disadvantages. However, caution is needed since renal functions should be monitored and sucrose-containing products should be avoided.

The precise mechanism of IVIG action in lupus nephritis is very complex.[68] Apart from the mechanisms common to all IVIG responsive patients (described at the beginning of this chapter), high IgG serum levels obtained after IVIG treatment could produce an antibody-excess state capable of dissociating IgG deposits. Thus, IVIG is able to interfere with the depositions of anti-DNA antibodies by solubilizing immune complexes. Another possible explanation is the inhibitory effect of antiidiotypic antibodies on the spontaneous secretion of anti-dsDNA by peripheral B lymphocytes. Furthermore, regulatory T cells may recognize antiidiotypic antibodies or a complex of idiotype–antiidiotypic antibodies, and produce anti-inflammatory cytokines that ameliorate the immune response.

Table 22.2 Major studies dealing with IVIG administration in lupus-related glomerulonephritis

Reference	Description	Results
Improvement of histological and immunological change in steroid and immunosuppressive drug-resistant lupus nephritis by high-dose intravenous gamma globulin. Lin et al.[70]	Nine patients with steroid and cyclophosphamide-resistant lupus nephritis (WHO class IV and V) were treated with high-dose IVIG.	Three-fifth cases of class IV lupus nephritis had a good response with decreased proteinuria and creatinine, increase in C3 and C4 levels, and decrease in glomerular IgG deposits in repeat biopsy. The other patients had partial response.
Intravenous immuno-globulin treatment in lupus nephritis. Levi et al.[71]	Seven lupus nephritis patients (membranous or membranoprolif-erative glomerulonephritis per biopsy) who failed to respond to prednisone and cyclophosphamide were treated with high-dose IVIG (2 g/kg divided for 5 days).	Five patients were treated with 1–2 courses of IVIG. The therapy resulted in reversal of nephritic syndrome – elevation of plasma albumin, decrease in plasma choles-terol, resolution of edema, and reduction of proteinuria. The therapeutic effect lasted for at least 6 months. two patients received six courses of IVIG. One achieved full disappearance of the nephritic syndrome, the other achieved partial response.
Intravenous immuno-globulin compared with cyclophosphamide for proliferative lupus nephritis. Boletis et al.[72]	A pilot randomized trial, aimed to assess the safety and efficacy of maintenance therapy with monthly IVIG compared with cyclophosph-amide in patients with proliferative lupus nephritis. Fourteen patients participated, five received IVIG, nine received cyclophosphamide.	There was no significance difference between the two groups. IVIG is as effective and safe as cyclophosph-amide, and might be an alternative maintenance therapy in lupus nephritis.
A study of 20 SLE patients with intrave-nous immunoglobulin – clinical and serologic response. Levy et al.[57]	Twenty SLE patients were treated with 2 g/kg IVIg monthly, in a 5-day schedule (1–8 courses). Five of the patients suffered from proteinuria.	Four-fifth patients responded with a decrease in proteinuria, but in three of them, there was only a slight or temporary reduction.
High-dose intravenous gamma globulin in systemic lupus erythematosus. Oliet et al.[73]	A case report. A 21-year-old woman with SLE and lupus nephritis, who failed treatment with MP, steroids and cyclophos-phamide, received IVIG 400/mg/kg/day for 5 days.	Proteinuria decreased from 3.6 to 0.7gr/day.
Treatment of systemic lupus erythematosus by prolonged administration of high-dose intravenous immunoglobulin: report of two cases. Winder et al.[74]	Two patients with life-threatening manifestations of SLE (one with lupus nephritis), unresponsive to corticosteroid and immunosuppres-sive therapy, were treated with high-dose intravenous immuno-globulin (2 g/kg)	Improvement of renal functions, cytotoxic agent treatment was stopped, and steroids dosage lowered. Exacerbation of lupus nephritis occurred after 10 months of IVIG therapy.

22.5
IVIG in Unresponsive Serositis

Apart from pericarditis, IVIG treatment can be useful in other persistent serositis. Meissner et al.[76] report of a 39-year-old woman who presented with a small pericardial effusion, bilateral pleural effusion and a small amount of fluid in the peritoneal cavity. On physical examination and laboratory finding, 6 of the 11 ACR criteria for lupus were met. Due to the severe clinical presentation, IVIG treatment was started (7 consecutive days of 400 mg/kg), in parallel to her previous treatment (including high-dose corticosteroids). Within 1 week after the treatment, the patient's condition improved dramatically. In another report, Sherer et al.[77] bring the case of a 48-year-old woman who was admitted with bilateral pleural effusions. The fluid was repeatedly drained and the patient was treated with a variety of immunomodulating agents, several pleural talcage, and pleurectomy, without any apparent response. During a 2.5-year period, the patient underwent an extensive diagnostic workup that disclosed elevated serum antinuclear antibodies, serum anti-dsDNA antibodies, pleural fluid anti-dsDNA, and decreased pleural fluid C3 and C4, but no other criteria for lupus were met. Due to the failure of all traditional treatment, the patient received six courses of IVIG (2 g/kg body weight) in monthly intervals, followed by 4-month treatment with cyclosporine. This treatment resulted in gradual and eventually complete disappearance of the pleural effusion.

A similar case, with a transient response of lupus refractory pleural effusion to treatment with IVIG is described by Ben-Chitrit et al.[78]

22.6
Conclusion

In conclusion, the clinical discussion of the putative roles IVIG has in autoimmune conditions all imply that there are significant prospects in its future use in autoimmune conditions. The easiness of its administration on one hand and of course the improved safety profile on the other hand (particularly when compared to other therapeutical options that are often prescribed to patients with autoimmune conditions) turn this option interesting and attractive. Larger clinical studies are warranted and presumably at least in several conditions will be executed.

References

1. Arnson Y, Shoenfeld Y, Amital H. Intravenous immunoglobulin therapy for autoimmune diseases. *Autoimmunity*. 2009;42(6):553-560.
2. Fehr J, Hofmann V, Kappeler U. Transient reversal of thrombocytopenia in idiopathic thrombocytopenic purpura by high-dose intravenous gamma globulin. *N Engl J Med*. 1982;306(21):1254-1258.
3. Kimberly RP, Salmon JE, Bussel JB, Crow MK, Hilgartner MW. Modulation of mononuclear phagocyte function by intravenous gamma-globulin. *J Immunol*. 1984;132(2):745-750.

4. Bruhns P, Samuelsson A, Pollard JW, Ravetch JV. Colony-stimulating factor-1-dependent macrophages are responsible for IVIG protection in antibody-induced autoimmune disease. *Immunity*. 2003;18(4):573-581.

5. Mollnes TE, Hogasen K, De Carolis C, et al. High-dose intravenous immunoglobulin treatment activates complement in vivo. *Scand J Immunol*. 1998;48(3):312-317.

6. Basta M, Van Goor F, Luccioli S, et al. F(ab)′2-mediated neutralization of C3a and C5a anaphylatoxins: a novel effector function of immunoglobulins. *Nat Med*. 2003;9(4):431-438.

7. Klaesson S, Ringden O, Markling L, Remberger M, Lundkvist I. Immune modulatory effects of immunoglobulins on cell-mediated immune responses in vitro. *Scand J Immunol*. 1993;38(5):477-484.

8. Rossi F, Kazatchkine MD. Antiidiotypes against autoantibodies in pooled normal human polyspecific Ig. *J Immunol*. 1989;143(12):4104-4109.

9. Adib M, Ragimbeau J, Avrameas S, Ternynck T. IgG autoantibody activity in normal mouse serum is controlled by IgM. *J Immunol*. 1990;145(11):3807-3813.

10. Seite JF, Shoenfeld Y, Youinou P, Hillion S. What is the contents of the magic draft IVIG? *Autoimmun Rev*. 2008;7(6):435-439.

11. El-Shanawany T, Jolles S. Intravenous immunoglobulin and autoimmune disease. *Ann NY Acad Sci*. 2007;1110:507-515.

12. Bussel JB, Kimberly RP, Inman RD, et al. Intravenous gammaglobulin treatment of chronic idiopathic thrombocytopenic purpura. *Blood*. 1983;62(2):480-486.

13. Katz U, Achiron A, Sherer Y, Shoenfeld Y. Safety of intravenous immunoglobulin (IVIG) therapy. *Autoimmun Rev*. 2007;6(4):257-259.

14. Noutsias M, Pauschinger M, Poller WC, Schultheiss HP, Kuhl U. Immunomodulatory treatment strategies in inflammatory cardiomyopathy: current status and future perspectives. *Expert Rev Cardiovasc Ther*. 2004;2(1):37-51.

15. McNamara DM, Rosenblum WD, Janosko KM, et al. Intravenous immune globulin in the therapy of myocarditis and acute cardiomyopathy. *Circulation*. 1997;95(11):2476-2478.

16. Goland S, Czer LS, Siegel RJ, et al. Intravenous immunoglobulin treatment for acute fulminant inflammatory cardiomyopathy: series of six patients and review of literature. *Can J Cardiol*. 2008;24(7):571-574.

17. Bozkurt B, Villaneuva FS, Holubkov R, et al. Intravenous immune globulin in the therapy of peripartum cardiomyopathy. *J Am Coll Cardiol*. 1999;34(1):177-180.

18. McNamara DM, Holubkov R, Starling RC, et al. Controlled trial of intravenous immune globulin in recent-onset dilated cardiomyopathy. *Circulation*. 2001;103(18):2254-2259.

19. Gullestad L, Aass H, Fjeld JG, et al. Immunomodulating therapy with intravenous immunoglobulin in patients with chronic heart failure. *Circulation*. 2001;103(2):220-225.

20. Eleftheriou AE, Stamatelopoulos SF. Rapid recovery from acute, potentially lethal myocarditis. *J Int Med Res*. 2009;37(5):1522-1525.

21. Kato S, Morimoto S, Hiramitsu S, et al. Successful high-dose intravenous immunoglobulin therapy for a patient with fulminant myocarditis. *Heart Vessels*. 2007;22(1):48-51.

22. Haque A, Bhatti S, Siddiqui FJ. Intravenous immune globulin for severe acute myocarditis in children. *Indian Pediatr*. 2009;46(9):810-811.

23. Sherer Y, Levy Y, Shoenfeld Y. Marked improvement of severe cardiac dysfunction after one course of intravenous immunoglobulin in a patient with systemic lupus erythematosus. *Clin Rheumatol*. 1999;18(3):238-240.

24. Kuek A, Weerakoon A, Ahmed K, Ostor AJ. Adult-onset Still's disease and myocarditis: successful treatment with intravenous immunoglobulin and maintenance of remission with etanercept. *Rheumatology*. 2007;46(6):1043-1044.

25. Peterlana D, Puccetti A, Simeoni S, Tinazzi E, Corrocher R, Lunardi C. Efficacy of intravenous immunoglobulin in chronic idiopathic pericarditis: report of four cases. *Clin Rheumatol*. 2005;24(1):18-21.

26. Tona F, Bellotto F, Laveder F, Meneghin A, Sinagra G, Marcolongo R. Efficacy of high-dose intravenous immunoglobulins in two patients with idiopathic recurrent pericarditis refractory to previous immunosuppressive treatment. *Ital Heart J.* 2003;4(1):64-68.

27. Grenader T, Shavit L. Intravenous immunoglobulin in treatment of cardiac tamponade in a patient with systemic lupus erythematosus. *Clin Rheumatol.* 2004;23(6):530-532.

28. Aizawa-Yashiro T, Oki E, Tsuruga K, Nakahata T, Ito E, Tanaka H. Intravenous immuno-globulin therapy leading to dramatic improvement in a patient with systemic juvenile idiopathic arthritis and severe pericarditis resistant to steroid pulse therapy. *Rheumatol Int.* 2010. Epub.

29. Harel M, Shoenfeld Y. Intravenous immunoglobulin and Guillain-Barre syndrome. *Clin Rev Allergy Immunol.* 2005;29(3):281-287.

30. van Doorn PA, Kuitwaard K, Walgaard C, van Koningsveld R, Ruts L, Jacobs BC. IVIG treat-ment and prognosis in Guillain–Barre syndrome. *J Clin Immunol.* 2010;30(suppl 1):74-78.

31. van Doorn PA, Ruts L, Jacobs BC. Clinical features, pathogenesis, and treatment of Guillain-Barre syndrome. *Lancet Neurol.* 2008;7(10):939-950.

32. The Guillain-Barre syndrome Study Group. Plasmapheresis and acute Guillain-Barre syn-drome. *Neurology.* 1985;35(8):1096-1104.

33. French Cooperative Group on Plasma Exchange in Guillain-Barre syndrome. Efficiency of plasma exchange in Guillain-Barre syndrome: role of replacement fluids. *Ann Neurol.* 1987; 22(6):753-761.

34. French Cooperative Group on Plasma Exchange in Guillain-Barre Syndrome. Plasma exchange in Guillain-Barre syndrome: one-year follow-up. *Ann Neurol.* 1992;32(1):94-97.

35. van der Meche FG, Schmitz PI. A randomized trial comparing intravenous immune globulin and plasma exchange in Guillain-Barre syndrome. Dutch Guillain-Barre study group. *N Engl J Med.* 1992;326(17):1123-1129.

36. Bril V, Ilse WK, Pearce R, Dhanani A, Sutton D, Kong K. Pilot trial of immunoglobulin versus plasma exchange in patients with Guillain-Barre syndrome. *Neurology.* 1996;46(1): 100-103.

37. Hughes RAC, Swan AV. Randomised trial of plasma exchange, intravenous immunoglobulin, and combined treatments in Guillain-Barre syndrome. Plasma exchange/sandoglobulin Guillain-Barre Syndrome trial group. *Lancet.* 1997;349(9047):225-230.

38. Diener HC, Haupt WF, Kloss TM, et al. A preliminary, randomized, multicenter study com-paring intravenous immunoglobulin, plasma exchange, and immune adsorption in Guillain-Barre syndrome. *Eur Neurol.* 2001;46(2):107-109.

39. Raphael JC, Chevret S, Harboun M, Jars-Guincestre MC. Intravenous immune globulins in patients with Guillain-Barre syndrome and contraindications to plasma exchange: 3 days versus 6 days. *J Neurol Neurosurg Psychiatry.* 2001;71(2):235-238.

40. Gurses N, Uysal S, Cetinkaya F, Islek I, Kalayci AG. Intravenous immunoglobulin treatment in children with Guillain-Barre syndrome. *Scand J Infect Dis.* 1995;27(3):241-243.

41. Hughes RA, Raphael JC, Swan AV, van Doorn PA. Intravenous immunoglobulin for Guillain-Barre syndrome. *Cochrane Database Syst Rev.* 2006;(1):CD002063.

42. Robinson P, Anderson D, Brouwers M, Feasby TE, Hume H. Evidence-based guidelines on the use of intravenous immune globulin for hematologic and neurologic conditions. *Transfus Med Rev.* 2007;21(2 suppl 1):S3-S8.

43. Hughes RA, Wijdicks EF, Barohn R, et al. Practice parameter: immunotherapy for Guillain-Barre syndrome: report of the quality standards subcommittee of the American Academy of Neurology. *Neurology.* 2003;61(6):736-740.

44. Sonneville R, Klein IF, Wolff M. Update on investigation and management of postinfectious encephalitis. *Curr Opin Neurol.* 2010;23(3):300-304.

45. Sonneville R, Klein I, de Broucker T, Wolff M. Post-infectious encephalitis in adults: diagnosis and management. *J Infect.* 2009;58(5):321-328.

46. Ben-Nathan D, Lustig S, Tam G, Robinzon S, Segal S, Rager-Zisman B. Prophylactic and therapeutic efficacy of human intravenous immunoglobulin in treating West Nile virus infection in mice. *J Infect Dis*. 2003;188(1):5-12.

47. Diamond MS, Shrestha B, Marri A, Mahan D, Engle M. B cells and antibody play critical roles in the immediate defense of disseminated infection by West Nile encephalitis virus. *J Virol*. 2003;77(4):2578-2586.

48. Tesh RB, Arroyo J, Travassos Da Rosa AP, et al. Efficacy of killed virus vaccine, live attenuated chimeric virus vaccine, and passive immunization for prevention of West Nile virus encephalitis in hamster model. *Emerg Infect Dis*. 2002;8:1392-1397.

49. Makhoul B, Braun E, Herskovitz M, Ramadan R, Hadad S, Norberto K. Hyperimmune gammaglobulin for the treatment of West Nile virus encephalitis. *Isr Med Assoc J*. 2009;11(3): 151-153.

50. Haley M, Retter AS, Fowler D, Gea-Banacloche J, O'Grady NP. The role for intravenous immunoglobulin in the treatment of West Nile virus encephalitis. *Clin Infect Dis*. 2003; 37(6):e88-e90.

51. Nakajima M, Sakuishi K, Fukuda S, Fujioka S, Hashida H. Recovery from adult measles encephalitis immediately after early immunomodulation. *Clin Infect Dis*. 2008;47(1):148-149.

52. Van Dam CN, Syed S, Eron JJ, et al. Severe postvaccinia encephalitis with acute disseminated encephalomyelitis: recovery with early intravenous immunoglobulin, high-dose steroids, and vaccinia immunoglobulin. *Clin Infect Dis*. 2009;48(4):e47-e49.

53. Caramello P, Canta F, Balbiano R, et al. Role of intravenous immunoglobulin administration in Japanese encephalitis. *Clin Infect Dis*. 2006;43(12):1620-1621.

54. Chambert-Loir C, Ouachee M, Collins K, Evrard P, Servais L. Immediate relief of *Mycoplasma pneumoniae* encephalitis symptoms after intravenous immunoglobulin. *Pediatr Neurol*. 2009;41(5):375-377.

55. Sherer Y, Levy Y, Langevitz P, Lorber M, Fabrizzi F, Shoenfeld Y. Successful treatment of systemic lupus erythematosus cerebritis with intravenous immunoglobulin. *Clin Rheumatol*. 1999;18(2):170-173.

56. Tomer Y, Shoenfeld Y. Successful treatment of psychosis secondary to SLE with high dose intravenous immunoglobulin. *Clin Exp Rheumatol*. 1992;10(4):391-393.

57. Levy Y, Sherer Y, Ahmed A, et al. A study of 20 SLE patients with intravenous immunoglobulin – clinical and serologic response. *Lupus*. 1999;8(9):705-712.

58. Granata T. Rasmussen's syndrome. *Neurol Sci*. 2003;24(suppl 4):S239-S243.

59. Hart YM, Cortez M, Andermann F, et al. Medical treatment of Rasmussen's syndrome (chronic encephalitis and epilepsy): effect of high-dose steroids or immunoglobulins in 19 patients. *Neurology*. 1994;44(6):1030-1036.

60. Wise MS, Rutledge SL, Kuzniecky RI. Rasmussen syndrome and long-term response to gamma globulin. *Pediatr Neurol*. 1996;14(2):149-152.

61. Krauss GL, Campbell ML, Roche KW, Huganir RL, Niedermeyer E. Chronic steroid-responsive encephalitis without autoantibodies to glutamate receptor GluR3. *Neurology*. 1996;46(1):247-249.

62. Leach JP, Chadwick DW, Miles JB, Hart IK. Improvement in adult-onset Rasmussen's encephalitis with long-term immunomodulatory therapy. *Neurology*. 1999;52(4):738-742.

63. Arias M, Dapena D, Arias-Rivas S, et al. Rasmussen encephalitis in the sixth decade: magnetic resonance image evolution and immunoglobulin response. *Eur Neurol*. 2006;56(4):236-239.

64. Granata T, Fusco L, Gobbi G, et al. Experience with immunomodulatory treatments in Rasmussen's encephalitis. *Neurology*. 2003;61(12):1807-1810.

65. Geschwind MD, Tan KM, Lennon VA, et al. Voltage-gated potassium channel autoimmunity mimicking creutzfeldt-jakob disease. *Arch Neurol*. 2008;65(10):1341-1346.

66. Mittal M, Hammond N, Lynch SG. Immunotherapy responsive autoimmune subacute encephalitis: a report of two cases. *Case Rep Med*. 2010;2010:837371.

67. Fumal A, Jobe J, Pepin JL, et al. Intravenous immunoglobulins in paraneoplastic brainstem encephalitis with anti-Ri antibodies. *J Neurol*. 2006;253(10):1360-1361.
68. Rauova L, Lukac J, Levy Y, Rovensky J, Shoenfeld Y. High-dose intravenous immunoglobulins for lupus nephritis – a salvage immunomodulation. *Lupus*. 2001;10(3):209-213.
69. Monova D, Belovezhdov N, Altunkova I, Monov S. Intravenous immunoglobulin G in the treatment of patients with chronic glomerulonephritis: clinical experience lasting 15 years. *Nephron*. 2002;90(3):262-266.
70. Lin CY, Hsu HC, Chiang H. Improvement of histological and immunological change in steroid and immunosuppressive drug-resistant lupus nephritis by high-dose intravenous gamma globulin. *Nephron*. 1989;53(4):303-310.
71. Levy Y, Sherer Y, George J, et al. Intravenous immunoglobulin treatment of lupus nephritis. *Semin Arthritis Rheum*. 2000;29(5):321-327.
72. Boletis JN, Ioannidis JP, Boki KA, Moutsopoulos HM. Intravenous immunoglobulin compared with cyclophosphamide for proliferative lupus nephritis. *Lancet*. 1999;354(9178):569-570.
73. Oliet A, Hernandez E, Gallar P, Vigil A. High-dose intravenous gamma-globulin in systemic lupus erythematosus. *Nephron*. 1992;62(4):465.
74. Winder A, Molad Y, Ostfeld I, Kenet G, Pinkhas J, Sidi Y. Treatment of systemic lupus erythematosus by prolonged administration of high dose intravenous immunoglobulin: report of 2 cases. *J Rheumatol*. 1993;20(3):495-498.
75. Orbach H, Tishler M, Shoenfeld Y. Intravenous immunoglobulin and the kidney – a two-edged sword. *Semin Arthritis Rheum*. 2004;34(3):593-601.
76. Meissner M, Sherer Y, Levy Y, Chwalinska-Sadowska H, Langevitz P, Shoenfeld Y. Intravenous immunoglobulin therapy in a patient with lupus serositis and nephritis. *Rheumatol Int*. 2000;19(5):199-201.
77. Sherer Y, Langevitz P, Levy Y, Fabrizzi F, Shoenfeld Y. Treatment of chronic bilateral pleural effusions with intravenous immunoglobulin and cyclosporin. *Lupus*. 1999;8(4):324-327.
78. Ben-Chetrit E, Putterman C, Naparstek Y. Lupus refractory pleural effusion: transient response to intravenous immunoglobulins. *J Rheumatol*. 1991;18(10):1635-1637.

Life-Threatening Complications of Biological Therapies

23

Ana Campar and David A. Isenberg

Abstract The last decade was characterized by the successive introduction of several biological agents for the treatment of autoimmune rheumatic diseases (ARD). Randomized controlled trials (RCT) proved them to have globally acceptable safety and tolerability profiles. However, life-threatening complications are rare events and RCT are underpowered to detect them. As these drugs became more widely prescribed in clinical practice, and particularly, having the information from multiple national biologics registries available, serious adverse events became perceptible. Infection remains the major concern, but other serious and life-threatening complications have emerged, such as malignancies, congestive heart failure, demyelinating disorders, and drug-induced autoimmune syndromes. Several of these are correlated with either the underlying disease or concomitant immunosuppressive medication. Most of them can be avoided by the adoption of preventive measures and an early proper management might significantly change the outcome. Awareness of the possible serious side effects is of utmost importance for a safer use of biological agents.

In this chapter, we aim to describe the most commonly reported life-threatening complications of biological therapies in the literature – including those with antitumor necrosis factor agents, rituximab, abatacept, tocilizumab, and anakinra. Risk groups are identified and strategies for the prevention and initial management are included.

Key words Autoimmune diseases • Biologics • Complications • Demyelinating disorders • Drug-induced autoimmune syndromes • Heart failure • Infections • Malignancies • Management • Prevention

A. Campar (✉)
Internal Medicine Department, Santo António
Hospital, 4099-001 Porto, Portugal
e-mail: anaccampar@hotmail.com

M.A. Khamashta and M. Ramos-Casals (eds.), *Autoimmune Diseases*,
DOI: 10.1007/978-0-85729-358-9_23, © Springer-Verlag London Limited 2011

23.1
Introduction

Improved understanding of the immunopathology of various autoimmune rheumatic diseases (ARD), combined with biopharmaceutical development, has led to the introduction of biological therapeutics. These agents target specific components of the immune response (e.g., cytokines, immune cells) that are central to the etiology of the disease process. Biological therapy has brought a paradigm shift in the management of several ARD decreasing the disability and improving quality of life and health outcomes. Biological agents include those that interfere with cytokine function (antitumor necrosis factor-α agents [anti-TNF-α], Tocilizumab, Anakinra); deplete B cells (Rituximab); and downregulate T-cell stimulation (Abatacept) (Table 23.1).[1] The most widely used are TNF-α antagonists.

These therapies have demonstrated acceptable safety and tolerability profiles during randomized controlled trials (RCT). However, RCT are underpowered to detect specific risks (particularly rare events) due to short duration of follow-up, relatively small number of patients studied, and exclusion of those with risk factors for complications. During post-approval surveillance, increased risks of serious infections (including opportunistic), malignancies, congestive heart failure, demyelinating disorders, and drug-induced autoimmune syndromes have been reported.[2-4] Nonetheless, these findings have been inconsistent and the reported risks and frequencies differ widely (Table 23.2).[5-11] Recognized limitations of the different sources of safety data (post-marketing surveillance reports, national registries and meta-analyses), such as lack of a control group and channeling or confounding by indication bias, underlie this variability.[12,13] Different mechanisms of drug action and their diverse pharmacokinetics and pharmacodynamics characteristics influence their safety profile, including the risk of serious adverse events (SAE) (Table 23.1). Patients with ARD have a higher mortality compared to general population, due to increased susceptibility to infections, malignancy, and cardiovascular disorders.[14-17] The underlying immune deregulation of these diseases, the concomitant immunosuppression by conventional disease-modifying antirheumatic drugs (DMARD) and steroids, and the frequent existence of comorbidities are recognized as major factors. These complex interactions make it difficult to ascribe complications solely to biological agents.

Infection remains the major concern of biological therapy, but other – some unexpected – serious complications have emerged as these agents became more widely prescribed. Overall, SAE appear to be rare (Table 23.2), but some are life-threatening, requiring judicious selection of candidates, pretreatment screening and eventual prophylactic measures, close observation during therapy, and careful attention to patient education.

23.2
Life-Threatening Complications of Biological Therapies

In safety reports of biological agents, complications that threaten life or function of a patient are often not specifically analyzed and rather are included in a broader category of SAE, i.e., those that require admission to hospital, are fatal or life-threatening, or result

Table 23.1 Biological therapies most used in autoimmune rheumatic diseases

Biologic agent	Target/affinity	Immune actions	Half-life	Administration	Approved indications[a]
Etanercept (humanized fusion protein)	TNF[b]-α, lymphotoxin-α (TNF-β). Soluble TNF-α	Decreases circulating TNF-α; partial blockade; no lysis of TNF-expressing cells	4 days	Subcutaneous injection of 25 mg/kg twice per week or 50 mg/kg once a week	RA[c], JIA[d], PsA[e], AS[f], plaque psoriasis
Infliximab (chimeric mAb[g])	TNF-α. Soluble and membrane TNF-α	Monocyte and T-cell apoptosis; lysis of TNF-expressing cells	9 days	Infusion of 3–5 mg/kg at 0, 2, 6 weeks and then every 6–8 weeks	RA, AS, PsA, Crohn's disease, ulcerative colitis, plaque psoriasis
Adalimumab (humanized mAb)	TNF-α. Soluble and membrane TNF-α	Lysis of TNF-expressing cells; possible effects on apoptosis, monocytes, and natural killer cells	14 days	Subcutaneous injection of 40 mg every 2 week	RA, PsA, AS, Crohn's disease
Rituximab (chimeric mAb)	CD20-positive B cells	Lysis of CD20-expressing pre-B lymphocytes and mature B lymphocytes; potential modulation of T-cell immunity	3.5–17 days	Two infusions (1 gr) with 2 week-interval	RA
Abatacept (humanized fusion protein)	Selective modulation of CD80/86:CD28 costimulatory signal required for full T-cell activation	Modulates T-cell activation, by inhibiting the "second signal" between T cells and APC[h]	8–25 days	Infusion of 8–10 mg/kg at 0, 2, 4 weeks and then every 4 weeks	RA
Tocilizumab (humanized mAb)	IL-6 receptor	Competitive blocking of IL-6 receptor	5–10 days	Infusion of 4 or 8 mg/kg every 4 weeks	RA; in Japan also: polyarticular or systemic-onset JIA, multicentric Castleman's disease

(continued)

Table 23.1 (continued)

Biologic agent	Target/affinity	Immune actions	Half-life	Administration	Approved indications[a]
Anakinra (recombinant human protein)	IL-1 receptor	Competitive blocking of IL-1 receptor; signal blockade	4–6 h	Daily subcutaneous injection	RA, JIA, Adult-onset Still's disease, CAPS[i]

[a]Approved indications for autoimmune diseases as defined by United States Food and Drug Administration (FDA) and European Medicines Agency (EMEA)
[b]Tumor necrosis factor
[c]Rheumatoid arthritis
[d]Juvenile idiopathic arthritis
[e]Psoriatic arthritis
[f]Ankylosing spondylitis
[g]Monoclonal antibody
[h]Antigen-presenting cells
[i]Cryopyrin-associated periodic syndromes

Table 23.2 Serious adverse events of biological agents as estimated in selected studies

Author (reference)	Biological agent	Disease/number of patients included (n)	Serious adverse events
Leombruno et al.[5]	Anti-TNF[a]-α agents	RA[b]; $n=5,759$ (meta-analysis of 18 RCT[c])	13.9% (anti-TNF at recommended doses) vs 11.8% (control group); OR[d] 1.11 (95% CI[e], 0.94–1.32); RR[f] 0.94 (95% CI, 0.77–1.15)
Dixon et al.[6]	Anti-TNF-α agents	RA; $n=7,664$	53.2 per 1,000 patient-years (anti-TNF) vs 41.4 per 1,000 person-years (DMARD); adjusted* IRR[g] 1.03 (95% CI, 0.68–1.57)
Cohen et al.[7]	Rituximab	RA; $n=520$	7% – 5.3 per 100 patient-years (1 g dose) vs 10% (control group)
Keystone et al.[8]	Rituximab (additional courses)	RA; $n=1,039$ (course 1), 571 (course 2), 191 (course 3), 40 (course 4)	1.5 (0.5–2.9), 1.2 (0.5–2.4), 1.1(0.2–8.0) and 8.0(1.1–56.8)** per 100 patient-years during courses 1,2,3 and 4 (respectively) (95% CI)
Sibilia and Westhovens et al.[9]	Abatacept	RA; $n=1,955$	14% (10 mg/kg dosage) vs 12.5% (control group)
Emery et al.[10]	Tocilizumab	RA; $n=499$	6.3% (8 mg/kg dose group), 7.4% (4 mg/kg dose group) vs 11.3% (control group)
Fleischmann et al.[11]	Anakinra	RA; $n=1,346$	26.5–27.7 per 100 patient-years (3 years) vs 22.3 per 100 person-years (placebo)

[a]Tumour necrosis factor
[b]Rheumatoid arthritis
[c]Randomized controlled trials
[d]Odds ratio
[e]Confidence interval
[f]Risk ratio
[g]Psoriatic arthritis
[h]Incidence rate ratio
*Adjusted for age, sex, disease severity, comorbidity, extraarticular manifestations, steroid use, and smoking
**Rates for course 4 were based on a limited number of patients (12.5 patient-years), and the amount of follow-up was considered by the authors of the study to be insufficient to provide meaningful data and reliably estimate a serious adverse event rate

in persistent or significant disability. Causes of mortality are also frequently not specified. Thus, detailed analysis on life-threatening events is restricted.

Most of the data on SAE of biologics refer to anti-TNF agents and less to Rituximab; so, we focus on these here, with references to other biological agents (Abatacept, Tocilizumab and Anakinra) as appropriate. With respect to ARD, most safety reports refer to patients with rheumatoid arthritis (RA), with less focus on other diseases.

Table 23.3 Potential life-threatening complications of biological therapy

Infections
  Serious and life-threatening infections
    Postoperative infectious complications
  Opportunistic infections
    Tuberculosis
    Nontuberculous mycobacteria infections
    Invasive fungal infections
    Other granulomatous infections
    Viral infections
    Reactivation of chronic viral infections

Malignancies (melanoma)

Anaphylactic reactions
  Serum-sickness-like reactions

Cardiovascular complications

Autoimmune diseases induced by biological agents
  Vasculitis
  Systemic lupus erythematosus
  Interstitial lung disease

Demyelinating disorders

Other serious complications
  Cytopenias
  Hepatotoxicity
  Pulmonary complications
  Gastrointestinal perforation

Most frequent life-threatening complications can be included in six broad categories (Table 23.3). Other less frequent potentially fatal adverse events have also been described.

23.2.1
Infections

Infection remains one of the leading causes of morbidity and mortality in autoimmune diseases, particularly RA and systemic lupus erythematosus (SLE), and these patients appear to have increased baseline susceptibility for infection, including serious and opportunistic infections.[14-17] In patients with RA, a twofold increased incidence of infections was estimated in the prebiologics era.[14,18] In SLE, infection is responsible for approximately 25% of all deaths. The prevalence of life-threatening infections appears to be highest within the first 5 years of the disease onset.[15-17] Immunosuppressive therapy, including steroids, also plays a key role.[15,16]

The potential from biological therapies to increase infection risk has been a major concern. They have been associated with a widely variable increased incidence of severe and non-severe infections. An increased incidence of TB and opportunistic infections associated with biologic treatments is evident, and some are fatal. Likewise, new infections or reactivation of latent viral infections resulting in serious complications or death are also concerning. Concomitance of ARD and chronic viral diseases can be a major problem when additional immunosuppression is added. However, screening strategies and prophylactic measures are effective in reducing these potentially life-threatening complications.

23.2.1.1
Serious and Life-Threatening Infections

Life-threatening infections are included in a broader category of "serious infections," i.e., those fulfilling the criteria for SAE or requiring intravenous antibiotics. Incidence rates of serious infection vary among the studies, and no firm conclusion exists about the overall increased risk of infection in patients on biologics (Table 23.4).[5-7,10,18-26]

An increased risk for serious infections is apparent in patients on anti-TNF therapy (with odds ratios (OR) varying from 1.22 to 2.16), particularly in the first 3 months of treatment and at specific sites of infection (notably the lower respiratory tract and skin/soft tissue) (Table 23.4). Common pathogens prevail (most frequently *Streptococcus pneumoniae* and *Staphylococcus aureus*, respectively). This risk appears to be somewhat higher with anti-TNF monoclonal antibodies (particularly Infliximab), compared to Etanercept, although not all studies agree.[6,20] The large induction dose of Infliximab, Etanercept's lower half-life, and different mechanistic properties between the two anti-TNF antibodies might account for these differences.[6,18,22,26] Life-threatening infections are more common in patients with risk factors (Table 23.5)[18,26] and usually result from disseminated disease and/or severe pulmonary infections progressing to respiratory failure. A common feature in fatal cases is the paucity of signs or symptoms indicating the severity of developing infections. Pneumococcal pneumonias can rapidly progress to fatal acute respiratory distress syndrome (ARDS) and septic shock. Atypical clinical presentation poses a problem in the differential diagnosis with a flare of the underlying disease, as clinical and laboratory signs of infection might be "blunted" in patients on anti-TNF therapy (e.g., absence of fever and elevated acute inflammatory markers). Occasionally, both problems are present. Distinguishing pneumonia and interstitial lung disease secondary to lung involvement and infectious meningitis/encephalitis and central nervous system (CNS) involvement of the diseases can be hard. Estimated death rates attributed to serious infections are generally not available, as these are generally calculated for total SAE. The risk for perioperative infections has rarely been addressed: Two studies showed that therapy interruptions before surgery did not significantly decrease the risk for infectious complications, though a recent study suggested that this risk was twofold lower in patients who stopped the drug for 28 days pre-surgery.[27-29]

Few studies have analyzed rates of serious infections in patients treated with other biologic agents. Results from major RCT in patients with RA[7,8,30,31] and other ARD[32] treated with Rituximab did not show a significant increase in serious infections. Infections of the lower respiratory tract seem more frequent, but are rarely severe. Even the presence of hypogammaglobulinemia (which only occurs with repeated cycles of Rituximab) does not correlate with a significant increase in serious infections. However, levels of the immunoglobulin (Ig) of the IgG isotype below 500 mg/dL are a concern (particularly if sustained for long periods).[33,34] In case reports of patients with severe pneumonia, concomitant immunosuppressives are invariably being taken. Nonetheless, the biologic effects post-Rituximab on memory B cells and Ig levels, with the concomitant modulation of T-cell immunity, require further investigation.[34]

Table 23.4 Rates of serious (including life-threatening) infections in patients with autoimmune rheumatic diseases according to selected published studies and meta-analyses

Author (reference)	Biological agent	Population studied	Number of patients included (n)	Serious infections
Bongartz et al.[19]	Anti-TNF-α antibodies (Infliximab and Adalimumab)	RA[b]	n=5,014 with 3–12 months of follow-up; meta-analysis of 9 RCT[c]	OR[d] 2.0 (95% CI[c], 1.3–3.1) in patients treated with anti-TNF antibodies compared to RA controls
Leombruno et al.[5]	Anti-TNF agents (all)	RA	n=8,808 with 7,846 years of follow-up; meta-analysis of 18 RCT	In patients treated with anti-TNF antibodies compared to RA controls: at recommended doses: OR 1.21 (95% CI, 0.89–1.63); at higher doses: OR 2.07 (95% CI, 1.31–3.26)
Listing et al.[20]	Anti-TNF-α agents (Infliximab and Etanercept)	RA	n=858 with a median follow-up<1 year	In patients treated with anti-TNF antibodies compared to RA controls: adjusted RR[f]: 2.31 (95% CI, 1.4–3.9) for Etanercept vs 3.01 (95% CI, 1.8–5.2) for Infliximab
Dixon et al.[6]	Anti-TNF-α agents (all)	RA	n=8,973 (7,664 in the anti-TNF cohort); median follow-up 1.26 years	Overall serious infections: IRR[g] 1.03 (95%CI, 0.68–1.57) Severe skin/soft tissue infection: IRR 4.28 (95% CI, 1.06–17.17) compared to RA control group
Dixon et al.[21]	Anti-TNF-α agents (all)	RA	n=10,755 (8,659 in the anti-TNF cohort, 2096 in the control group)	*According to "at-risk" period:* for the whole treatment period – adjusted IRR 1.22 (95% CI, 0.88–1.69); first 90 days after starting the treatment – adjusted IRR 4.6 (95% CI, 1.8–11.9) *According to the anti-TNF agent:* for Infliximab: 95.4/1,000 person-years (95% CI, 75.0–119.2), for adalimumab: 59.9/1,000 person-years (95% CI, 39.8–85.9), for Etanercept: 60.0/1,000 person-years (95% CI, 45.5–77.4)
Askling et al.[22]	Anti-TNF-α agents (all)	RA	n=44,946 (4,167 in the anti-TNF cohort); 7,776 person-years of follow-up	*Rate of hospitalization (anti-TNF cohort vs RA controls) according to period of treatment:* first year – adjusted RR 1.43 (95% CI, 1.18–1.73); second year – adjusted IRR 1.15 (95% CI, 0.88–1.51); after 2 or more years: 0.82 (95% CI, 0.62–1.08)
Curtis et al.[23]	Anti-TNF-α agents (Etanercept and Infliximab)	RA	n=5,195 (Infliximab-treated 850, Etanercept-treated 1,412, control group 2,933)	*According to the anti-TNF agent:* adjusted IRR 2.4 (95% CI, 1.23–4.68) vs 1.61 (95% CI, 0.75–3.47) for Infliximab versus Etanercept (respectively)

Study	Agent	Disease	n / follow-up	Results
Lichtenstein et al.[24]	Anti-TNF-α agent (Infliximab)	Crohn's disease	n = 6,290 patients; follow-up 10,000 patient-years; mean follow-up 1.9 years	No increased risk for serious infection (OR, 0.99; 95% CI, 0.64–1.54) Annualized incidence rate within the first 3 months: 1.3% vs 0.7% during the rest of the time
Salliot et al.[25]	Rituximab	RA	n = 1,143 (745 treated with Rituximab, 398 in the control group) (meta-analysis of 3 RCT)	2.3% (Rituximab) vs 1.5% (control group); pooled OR 1.45 (95% CI, 0.56–3.73)
Cohen et al.[7]	Rituximab	RA	n = 520 (311 treated with Rituximab, 209 in the control group)	Incidence rate: 5.2 (Rituximab) vs 3.7 (control group) per 100 patient-years
Emery et al.[10]	Tocilizumab	RA	n = 499	6.3% (Tocilizumab 8 mg/kg), 7.4% (Tocilizumab 4 mg/kg) vs 11.3% (control group)
Salliot et al.[25]	Abatacept	RA	n = 2,945 (1,960 treated patients, 985 in the control) (meta-analysis of 5 RCT)	2.5% (Abatacept) vs 1.8% (control group); pooled OR 1.35 (95% CI, 0.78–2.32)
Salliot et al.[25]	Anakinra	RA	n = 2,791 (2,062 treated patients, 729 in the control group) (meta-analysis of 4 RCT)	1.4% (Anakinra) vs 0.5% (control group); pooled OR 2.75 (95% CI, 0.90–8.35)

[a]Tumour necrosis factor
[b]Rheumatoid arthritis
[c]Randomized controlled trials
[d]Odds ratio
[e]Confidence interval
[f]Rate ratio
[g]Incidence rate ratio

Table 23.5 Risk factors associated with serious infections in patients treated with biological therapy

Type of serious infections	Risk factors
Common infections	– Comorbidities (e.g., diabetes mellitus, chronic lung disease, chronic renal failure) – Previous splenectomy – Concomitant immunosuppressive medication (particularly steroids) – Immunodeficiency (primary or acquired) – Hypogammaglobulinemia (primary or acquired – e.g., Rituximab) severe (IgG[a] < 500 mg/dL) or prolonged – Elderly – Active underlying autoimmune disease
Opportunistic infections (global risks for all opportunistic infections)	– Immunosuppression: primary or acquired (e.g., exposure to immunosuppressive medication – particularly steroids, HIV[b] infection, transplanted persons) – Comorbidities (chronic renal failure, diabetes mellitus, chronic heart failure, chronic lung disease)
– Tuberculosis	– Birth or extended living in high-endemic country for TB[c] – Risk contacts for TB (recent contact with an active case, history of substance abuse, incarceration, living in homeless shelter or nursing home or contact with persons in these conditions; recent travel in endemic areas) – Occupational exposure to TB (employment in health care system) – Chest radiograph abnormalities (chronic lung disease – particularly silicosis, signs suggestive of previous TB)
– Nontuberculous mycobacteria infections	– Risk exposure (e.g., fishing)
– Invasive fungal infections	– Colonization with pathogenic fungi – History of invasive aspergillosis or other mold infections – Environmental exposure – High-risk travel in endemic area (e.g., histoplasmosis, coccidioidomycosis) – High-risk outdoor activities (e.g., spelunking, cleaning chicken coops, disturbing soil beneath bird-roosting sites) – Occupational exposure (e.g., construction) – Chronic neutropenia and renal dysfunction
– Other granulomatous infections	– Elderly, children, pregnant women, and presence of lymphocytopenia (for *Listeria*) – Exposure to air-conditioning devices (for *Legionella*) – Risky dietary habits (e.g., unpasteurized dairy products, raw eggs or meat, precooked meats, soft cheeses) (for *Salmonella* and *Listeria*)
– Viral infections	– CD4[+] T lymphopenia (particularly if <200 cells/mm³)

[a]Immunoglobulin isotype G
[b]Human immunodeficiency virus
[c]Tuberculosis

Data published on Abatacept indicate an increased risk of serious infection limited to subsets of patients treated concomitantly with another biologic.[35] However, a slightly increased risk for hospitalization with infection was found in a large cohort of patients treated with Abatacept compared to biologic-naïve RA cohorts.[36]

A recent meta-analysis (from 12 RCT performed with Rituximab, Abatacept and Anakinra) did not show an increase of serious infections with Rituximab or Abatacept. Anakinra's increased risk was correlated to the presence of comorbidities.[25]

Studies on Tocilizumab safety did not report an increase in serious infections compared to biologic-naïve RA controls.[10]

Prevention and management: Immunization against *Pneumococcus* is recommended before (2–3 weeks) the initiation of anti-TNF treatment. Exclusion of hypogammaglobuline-mia is warranted for candidates to biological therapy (particularly Rituximab) and the evaluation should be repeated before additional courses or in the event of an active infection. A high level of suspicion for infection is necessary, particularly in patients with baseline risk factors (Table 23.5).[18,26] Once symptoms become clinically overt, severe sepsis must be anticipated and immediate discontinuation of the biological therapy (anti-TNF agents) is essential as well as prompt evaluation. Appropriate preemptive antibiotic therapy should be initiated until infection is definitely ruled out. Support treatment with intravenous Ig (IVIg) might be provided as an individual case decision and according to other risk factors.[33]

23.2.2
Opportunistic Infections

As set out above, patients with ARD are inherently prone to infections with opportunistic agents, including mycobacteria, atypical bacteria, virus, fungi, and parasites. The risk increases with biological therapy (Table 23.6).

23.2.2.1
Tuberculosis

For patients with RA, in the prebiologics era, estimated increased risks of Tuberculosis (TB) vary among the studies (between two and up to ninefold)[18,37] and mirror the background prevalence in different countries. In some, where tuberculosis is endemic, the incidence of infection among SLE patients exceeds 5% and commonly it presents in the miliary form with high mortality.[38] Immunosuppressive therapy and notably steroids are known to be associated with miliary or disseminated TB.

TB remains the most frequent opportunistic infection associated with the use of biological therapy, particularly with TNF-α inhibitors (Table 23.7).[37,40-43] TNF is essential to immune defense playing a major role in the recruitment of inflammatory cells to the site of infection and in the granuloma formation and maintenance, which is necessary for containment of intracellular infections. Being born in a TB-endemic country is a major risk factor, which may be elevated up to ~10-fold (OR 10.35; 95% CI, 2.40–44.55).[43] Other frequent

Table 23.6 Most commonly reported opportunistic infections and etiologic agents complicating the use of biological therapy

Opportunistic infections	Etiologic agents (most common)
Tuberculosis infection	*Mycobacterium tuberculosis*
Nontuberculous mycobacteria infections	Nontuberculous mycobacteria (*M. avium species, M. chelonae, M. marinum, M. abscessus*)
Invasive fungal infections	*Histoplasma capsulatum* (endemic areas)[a] *Aspergillus* species *Candida* species *Pneumocystis jirovecii* *Cryptococcus neoformans* *Coccidioides* species (endemic areas)[a] *Zygomycetes* species
Other granulomatous infections (atypical and intracellular bacteria)	*Listeria monocytogenes* *Nocardia* species *Salmonella* species *Legionella* species
Viral infections (disseminated cytomegalovirus infection, herpes zoster, primary varicella-zoster infection)	Cytomegalovirus Varicella-zoster virus
Progressive multifocal leukoencephalopathy	JC virus

[a]Regions in the Ohio and Mississippi River valleys (interior central states of United States of America)

risk factors include older age and concomitant use of corticosteroids (Table 23.5).[40,43] The clinical presentation can be atypical and is dominated by extrapulmonary disease, occurring in 60–70% of cases, with a significant percentage (>25%) of these presenting disseminated TB. Unusual sites of infection (e.g., meningoencephalitis, gastrointestinal, spondylodiscitis) are also more commonly seen. Most cases of TB occur soon after the initiation of treatment, especially with Infliximab. However, a significant number of disseminated TB cases in patients treated with Adalimumab occurred after therapy has been stopped (>3 months).[43]

Whether the risk of TB infection is a class effect of the anti-TNF agents is still debated, although most studies conclude that treatment with anti-TNF monoclonal antibodies confers a higher risk of this complication (up to three- to fourfold in most reports) (Table 23.7).[37,40,44] Different drug pharmacokinetics/pharmacodynamics and mechanisms of action (e.g., antibodies' apoptosis-inducing activity, different avidities of the agents for soluble *versus* transmembrane TNF, and the irreversibly high and fast binding to TNF exhibited by Infliximab compared with Etanercept) potentially explain the dissimilar risks of TB development.[44] A dissimilar action of the two types of anti-TNF agents on specific effector T cells and Treg cells has also been suggested.[43] In addition, differences in the time to develop TB are apparent. For Infliximab, most cases occur sooner after the treatment (first 90 days) than for Adalimumab and Etanercept (median interval above 1 year). These

Table 23.7 Risk of tuberculosis associated with antitumor necrosis factor α agents according to selected studies

Author (reference)	Source of data	Estimated risk of tuberculosis
Wolfe et al.[39]	United States of America national database	Latent TB[a] (before and post-introduction of Infliximab): 6.2 cases per 100,000 RA[b] patients *versus* 52.5 cases per 100,000 patient-years (respectively)
Dixon et al.[40]	BSRBR[c]	For Adalimumab: 144 events/100,000 person-years (pyrs); for Infliximab: 136/100,000 pyrs; for Etanercept: 39/100,000 pyrs. Compared to Etanercept: adjusted IRR[d] 3.1 (95% CI[e], 1.0–9.5) for Infliximab and 4.2 (95% CI, 1.4–12.4) for Adalimumab.
Gomez-Reino et al.[41]	Spanish national database (BIOBADASER[f])	Risk ratio of TB: 90.1 (95% CI, 58.8–146.0) for Infliximab-treated RA patients *versus* the general population and 19.9 (95% CI, 16.2–24.8) *versus* patients with RA treated with non-biologic therapy
Seong et al.[42]	Korean cohort	Adjusted RR[g] for TB of 30.1 (95% CI, 7.4–122.3) compared with the general population
Tubach et al.[43]	French national biologics registry (RATIO[h])	For all anti-TNF[i] agents: SIR[j] 12.2 (95% CI, 9.7–15.5) in patients with various autoimmune diseases For Infliximab: SIR 18.6 [95% CI, 13.4–25.8] and Adalimumab: SIR 29.3 [95% CI, 20.3–42.4] *versus* SIR 1.8 [95% CI, 0.7–4.3], for Etanercept
Askling et al.[37]	Swedish biologics register (ARTIS[k])	For Infliximab: 145 per 100 patient-years (95% CI, 58–129) *versus* Etanercept: 80 per 100 patient-years (95% CI, 16–232)

[a]Tuberculosis
[b]Rheumatoid arthritis
[c]British Society for Rheumatology Biologics Register
[d]Incidence rate ratio
[e]Confidence interval
[f]Spanish Society for Rheumatology Biologic Products Database ('*Base de Datos de Productos Biológicos de la Sociedad Española de Reumatología*')
[g]Rate ratio
[h]French Research Axed on Tolerance of Biotherapies registry,
[i]Tumor necrosis factor
[j]Standardized incidence ratio
[k]Antirheumatic Treatment in Sweden

differences suggest that Infliximab-related TB cases are particularly related to reactivation of latent TB, whereas the linearity of the TB infection curve until late phases of treatment with Etanercept is related to reactivation and probably to new infections.[44] Screening procedures for the diagnosis and proper treatment of latent TB before initiating anti-TNF therapy reduce significantly the incidence of the infection.[45,46] However, cutaneous anergy is more common in RA patients. Indeed, studies from the French registry report that two-thirds of TB cases during anti-TNF therapy occurred in patients with negative tuberculin skin testing (TST) at screening.[43]

The frequent atypical presentations, the potential false-negative screening tests, and the occurrence of TB after discontinuation of anti-TNF therapy warrant a high level of suspicion for the possibility of this infection, when using these drugs, particularly monoclonal antibodies.

Prevention and management: Screening for latent TB is mandatory before initiation of anti-TNF therapy. Careful assessment of risk factors is required (Table 23.5). The threshold for considering latent TB should be lowered in high-risk patients (considering as positive an induration ≥5 mm in the TST). Blood-based diagnostic assays, such as QuantiFERON-TB or T-Spot TB, have greater specificity and are preferred in patients previously vaccinated with bacille Calmette-Guérin (BCG), as false-negative TST results are more common among them. A diagnosis of latent TB warrants the exclusion of active infection before initiation of prophylactic medication. The optimal interval between initiation of preventive treatment and starting TNF blockers is unknown, but observational data suggest that initiating anti-TNF therapy after 1 month of prophylactic treatment for latent TB substantially decreases the risk of reactivation. Likewise, the lag period between initiation of treatment of active TB and starting anti-TNF agents is not defined, but this appears safe after 2 months of treatment for TB.[1] Precise guidelines on re-testing patients are not defined, but latest recommendations suggest that in areas of high TB prevalence, or in the event of potential TB exposure, repeat testing should be considered.

Few cases of TB infection associated with treatment with other biologic agents (Rituximab, Abatacept and Tocilizumab) have been described, and most studies report the absence of TB infections subsequently.[7,8,18,30,47,48] Most patients included had already been screened for latent TB for previous biological therapy (anti-TNF agents) and those with latent infection were excluded in most major RCT with newer biologics; this fact helps to explain the difference in incidence rates compared to anti-TNF agents. However, some studies included patients without previous screening for latent TB and the results have not shown an increased incidence of TB infection. Differences in the mechanism of action between these new agents and anti-TNF drugs might also cause variance in the risk. Screening for TB is now recommended before initiating treatment with Abatacept and Tocilizumab but not with Rituximab.[1]

23.2.2.2
Other Opportunistic Infections

Increasing incidence of other opportunistic serious infections has been seen in patients on biological therapy. Some carry high rates of mortality. Particularly, important high risk factors are inherent impairment in cellular immunity, especially CD4[+] T-cell lymphopenia, and prolonged immunosuppression, most notably with steroids.

Many pathogens causing opportunistic infections have been reported in patients receiving biological therapies (Table 23.6).[3,18,26] The most common are infections by mycobacteria other than TB, invasive fungal infections, and other granulomatous infectious diseases and viral infections.

Nontuberculous Mycobacteria (NTM)

Recent reports on NTM infections in patients receiving mostly anti-TNF agents, but also B-cell depletion therapy, have increased substantially.[18,49] These pathogens most frequently cause a serious infection, with nearly half of the patients presenting with extrapulmonary or disseminated disease. Admission to hospital is often needed, and relatively high mortality rates (9–15%) have been seen. In patients without disseminated disease, the most commonly affected organ is the lung, particularly in those with previous pulmonary disease. *Mycobacterium avium* is the most commonly reported pathogen. TNF inhibitors, and especially Infliximab, are the agents most frequently implicated agents. Unlike TB infection, much longer median periods (18–43 weeks) between the start of drug use and infection diagnosis are described. Whether this is due to newly acquired infections during biological therapy or to reactivation of pretreatment undiagnosed pulmonary infection, remains unclear. Most of the existing studies on NTM infections are based on data from spontaneous reporting; thus, the actual number of cases is likely to be underestimated.

Invasive Fungal Infections (IFI)

These opportunistic infections in patients on biological therapy have been reported increasingly in recent years.[4,18,26,44,50,51] Published information is limited mainly to case reports and case series, and most data are derived from voluntary reporting systems; so, the true incidence is unknown. The most common IFI is histoplasmosis, followed by aspergillosis, candidiasis, and pneumocystosis. Histoplasmosis and coccidioidomycosis occur mainly in patients living in, or coming from, high-endemic geographic regions in the Ohio and Mississippi River valleys (interior central states of United States of America). *Aspergillus* species are ubiquitous worldwide in the environment. Serious *Pneumocystis jirovecii* (formerly *Pneumocystis carinii*) infections have been linked to anti-TNF agents and more recently to B-cell depletion.[9,26] Concomitant immunosuppressive therapy is an additional major factor in nearly all cases of IFI.

Most of these infections involve the lung or present as disseminated disease. The clinical course, in patients on TNF blockers, is often serious or fulminant and the diagnosis might be challenging due to a paucity of early signs and symptoms of infection (a consistent feature of the descriptions) and the similarity of presentation of some cases to flares of underlying diseases. High rates of mortality are reported in patients receiving biologic treatment diagnosed with IFI, particularly with respect to aspergillosis, disseminated candidiasis, and cryptococcosis (ranging from 50% to 100%), and somewhat less with histoplasmosis (20%).[50,51] The time for recognition and treatment appears to influence significantly the clinical course and outcome. Host conditions (e.g., neutropenia, environmental exposure) are also determinant factors in the severity of IFI.[51] Infliximab is the biologic agent most commonly reported (an estimated increased risk of granulomatous infections 3.25-fold higher with Infliximab *versus* Etanercept is reported[26]), but all anti-TNF agents and the other biologic agents may be implicated. Most infections occurred soon after the start of treatment, particularly with Infliximab (median: ≤3 infusions).[26,50,51]

Close surveillance, a high level of suspicion, and prompt treatment of these life-threatening complications are essential, particularly in high-risk populations (Table 23.5).

Prevention and management: To date, there is no reliable method to screen patients before starting anti-TNF therapy, to predict their risk for IFI, partially because most of them are *de novo* infections. Screening for risk factors is essential (Table 23.5). Patients on treatment are recommended to avoid high-risk activities associated with the endemic mycosis in their geographic areas (Table 23.5).[50,51] Physicians should maintain a high level of suspicion for the possibility of IFI, particularly when patients present with respiratory and/or atypical symptoms. Discontinuation of TNF antagonists is warranted and targeted anti-fungal therapy should be started promptly in a patient with signs of serious infection, not improving while on appropriate antibiotics for common infections, particularly if no pathogen is isolated. Uncertainty remains about when the high-risk period abates after TNF blockade, and thus the question of when it is safe to restart these drugs (if at all) cannot be answered easily.

Other Granulomatous Infections

Intracellular bacteria, such as *Listeria*, *Salmonella Nocardia*, and *Legionella* species (among others), have been linked to disseminated life-threatening infections in patients treated with anti-TNF therapy.[4,18,26,47] *Listeria* infection was found to occur at a higher incidence among patients on this therapy when compared to healthy and biologic-naïve RA populations in Spain. Estimated rate ratio (RR) for acquiring *Legionella* pneumonia in patients treated with TNF antagonists was between 16.5 and 21.0 in a recent French study.[18] For most other pathogens, however, there are no studies comparing frequencies of infection in patients receiving biologics to those given conventional DMARD.

Viral Infections

Serious viral infections, including primary varicella, herpes zoster, and cytomegalovirus infections, have been reported, especially after treatment with anti-TNF monoclonal antibodies and, to a lesser extent, Rituximab. Fatal or life-threatening cases are related to disseminated disease or involvement of major internal organs (e.g., pneumonia, fulminant hepatitis).[4,48,52] Influenza can also cause serious infections in these patients and is associated with secondary bacterial infections, which may progress to sepsis.[26]

An FDA alert in 2006 about the possibility of Progressive Multifocal Leukoencephalopathy (PML) in patients with ARD receiving B-cell depletion raised an additional concern. PML is a rare, serious, and usually fatal demyelinating disease, which occurs upon reactivation of JC virus, predominantly in severely immunosuppressed populations (such as persons infected with human immunodeficiency virus (HIV)). Up to 92% of the adult population is seropositive for JC virus, without clinical disease. However, recent reviews found that immunosuppressed persons other than HIV-positive, notably those with ARD, may have an intrinsically raised risk of developing PML. It appears that SLE patients are at the highest risk.[53]

As a complication of Rituximab therapy, it was first described in oncology. More recently, five cases of PML have been reported (as of February 2010): two in patients with

SLE and one case each in other three different ARD.[54,55] Median time from last Rituximab dose to PML diagnosis was 5.5 months, and the median time to death was 2 months. The mortality rate reached 90%. CD4$^+$ T lymphopenia was associated with cases occurring sooner after the treatment and carrying higher mortality.[54] All patients were receiving concomitant immunosuppressive therapy, at varying intensities. The link between Rituximab use and the development of PML is unclear, as more than 20 patients with SLE *not* taking Rituximab have been reported to develop PML. Close surveillance remains necessary though, as early diagnosis is crucial. However, differentiating PML from the new-onset or exacerbation of CNS complications in various ARD can be difficult, such as in acute neuropsychiatric SLE or CNS vasculitis.[53,54]

Despite the possibility of underlying undiagnosed PML as the etiology of some cases of demyelinating disorders occurring in patients on anti-TNF therapy, so far, there are no reports of confirmed PML associated with these agents.[56]

Prevention and management: Influenza vaccination should be provided to candidates to anti-TNF and Rituximab therapies. CD4$^+$ T lymphopenia <200/mm^3 precludes B-cell depletion therapy. New-onset or aggravated neurological symptoms and signs in patients on biological therapy should raise the possibility of PML as a potential cause. Neuroimaging studies and a Neurology opinion can help in the differential diagnosis. The gold standard for the definitive diagnosis relies on brain biopsy with histological and virological examinations. However, less invasive detection of JC virus DNA (by protein chain reaction analysis) of the cerebrospinal fluid has a high specificity (though lower sensitivity), being the most commonly used test. Prompt efforts at immune reconstitution may improve survival rates, as currently available antiviral treatment appears essentially ineffective.[54,55]

23.2.3
Reactivation of Chronic Viral Infections

Hepatitis B virus (HBV) reactivation with hepatic failure or fulminant hepatitis (resulting in death or hepatic transplantation) has been reported following Rituximab and anti-TNF therapy (particularly with Infliximab).[26,47,57,58] Cases reported include patients who were inactive or occult carriers (hepatitis B surface antigen (HBsAg)-negative, HBsAg antibody-positive).[58] With Rituximab, this complication has been seen more frequently, but not exclusively, in cancer patients on concomitant chemotherapy. The median time to diagnosis of hepatitis is approximately 4 months after initiation of treatment and approximately 1 month after the last dose. In patients on anti-TNF therapy, HBV reactivation more often occurs after the second or third treatments, but surprisingly it has also been seen (though less frequently) after the discontinuation of treatment.[58] Concomitant immunosuppressives were invariably present, making a causal relationship with biologics less clear-cut.

Prevention and management: Hepatitis B virus status should be assessed before treatment with anti-TNF and Rituximab therapy. Both are usually contraindicated, if active infection is detected and should be used with caution in inactive HBsAg carriers.[1,58] These patients should be closely monitored for clinical and laboratory signs of active hepatitis, as the risk of reactivation seems to be high. Although the prophylactic treatment (specifically with lamivudine) is not agreed, much evidence suggests its efficacy in significantly reducing this risk during both biological therapies and it probably should be given for a long time after TNF inhibitors are discontinued.[57,58]

Anti-TNF and Rituximab therapies have been both used safely for the treatment of hepatitis C virus (HCV)–induced cryoglobulinemic vasculitis (more frequently with concomitant antiviral therapy) and in HIV patients (anti-TNF agents), without complications.[26,59-61]

23.3
Malignancies

Epidemiological studies have demonstrated an increased baseline incidence of malignancies in several ARD.[14,62] In RA patients, cancer is estimated to be the second most common cause of mortality, and lymphoma has a prevalence twice as high as healthy controls. Lung and skin cancers are also more prevalent. This risk seems to be correlated with the disease severity. In SLE, the risk of lymphoma (notably non-Hodgkin lymphoma) is also significantly increased (estimated prevalence rates up to fourfold), and to a lesser extent lung cancer (though in this case, smoking appears to be a more important risk factor).[62] The relative contribution of DMARDs seems to be modest, with cyclophosphamide being the most likely "culprit."

Does biologic therapy carry a potential increased cancer risk? While earlier studies and meta-analysis of RCT[5,19,63] indicated the possibility of an increased risk of several types of cancer, and particularly of lymphoma, in patients treated with anti-TNF therapy (particularly with higher doses), observational data and posterior studies (which included larger cohorts and longer follow-up periods) have not been able to replicate these findings.[64-66] Overall and based on the results of the most reliable latest studies, the use of TNF antagonists appears to be associated with slightly increased risk only of skin malignancies (namely, non-melanotic skin cancer OR 1.5, 95% CI 1.2–1.8 and melanoma OR 2.3, 95% CI 0.9–5.4).[66] This increased risk appears to affect predominantly patients with previous history of melanoma. Patients with low risk for malignancy treated with TNF blockers do not seem to be at an increased risk for other solid cancers nor for any major further increase in the already elevated lymphoma occurrence in RA. No trend toward an increased incidence or relative risk seems to exist over time (6 years posttreatment) either.[64]

23.3.1
Prevention

At present, cancer screening in all candidates for anti-TNF therapy is essential. In those with recent history (<5 years) of treated malignancy or current diagnosed cancer, other treatment options should be considered. Vigilance during therapy for the occurrence of malignancies (including recurrence of solid tumors) remains appropriate in patients with risk factors for cancer (e.g., smokers, chronic obstructive pulmonary disease, remote history of skin cancers).[1]

There is no convincing evidence of an increased risk of malignancies in patients treated with the new biological agents (Rituximab, Abatacept, Tocilizumab).[48,67,68] Larger studies and with longer follow-up periods are needed however.

23.4
Serious Anaphylactic Reactions

Severe anaphylactic reactions are rare events during therapy with biologic agents, but if they do occur, are potentially life threatening. Most data comes from case reports and RCT. Few of the meta-analyses and post-approval studies have analyzed this problem.

Anti-TNF agents are the most frequently implicated, particularly Infliximab.[2,4] Acute severe infusion reactions are more common (up to 2–3%). They occur during the administration of the drug and usually present with symptoms of bronchospasm, hypotension, and erythematous rash, that may evolve to anaphylactic shock with respiratory failure. In such instances, therapy should be stopped and supportive or emergent care should be administered until patient stabilisation. Infliximab infusions should thus be given with trained medical personnel in attendance with access to parenteral corticosteroids, diphenhydramine, and epinephrine. Delayed hypersensitivity infusion reactions (occurring 2–12 days after infusion) are more rare (<1%) and seem to be mediated by different pathophysiological mechanisms (involving immunoglobulin E). Clinical features are similar to those described for acute reactions, but rapidly progressing interstitial lung disease with ARDS and respiratory failure seem more common. Most events occurred with the third or fourth infusion. Histologically available data revealed eosinophilic pneumonia, and human antichimeric antibodies (HACA) also appear to be common.[4] Most reports refer to patients with Crohn's disease with long treatment-free intervals, but similar reactions in patients with other autoimmune diseases treated with Infliximab are recognized. Mortality rates are not reported but fatal cases have been described and most needed admission to intensive care units. Other anti-TNF agents have not been associated with this type of life-threatening reactions.

Severe acute reactions to Rituximab have been described mainly in oncology. A cytokine release syndrome appears to be the cause, resulting in severe pulmonary and cardiovascular infusion–related events, within 24 h of the drug administration. In patients with ARD, few rare fatal cases of ARDS and cardiogenic shock have occurred, despite the administration of pre-medication.[69]

In RA patients treated with Abatacept, extremely rare cases of severe, but not fatal, infusion reactions are reported with hypotension and bronchospasm.

23.4.1
Serum-Sickness-Like Reactions

This type of delayed hypersensitivity reaction may be associated with rapidly progressing severe complications of biologics and have been reported most frequently with B-cell depletion therapy. The differential diagnosis with flares of the underlying disease can be difficult, as the clinical presentation is frequently nonspecific. In patients on anti-TNF agents (mainly Infliximab), this SAE is often associated with the development of antibodies against Infliximab.[2]

With Rituximab, the association with HACA is not as clear-cut. In SLE, HACA (with an estimated prevalence around 9%) seem important in the development of this complication and are associated with previous low-dose treatment and absence of pre-medication. Serum-sickness reactions are particularly frequent in Rituximab-treated patients with Sjögren's syndrome (SS) (10–20%) and those with HCV-induced vasculitis also seem susceptible. Identified risk factors include prominent hypergammaglobulinemia and high baseline cryocrit. A short period (e.g., 5 days) of intermediate dose of oral steroids following the drug infusion for SS patients and plasma exchange treatment prior to infusion in HCV-induced vasculitis are suggested to prevent this complication in high-risk patients.[70,71]

23.5
Cardiovascular Complications

Cardiovascular disease plays a major role in the increased morbidity and mortality associated with ARD. It is the most common cause of death among RA patients and one of the leading causes in SLE, particularly late in the disease course.[14,17,72-74] Traditional cardiovascular risk factors (such as smoking, diabetes, hypertension, and obesity) cannot explain this increased risk, alone.[74] Although the use of corticosteroids is an important risk factor, chronic systemic inflammation is assumed to play an important role, partly through the action of pro-inflammatory cytokines. TNF-α is a mediator of endothelial dysfunction, vascular instability, and disease progression in atherosclerosis and is known to contribute to the progression of heart failure.[73,74] However, Etanercept and Infliximab treatments for severe heart failure have not been successful.[73]

The issue of prescribing anti-TNF agents to patients with diagnosis of or risk factors for heart failure is controversial. There have been several post-marketing reports of new-onset and worsening of congestive heart failure (CHF) in patients receiving anti-TNF therapy, including cases of *de novo* CHF in young patients without identifiable cardiovascular risk factors.[2,3] The median interval from the first dose of TNF antagonist to a diagnosis of new-onset or exacerbation of CHF was 3.5–4 months (ranging from 24 h to several months). In some cases, symptoms and signs of CHF disappeared completely with the discontinuation of the drug, suggesting a potential causative role for TNF antagonists. Rare fatalities were also reported.

Recent studies indicate that anti-TNF treatment in patients with RA is more likely to be beneficial than harmful with respect to the risk of CHF (through suppression of inflammation), particularly if there is no concomitant therapy with corticosteroids.[73] Furthermore, it was also shown that TNF inhibition does not increase the risk of exacerbating prevalent CHF and it may produce an early (by 6 months) reduction in myocardial infarction in those patients that respond to treatment.[73,74]

Prevention and management: In patients with history of advanced CHF (New York Heart Association (NYHA) class III or IV), consideration of other treatment options seems the best approach and anti-TNF agents should be used with caution in patients with milder CHF with close monitoring for their cardiac status during therapy, particularly if higher doses are used.[1]

Patients with preexisting cardiac arrhythmias and angina have had recurrences of these events during Rituximab infusions. Arrhythmias reported include ventricular tachycardia, supraventricular tachycardia, and trigeminy. Angina and myocardial infarction have been rarely reported following its administration. Rare, fatal heart failure with symptomatic onset weeks after Rituximab has occurred. It remains unknown what, if any, role the drug had in these incidents. Patients with ARD who develop significant cardiopulmonary events should have Rituximab discontinued, and it should be used with caution in those with severe CHF (NYHA class IV).[1]

No significant increased short-term risk of serious cardiovascular events has been reported, so far, in association with Abatacept and Tocilizumab.[9,48]

23.6
Autoimmune Diseases Induced by Biological Therapies

Although a variety of autoantibodies have been noted to develop after the introduction of TNF-α blockers,[3,4,75,76] the appearance of clinical autoimmune syndromes is much less frequent (vasculitis up to 3.9%, lupus <0.5%). Most cases are mild diseases, which resolve after discontinuation of the drug.[2,4,75] Nevertheless, a growing number of reports of autoimmune processes related to TNF antagonists use have documented rare cases with serious, life-threatening or even fatal complications.[75] The most frequent clinical presentations consist of vasculitis – with an impressive ~25% having extracutaneous involvement (peripheral and central nervous system, renal and lung) – lupus-like syndromes and SLE (with articular, cutaneous, and constitutional symptoms, being the most common features) and interstitial lung disease (ILD). Less frequent clinical features include inflammatory myopathies, antiphospholipid syndrome, and autoimmune hepatitis.[75] The three anti-TNF agents display different risks for the diverse autoimmune disorders, with Infliximab being the most frequently implicated, except for vasculitis where Etanercept has the strongest association. The interval between administration of the drug and the appearance of the autoimmune syndrome varies between 6 and 10 months. Generally, these disorders are self-limiting after stopping anti-TNF therapy but may require corticosteroids and immunosuppressive treatment.[75,76] However, significant morbidity and mortality has also been seen. Reported causes of death were related to renal involvement of vasculitis, with rapidly progressive anti-neutrophil cytoplasmic antibodies (ANCA)-positive glomerulonephritis, and relentless progression of interstitial lung disease.[75] A case series found a significant poor prognosis in patients with induced ILD in spite of cessation of anti-TNF therapy and initiation of corticosteroids and immunosuppressives, with more than one half of patients showing no resolution and ~33% dying.[75]

Precise etiopathogenic link between these autoimmune diseases and TNF blockade remains unclear. An underlying predisposition of some patients for a second autoimmune disease (particularly in RA), given that some of them already had these autoantibodies prior to the anti-TNF therapy and the contribution or synergistic action of concomitant medication (particularly methotrexate in ILD) are confounding factors.[75,76] With respect to lupus, some authors refer to a new concept – anti-TNF-induced lupus (ATIL) – as being apparently distinct from classical drug-induced lupus (DIL) and with a phenotype more similar to idiopathic SLE (namely: cerebral and renal involvement and anti-double-stranded DNA (dsDNA) antibodies are more common, while anti-histone antibodies are less frequent, when compared to classical DIL).[76]

Prevention and management: Careful clinical and immunological screening for features suggestive of the existence of undiagnosed autoimmune disease prior to and during anti-TNF therapy is important. Screening of candidates for underlying ILD is recommended, particularly in those receiving methotrexate. Anti-TNF agents should not be used in patients with preexisting interstitial pulmonary disorders. Confirmation of an autoimmune disease induced by these agents should be followed by the drug withdrawal, unless the symptoms are very mild.[75]

The other biological therapies (Rituximab, Abatacept, Tocilizumab) have rarely been reported to induce autoantibody formation or clinical manifestations (e.g., skin vasculitis with Rituximab). Serious/life-threatening autoimmune syndromes do not appear to be associated with their use.[1,9]

23.7
Demyelinating Disorders

Concerns about potential serious neurological adverse events have been raised since the first reports on demyelinating disorders occurring in patients treated with anti-TNF antagonists a decade ago.[77] Several reports have since described the new-onset or exacerbation of both peripheral and central demyelinating disorders in small numbers of patients receiving anti-TNF therapy.[1-4] These include new-onset optic neuritis, *de novo* multiple sclerosis (MS), recurrence or flare of MS, encephalitis, myelitis, Guillain–Barré syndrome, chronic inflammatory demyelinating polyneuropathy, neuropathy, transverse myelitis, and leukoencephalopathy, while receiving either three of the anti-TNF agents. Etanercept has been the most often drug implicated, particularly in CNS adverse events. The mean time to symptom onset from initiation of therapy is 5 months, ranging from 1 week to 15 months.[77] Most cases show changes in magnetic resonance imaging consistent with demyelination. Other than a prior history of MS or other demyelinating diseases, no predictive factors have been identified and cases exist in patients with no history of neurological disorder.[3] In most cases, symptoms improve or resolve with cessation of therapy, but rarely neurological deficits persist. The etiopathogenesis of these demyelinating disorders occurring in patients receiving TNF inhibitors is not fully understood.

Apart from the PML cases reported in association with Rituximab (see Sect. 23.2.2.2.4), no other serious neurological adverse events have been reported in patients on the other biological agents.

Prevention and management: Anti-TNF therapy should be avoided in patients with history of central demyelinating disorders and used with caution in those with a positive family history. Patients should be carefully monitored for the development of neurological symptoms and signs while receiving TNF antagonists and these should be discontinued when clinical signs of white matter injury appear. It is probably not safe to continue to use or readminister the drug to patients who develop significant CNS adverse reactions.[1,3,77] Some authors also recommend an evaluation for JC virus infection, when features of leukoencephalopathy predominate, although, so far, confirmed PML has not been associated with TNF blockers use.[57,78]

23.8
Other Serious Complications Associated with Biological Agents

Other, rarer but potentially life-threatening, adverse events have been reported in association with the use of biologics. Some of these were unexpected and only revealed in post-marketing surveillance reports.

23.8.1
Cytopenias

Pancytopenias or cytopenias of only one cell lineage (especially thrombocytopenia) have rarely been ascribed to all anti-TNF agents use and isolated cases of aplastic anemia were also seen with Etanercept.[1-4] A minority of these resulted in death. Cytopenias developed more frequently in few weeks after therapy initiation (but the interval time can be as long as 30 weeks) and usually resolved with discontinuation of the drug. However, some patients required corticosteroids or IVIg for treatment. The reasons linking the cytopenias and TNF blockade remain unclear and concomitant medication or other comorbidities may also be responsible.[3] Periodic monitoring (every 3–6 months) of blood cell counts is suggested as well as close surveillance for clinical features of blood dyscrasias.[2]

Severe (grade 3 or 4) cytopenias (most commonly lymphopenia) following Rituximab administration have been observed essentially in oncology, where confounding factors for the etiology (including concomitant chemotherapy and reactivation of Parvovirus B19 infection) are important.[26] However, a specific complication of this biological agent – late-onset neutropenia (LON) – has been recognized and reported in patients receiving B-cell depletion for the treatment of ARD.[79] It occurs usually 40 days (or more) after the last dose of rituximab (ranging from 2 to 6 months) and the median duration is 10 days. In some cases, it can be accompanied by serious complications, such as febrile severe neutropenia (requiring growth-factor support) or serious infections. The underlying mechanism is unknown. Some authors report that patients with autoimmune blistering skin diseases (particularly Pemphigus vulgaris) might be more susceptible.[79]

Neutropenia has been frequently reported following treatment with Tocilizumab but severe neutropenia is rare (<1%) and it has been demonstrated not to be associated with increased likelihood of developing serious infection.[1]

23.8.2
Hepatotoxicity

Rare reports of liver failure or severe hepatic toxicity have been associated with TNF inhibitors use (particularly Infliximab). The most serious include cases of acute liver failure and fulminant hepatitis, which occurred between 2 weeks and over a year after initiation of therapy and less frequently after its discontinuation.[1,2,4] Some cases were fatal or required liver transplantation.[2,4] The etiology is not clear and confounding factors or hepatoxin exposure (e.g., sepsis, TB, isoniazid and other hepatotoxic drugs, alcohol hepatitis) may play a role. Severe or fatal reactivation of hepatitis B virus (HBV) in chronic carriers was the attributed cause in some cases (see Sect. 23.2.3).[4,57] However, in some patients, no other cause could be identified, thus suggesting a causative role for anti-TNF therapy.[2] TNF inhibitors should be stopped in patients with significant elevation of liver enzymes (>5 times the upper limit of normal).[1,4,57]

Fatal cases of fulminant hepatitis have also been reported in patients treated with Rituximab, but virtually all are associated with reactivation of HBV infection (see Sect. 23.2.3).

23.8.3
Pulmonary Complications

Rare instances of acute, severe and sometimes fatal interstitial lung disease (ILD) have been reported in patients using all TNF-α inhibitors.[1,80] Most patients had underlying previous mild or asymptomatic lung disease and/or were receiving pneumotoxic agents (e.g., methotrexate) concomitantly. However, cases without these risk factors have also been reported. Most cases occur after the second or third treatments. Histologically, usual interstitial pneumonia (UIP) has been the most frequent finding, particularly in the fatal cases[80]; less frequently, bronchiolitis obliterans organizing pneumonia (BOOP) has been found. The pathophysiology of the pulmonary insult is unknown, and in some cases, it may be autoantibody mediated. Caution and close screening before and after initiation of anti-TNF therapy is recommended, particularly in patients with previous history of lung disease and/or concomitant pneumotoxic medication. However, excluding an infectious complication (with particular focus for atypical pathogens) is mandatory before assuming any other diagnosis,[81] particularly if treatment with corticosteroids is being considered.

Cases of drug-induced lung disease have also been reported in association with Rituximab therapy and with significant mortality (18%).[69] Three "time-to-onset" patterns were documented. The most common presentation was acute/subacute hypoxemic BOOP, starting 2 weeks after the last infusion, usually resolving upon starting glucocorticoid therapy. Other cases referred to acute (within a few hours) ARDS (probably related to an infusion reaction) and delayed macronodular organizing pneumonia. The pathogenic mechanisms are not clear and most probably differ among the cases with different "time-to-onset." Monitoring during and after the Rituximab infusion is recommended, particularly in those patients with reversible "allergic-like" respiratory symptoms in previous administrations.

23.8.4
Gastrointestinal Perforation

Rare cases of upper and lower gastrointestinal perforation in patients treated with Tocilizumab have been reported. Some of these were fatal.[1,82] Risk factors are comorbidities (particularly, history of diverticulosis/diverticulitis and peptic ulcer) and concomitant medication (mostly corticosteroids and nonsteroidal anti-inflammatory drugs).

The relative risk is still not well characterized. Caution is recommended when considering the use of Tocilizumab in patients with history of diverticulitis or intestinal ulceration and, during therapy, prompt evaluation of patients with suggestive symptoms should ensue.[1,82]

23.9
Summary

Biological therapy is generally safe, particularly when compared to conventional DMARD therapy. Serious adverse events appear to be rare, but are potentially associated with life-threatening conditions. Several of these are correlated with either the underlying disease *per se* or the concomitant medication use. Most of them can be avoided by the judicious selection of candidates and adoption of preventive/prophylactic measures. The outcome may be significantly changed by close vigilance and an early proper management. Awareness of the possible serious side effects when using biological therapy is the first essential step for its safer use in patients with autoimmune diseases.

References

1. Furst DE, Keystone EC, Fleischmann R, et al. Updated consensus statement on biological agents for the treatment of rheumatic diseases. *Ann Rheum Dis*. 2010;69(suppl I):i2-i29.
2. Cush JJ. Safety overview of new disease-modifying antirheumatic drugs. *Rheum Dis Clin N Am*. 2004;30:237-255.
3. Hyrich KL, Silman AJ, Watson KD, et al. Anti-tumour necrosis factor α therapy in rheumatoid arthritis: an update on safety. *Ann Rheum Dis*. 2004;63:1538-1543.
4. Reddy JG, Loftus EV. Safety of infliximab and other biologic agents in the inflammatory bowel diseases. *Gastroenterol Clin N Am*. 2006;35(4):837-855.
5. Leombruno JP, Einarson TR, Keystone EC. The safety of anti-tumour necrosis factor treatments in rheumatoid arthritis: meta and exposure adjusted pooled analyses of serious adverse events. *Ann Rheum Dis*. 2009;68:1136-1145.
6. Dixon WG, Watson K, Lunt M, et al. Rates of serious infection, including site-specific and bacterial intracellular infection, in rheumatoid arthritis patients receiving anti-tumour necrosis factor therapy: results from the British Society for Rheumatology Biologics Register. *Arthritis Rheum*. 2006;54:2368-2376.
7. Cohen SB, Emery P, Greenwald MW, et al. Rituximab for rheumatoid arthritis refractory to anti-tumor necrosis factor therapy: results of a multicenter, randomized, double-blind, placebo-controlled, phase III trial evaluating primary efficacy and safety at twenty-four weeks. *Arthritis Rheum*. 2006;54:2793-2806.
8. Keystone E, Fleischmann R, Emery P, et al. Safety and efficacy of additional courses of rituximab in patients with active rheumatoid arthritis: an open-label extension analysis. *Arthritis Rheum*. 2007;56:3896-3908.
9. Sibilia J, Westhovens R. Safety of T-cell co-stimulation modulation with abatacept in patients with rheumatoid arthritis. *Clin Exp Rheumatol*. 2007;25:S46-S56.
10. Emery P, Keystone E, Tony HP, et al. IL-6 receptor inhibition with tocilizumab improves treatment outcomes in patients with rheumatoid arthritis refractory to anti-tumour necrosis factor

biologicals: results from a 24-week multicentre randomised placebo-controlled trial. *Ann Rheum Dis*. 2008;67(11):1516-1523.

11. Fleischmann RM, Tesser J, Schiff MH, et al. Safety of extended treatment with anakinra in patients with rheumatoid arthritis. *Ann Rheum Dis*. 2006;65(8):1006-1012.

12. Fisher MC, Greenberg JD. Assessing infection risk with biologic agents in RA: methodological challenges. *Nat Rev Rheumatol*. 2009;5:288-291.

13. Hyrich KL. Assuming the safety of biological therapies in rheumatoid arthritis: the challenge of study design. *J Rheumatol*. 2005;32(suppl):48-50.

14. Gabriel SE, Michaud K. Epidemiological studies in incidence, prevalence, mortality and comorbidity of the rheumatic diseases. *Arthritis Res Ther*. 2009;11(3):229.

15. Goldblatt F, Chambers S, Rahman A, et al. Serious infections in British patients with systemic lupus erythematosus: hospitalisations and mortality. *Lupus*. 2009;18:682-689.

16. Ruiz-Irastorza G, Olivares N, Ruiz-Arruza I, et al. Predictors of major infections in systemic lupus erythematosus. *Arthritis Res Ther*. 2009;11:R109.

17. Bernatsky S, Boivin JF, Joseph L, et al. Mortality in systemic lupus erythematosus. *Arthritis Rheum*. 2006;54(8):2550-2557.

18. Martin-Mola E, Balsa A. Infectious complications of biologic agents. *Rheum Dis Clin N Am*. 2009;35:183-199.

19. Bongartz T, Sutton AJ, Sweeting MJ, et al. Anti-TNF antibody therapy in rheumatoid arthritis and the risk of serious infections and malignancies: systematic review and meta-analysis of rare harmful effects in randomised controlled trials. *JAMA*. 2006;295:2275-2285.

20. Listing J, Strangfeld A, Kary S, et al. Infections in patients with rheumatoid arthritis treated with biologic agents. *Arthritis Rheum*. 2005;52:3403-3412.

21. Dixon DG, Symmons DP, Lunt M, et al. Serious infections following anti-tumor necrosis alpha therapy in patients with rheumatoid arthritis: lessons from interpreting data from observational studies. *Arthritis Rheum*. 2007;56:2896-2904.

22. Askling J, Fored CM, Brandt L, et al. Time-dependent increase in risk of hospitalisation with infection among Swedish RA patients treated with TNF antagonists. *Ann Rheum Dis*. 2007;66:1339-1344.

23. Curtis JR, Xi J, Patkar N, et al. Drug-specific and time-dependent risks of bacterial infections among patients with rheumatoid arthritis who were exposed to tumor necrosis factor alpha antagonists. *Arthritis Rheum*. 2007;56:4226-4227.

24. Lichtenstein GR, Cohen RD, Feagan BG, et al. Serious infections and mortality in association with therapies for Crohn's disease: TREAT registry. *Clin Gastroenterol Hepatol*. 2006;4:621-630.

25. Salliot C, Dougados M, Gossec L. Risk of serious infections during rituximab, abatacept and anakinra treatments for rheumatoid arthritis: meta-analyses of randomized placebo-controlled trials. *Ann Rheum Dis*. 2009;68:25-32.

26. Saketkoo LA, Espinoza LR. Impact of biologic agents on infectious diseases. *Infect Dis Clin N Am*. 2006;20:931-961.

27. Dixon WG, Lunt M, Watson K, et al. Anti-TNF therapy and the risk of serious postoperative infection: results from the BSR biologics register (BSRBR). *Ann Rheum Dis*. 2007;66(Suppl II):118.

28. Askling J, Dixon W. The safety of anti-tumour necrosis factor therapy in rheumatoid arthritis. *Curr Opin Rheumatol*. 2008;20:138-144.

29. Bongartz T. Elective orthopedic surgery and perioperative DMARD management: many questions, fewer answers, and some opinions. *J Rheumatol*. 2007;34:653-655.

30. Emery P, Fleischmann R, Filipowicz-Sosnowska A, et al. The efficacy and safety of rituximab in patients with active rheumatoid arthritis despite methotrexate treatment: results of a phase IIB randomized, double-blind, placebo-controlled, dose-ranging trial. *Arthritis Rheum*. 2006;54:1390-1400.

31. Strangfeld A, Hierse F, Listing J, et al. RA patients treated with rituximab. Routine care data of the German Biologics Register RABBIT. *Arthritis Rheum*. 2008;58(Suppl):S305.

32. Fleischmann RM. Safety of biologic therapy in rheumatoid arthritis and other autoimmune diseases: focus on rituximab. *Semin Arthritis Rheum.* 2009;38(4):265-280.
33. Looney RJ, Srinivasan R, Calabrese LH. The effects of rituximab on immunocompetency in patients with autoimmune rheumatic disease. *Arthritis Rheum.* 2008;58(1):5-14.
34. Quartuccio L, Lombardi S, Fabris M, et al. Long-term effects of rituximab in rheumatoid arthritis: clinical, biologic and pharmacogenetics aspects. *Ann NY Acad Sci.* 2009;1773:692-700.
35. Smitten A, Covucci A, Simon T. Descriptive analysis of serious infections, hospitalised infections and malignancies over time in the abatacept clinical developmental program: a safety update with 10,000 person-years of exposure. *Ann Rheum Dis.* 2008;67(Suppl 2):338.
36. Hochberg MC, Simon TA. Safety of abatacept in patients with rheumatoid arthritis. *Ann Rheum Dis.* 2008;67(suppl 2):36.
37. Askling J, Fored CM, Brandt L, et al. Risk and case characteristics of tuberculosis in rheumatoid arthritis associated with tumor necrosis factor antagonists in Sweden. *Arthritis Rheum.* 2005;52:1986-1992.
38. Iliopoulos AG, Tsokos GC. Immunopathogenesis and spectrum of infections in systemic lupus erythematosus. *Semin Arthritis Rheum.* 1996;25(5):318-336.
39. Wolfe F, Michaud K, Anderson J, et al. Tuberculosis infection in patients with rheumatoid arthritis and the effect of infliximab therapy. *Arthritis Rheum.* 2004;50:372-379.
40. Dixon WG, Hyrich KL, Watson KD, et al. Drug-specific risk of tuberculosis in patients with rheumatoid arthritis treated with anti-TNF therapy: results from the British Society for Rheumatology Biologics Register (BSRBR). *Ann Rheum Dis.* 2009;69(3):522-528. doi:doi:10.1136/ard.2009.118935.
41. Gomez-Reino JJ, Carmona L, Valverde VR, et al. Treatment of rheumatoid arthritis with tumor necrosis factor inhibitors may predispose to significant increase in tuberculosis risk: a multicenter active-surveillance report. *Arthritis Rheum.* 2003;48:2122-2127.
42. Seong SS, Choi CB, Woo JH, et al. Incidence of tuberculosis in Korean patients with rheumatoid arthritis (RA): effects of RA itself and of tumor necrosis factor blockers. *J Rheumatol.* 2007;34:706-711.
43. Tubach F, Salmon D, Ravaud P, et al. Risk of tuberculosis is higher with anti-tumor necrosis factor monoclonal antibody therapy than with soluble tumor necrosis factor receptor therapy. The three-year prospective French Research Axed on Tolerance of Biotherapies Registry. *Arthritis Rheum.* 2009;60(7):1884-1894.
44. Furst DE, Wallis R, Broder M, et al. Tumor necrosis factor antagonists: different kinetics and/or mechanisms of action may explain differences in the risk for developing granulomatous infection. *Semin Arthritis Rheum.* 2006;36:159-167.
45. Gomez-Reino JJ, Carmona L, Angel DM. Risk of tuberculosis in patients treated with tumor necrosis factor antagonists due to incomplete prevention of reactivation of latent infection. *Arthritis Rheum.* 2007;57:756-761.
46. Carmona L, Gomez-Reino JJ, Rodriguez-Valverde V, et al. Effectiveness of recommendations to prevent reactivation of latent tuberculosis infection in patients treated with tumor necrosis factor antagonists. *Arthritis Rheum.* 2005;52:1766-1772.
47. Haroon N, Inman RD. Infectious complications of biological therapy. *Curr Opin Rheumatol.* 2009;21:397-403.
48. Nishimoto N, Miyasaka N, Yamamoto K, et al. Long-term safety and efficacy of tocilizumab, an anti-IL-6 receptor monoclonal antibody, in monotherapy in patients with rheumatoid arthritis (the STREAM study): evidence of safety and efficacy in a 5-year extension study. *Ann Rheum Dis.* 2009;68:1580-1584.
49. Winthrop KL, Chang E, Yamashita S, et al. Nontuberculous mycobacteria infections and anti-tumor necrosis factor-alpha therapy. *Emerg Infect Dis.* 2009;15(10):1556-1561.
50. Arnold TM, Sears CR, Hage CA. Invasive fungal infections in the era of biologics. *Clin Chest Med.* 2009;30:279-286.

51. Tsiodras S, Samonis G, Boumpas DT, et al. Fungal infections complicating tumor necrosis factor alpha blockade therapy. *Mayo Clin Proc*. 2008;50:1959-1966.

52. Strangfeld A, Listing J, Herzer P, et al. Risk of Herpes zoster in patients with rheumatoid arthritis treated with anti-TNF-α agents. *JAMA*. 2009;301:737-744.

53. Calabrese LH, Molloy ES, Huang D, et al. Progressive multifocal leukoencephalopathy in rheumatic diseases. Evolving clinical and pathologic patterns of disease. *Arthritis Rheum*. 2007;56(7):2116-2128.

54. Carson KR, Evens AM, Richey EA, et al. Progressive multifocal leukoencephalopathy after rituximab therapy in HIV-negative patients: a report of 57 cases from the research on adverse drug events and reports project. *Blood*. 2009;113:4834-4840.

55. Carson KR, Focosi D, Major EO, et al. Monoclonal antibody-associated progressive multifocal leukoencephalopathy in patients treated with rituximab, natalizumab and efalizumab: a review from the Research on Adverse Drug Events and Reports (RADAR) project. *Lancet Oncol*. 2009;10:816-824.

56. Roos JC, Ostor AJ. Anti-tumor necrosis factor alpha therapy and the risk of JC virus infection. *Arthritis Rheum*. 2006;54:381-382.

57. Calabrese LH, Zein NN, Vassilopoulos D. Hepatitis B virus (HBV) reactivation with immunosuppressive therapy in rheumatic diseases: assessment and preventive strategies. *Ann Rheum Dis*. 2006;65:983-989.

58. Zingarelli S, Frassi M, Bazzani C, et al. Use of tumor necrosis factor-alpha-blocking agents in hepatitis B virus-positive patients: report of 3 cases and review of the literature. *J Rheumatol*. 2009;36(6):1188-1194.

59. Ferri C, Ferracciolo G, Ferrari D, et al. Safety of anti-tumor necrosis factor-alpha therapy in patients with rheumatoid arthritis and chronic hepatitis C virus infection. *J Rheumatol*. 2008;35(10):1944-1949.

60. Terrier B, Saadoun D, Sène D, et al. Efficacy and tolerability of rituximab with or without PEGylated interferon alpha-2b plus ribavirin in severe hepatitis C virus-related vasculitis: a long-term follow-up study of thirty-two patients. *Arthritis Rheum*. 2009;60(8):2531-2540.

61. Cepeda EJ, Williams FM, Ishimori ML, et al. The use of anti-tumor necrosis factor therapy in HIV-positive individuals with rheumatic disease. *Ann Rheum Dis*. 2008;67(5):710-712.

62. Gayed M, Bernatsky S, Ramsey-Goldman R, et al. Lupus and cancer. *Lupus*. 2009;18:479-485.

63. Geborek P, Bladstrom A, Turesson C, et al. TNF blockers do not increase overall tumour risk in patients with rheumatoid arthritis, but may be associated with increased risk of lymphomas. *Ann Rheum Dis*. 2005;64:699-703.

64. Askling J, van Vollenhoven RF, Granath F, et al. Cancer risk in patients with rheumatoid arthritis treated with anti-tumor necrosis factor α therapies. Does the risk change with the time since start of treatment? *Arthritis Rheum*. 2009;60(11):3180-3189.

65. Askling J, Baecklund E, Granath F, et al. Anti-tumor necrosis factor therapy in rheumatoid arthritis and risk of malignant lymphomas: relative risks and time trends in the Swedish Biologics Register. *Ann Rheum Dis*. 2009;68:648-653.

66. Wolfe F, Michaud K. Biologic treatment of rheumatoid arthritis and the risk of malignancy. Analyses from a large US observational study. *Arthritis Rheum*. 2007;56(9):2886-2895.

67. van Vollenhoven RF, Emery P, Bingham CO 3rd, et al. Longterm safety of patients receiving rituximab in rheumatoid arthritis clinical trials. *J Rheumatol*. 2010;37(3):558-567.

68. Simon TA, Smitten AL, Franklin J, et al. Malignancies in the rheumatoid arthritis abatacept clinical development programme: an epidemiological assessment. *Ann Rheum Dis*. 2009;68:1819-1826.

69. Lioté H, Lioté F, Séroussi B, et al. Rituximab-induced lung disease: a systematic literature review. *Eur Respir J*. 2009;35(3):681-687.

70. Ramos-Casals M, Brito-Zerón P. Emerging biological therapies in primary Sjögren's syndrome. *Rheumatology*. 2007;46:1389-1396.

71. Sène D, Ghillani-Dalbin P, Amoura Z, et al. Rituximab may form a complex with IgM-Kappa mixed cryoglobulin and induce severe systemic reactions in patients with hepatitis C virus-induced vasculitis. *Arthritis Rheum.* 2009;60(12):3848-3855.
72. Gabriel SE. Heart disease and rheumatoid arthritis: understanding the risks. *Ann Rheum Dis.* 2010;69(suppl 1):i61-i64.
73. Listing J, Strangfeld A, Kekow J, et al. Does tumor necrosis factor α inhibition promote or prevent heart failure in patients with rheumatoid arthritis? *Arthritis Rheum.* 2008;58(3):667-677.
74. Dixon WG, Watson KD, Lunt M, et al. Reduction in the incidence of myocardial infarction in patients with rheumatoid arthritis who respond to anti-tumor necrosis factor α therapy. *Arthritis Rheum.* 2007;56(9):2905-2912.
75. Ramos-Casals M, Brito-Zerón P, Muñoz S, et al. Autoimmune diseases induced by TNF-targeted therapies. Analysis of 233 cases. *Medicine.* 2007;86:242-251.
76. Williams EL, Gadola S, Edwards CJ. Anti-TNF-induced lupus. *Rheumatology.* 2009;48(7): 716-720.
77. Mohan N, Edwards ET, Cupps TR, et al. Demyelination occurring during anti-tumor necrosis factor α therapy for inflammatory arthritides. *Arthritis Rheum.* 2001;44(12):2862-2869.
78. Roos JC, Ostör AJ. Neurological complications of infliximab. *J Rheumatol.* 2007;34:236-237.
79. Rios-Fernández R, Gutierrez-Salmerón MT, Callejas-Rubio JL, et al. Late-onset neutropenia following rituximab treatment in patients with autoimmune diseases. *Br J Dermatol.* 2007;157:1271-1272.
80. Ostör AJ, Chilvers ER, Somerville MF, et al. Pulmonary complications of infliximab therapy in patients with rheumatoid arthritis. *J Rheumatol.* 2006;33(3):622-628.
81. Roos JC, Chilvers ER. Interstitial pneumonitis and anti-tumor necrosis factor-α therapy. *J Rheumatol.* 2007;34:238-239.
82. van Vollenhoven RF, Keystone E, Furie R, et al. Gastrointestinal safety in patients with rheumatoid arthritis (RA) treated with tocilizumab in the Roche clinical trials database. Presented at: 73rd Annual Scientific Meeting of American College of Rheumatology (ACR); October 16–21, 2009; Philadelphia.

Index

M.A. Khamashta and M. Ramos-Casals (eds.), *Autoimmune Diseases*,
DOI: 10.1007/978-0-85729-358-9, © Springer-Verlag London Limited 2011

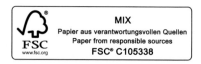
Printed by Books on Demand, Germany